THE
Livable Cities
ALMANAC

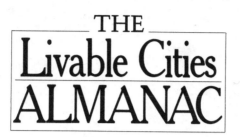

THE
Livable Cities
ALMANAC

John Tepper Marlin, Ph.D.

WITH
Andrea Kleine, Hans Bos, Anna DePalo, Gyorgy Feher,
Harriet Lowell, Linda Mattocks, Soo Mee Pak,
Gautam Rana, Robert Trager and Dawn A. Zuroff

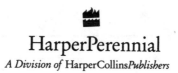

HarperPerennial
A Division of HarperCollins*Publishers*

Library of Congress Cataloging-in-Publication Data

Marlin, John Tepper.
    Livable cities almanac : how over 100 metropolitan areas compare in eco-
nomic health, air quality, water quality, crime rates, life expectancy, health
services, recreational opportunities, and more / John Tepper Marlin with Andrea
Kleine . . . [et al.].
    p. cm.
    Includes bibliographical references and index.
    ISBN 0-06-270035-9 (cloth ed.).—ISBN 0-06-273134-3 (paper ed.)
    1. Quality of life—United States—Statistics. 2. Urban health—United
States—Evaluation—Statistics. 3. Environmental health—United States—
Evaluation—Statistics. 4. Social indicators—United States. 5. Metropolitan
areas—United States—Statistics. I. Kleine, Andrea. II. Title.
HN60.M36 1992
306'.0973'021—dc20   91-16666

92 93 94 95 96 PS/HC 10 9 8 7 6 5 4 3 2 1

Contents

Acknowledgments

THANKS

- For helping with this project in its infancy in the mid–1980s and serving as an adviser: T. George Harris, founding editor of *Psychology Today* and *American Health Magazine*.
- For suggesting this book and serving as advisers: Joel Harnett, Publisher, Phoenix Home and Garden, and Arthur F. Rosenfeld, President, Maxwell Macmillan Professional Reference Publications, New York.
- For reviewing the plan for the book or portions of it: Dr. Michael Sacks, World Health Organization; Dr. Jeffrey Buckner, Mt. Sinai Medical Center, New York; Dr. Carter Dodge, Dartmouth Medical School; Fred Hart, Hart Environmental; Dr. Mitchell L. Moss, Director, New York University Urban Research Center; and Dr. Gerald Turino, Director, St. Luke's/Roosevelt Hospital Department of Medicine.
- For helpful advice on specialized topics: Ben Goldman, Karyn Feiden, Peter F. Rousmaniere, Jonathan Schorsch and Dr. Louis Slesin.
- For encouragement and superb editorial advice: Alice Tepper Marlin, my spouse; Carol Cohen and Nick Bakalar, my editors at Harper-Collins; F. Joseph Spieler, my agent; and Pat Vance, the book's copy editor.
- For serving as student interns on this project: in the summer of 1989, to develop the city questionnaires and initiate the survey process, Soo Mee Pak (New York University Medical School '92); in the spring and fall of 1990, to help with data analysis, Domenick

Bertelli (Harvard '92–'93), Hans Bos (NYU Graduate School of Public Administration '92) and Anke Schultz (NYU GSPA '92); in the second half of 1990 and spring of 1991, to pull together all the research, Anna DePalo (Harvard-Radcliffe '93), Gyorgy Feher (NYU MA '90), Harriet Lowell (NYU '92), Linda Mattocks (Columbia University pre–med program, '91), Gautam Rana (Wharton School, University of Pennsylvania, '91), Robert Trager (Fieldston School '91 and Middlebury College '95) and Dawn A. Zuroff (Barnard College '92); above all, in the final year of the process, to hammer out all the details, Andrea Kleine (NYU '91).

• Finally, for developing the technology that has boosted my productivity: the WordPerfect Corporation, Lotus (1-2-3 and Magellan), CyberSoft (StatMaster) and Zeos (the 386 Notebook computer, my traveling companion).

Introduction

A favorite Spanish toast is *salud, amor y pesetas*—"Health, love and money." Many add: "and the time to enjoy them all."

Increasingly, people recognize that their health is largely a matter of their own choosing. In the mid–1980s Surgeon General C. Everett Koop properly urged us all to refrain from smoking, from eating high–fat food, and from casual sex. While many joke that he has taken all the fun out of life, deep down we know that our bodies can suffer only so much abuse, and civilization has stretched us to the limit.

One choice we make is where to live and work, and most of us choose metropolitan areas. Computers and communications have in theory reduced our need for cities, yet we still cluster together to do business and socialize. Where we choose to be does seem to affect our health.

ARE CITIES INHERENTLY UNHEALTHY?

Over the years people have migrated to the big cities even though polls show people would rather live in small country towns. The post–World War II compromise was to live in suburbia and work in the city, but with commuting times up to three hours a day, the widespread separation of home from workplace has become a serious problem that has increased stress—a negative for health.

In some ways, cities are healthier than rural areas. For example, the quality of drinking water is high in most cities, while a significant fraction of rural dwellers drink from polluted wells. City-dwellers have prompt access to nearby emergency health services; rural-dwellers must resort to distant emergency rooms. While the air is polluted in many cities—ozone particularly continues to be a disturbing problem—country-dwellers are more threatened by insecticides and ticks. Congestion is much higher in the cities—an annoyance, but one that contributes to a lower rate of traffic fatalities than in the faster-moving vehicles on country roads and highways.

Above all, country-dwellers lack the range and challenge offered by the city's best jobs, as well as the companionship and constant stimulation of urban social and cultural life. From the perspective of mental health, cities offer diversion that potentially makes it easier to break dependence on cigarettes or alcohol. (Alcoholic over–indulgence is a common hazard in rural areas, especially during the inactive winters.)

HOW HEALTHY IS YOUR CITY?

This book shows people who can choose their city or neighborhood how to make the best choice from the perspective of health. It compares the environment (air and water quality), the disease and mortality rates, the availability of health services, and other criteria. It tells people with particular ailments which cities to avoid. It provides detailed information on *neighborhoods* in New York City.

Other books have ranked cities on numerous factors. *The Livable Cities Almanac* differs from them in at least four ways:

1. *We focus on health.* Our comparisons are made from the single perspective of health, instead of straying among many demographic, ethnic, fiscal and tourist topics.
2. *Our conclusions are presented succinctly and graphically.* We have condensed our findings into easily absorbed Things to Do and a rating system that is applied to each city or metro area.
3. *The book is balanced and carefully reviewed.* The book was reviewed by an advisory committee composed of doctors, urbanologists and other experts (see Acknowledgments). It seeks to provide a sober view of the importance of health and recreation services and the environment, properly considering lifestyle factors and preventive health care. Lifestyle factors depend greatly on the individual, but patterns emerge by looking at city data—for example, it is hard to get exercise in New York City, and some cities are more rigorous than others about requiring separate areas in public facilities for smokers and nonsmokers.
4. *Our data and analyses are carefully explained and annotated.* The reader does not have to take anything on faith.

The Livable Cities Almanac presents information on hazards that the reader may find alarming. However, our basic message is a favorable one—that individuals can take charge of their own futures by learning more about the health status of their homes and workplaces.

THE
Livable Cities
ALMANAC

CHAPTER ONE

Where You Live and Work

This book is about your health in relation to where you live and work—your neighborhood, your city or town, even your state and country.

Whether you seek advice on how to make your home or office healthier, or wish to evaluate different communities based on health, you will find ample information here. At the same time, we address questions that relate to the health of our nation and even our planet—for whatever affects the health of the planet ultimately affects our home and workplace.

WHICH CITY IS THE HEALTHIEST?

This is not a mystery story, so here on the first page are the results of decades of comparative research on city health. The healthiest U.S. metropolitan area is Honolulu, followed by Anchorage, Denver and Charlotte, N.C. The least healthy is Buffalo, followed by Toledo, Worcester and Newark, N.J. The rankings of all 100 are shown in Table 1-1.

How you use these conclusions depends on the details. In any city, as we shall see, some neighborhoods are much healthier than others, and how we handle our immediate surroundings—our workplace and home—may have more effect on our health than do the conditions of the larger community.

But our quest for a healthy place to live and work naturally begins with cities. A quick way to determine which cities are the healthiest is to ask: "In which cities do people live the longest?" That's what is behind Table 1-1. The first column shows how many people die in each metro area in relation to the area's average age.

Why is the average age important? Because when we identify the cities

TABLE 1-1
THE OVERALL HEALTH OF U.S. CITIES

Rank Metro Area	Deaths per 1,000	Residual Death Rate*	Rank Metro Area	Deaths per 1,000	Residual Death Rate*
1 Honolulu (Healthiest)	5.54	-3.42	51 Dayton	7.66	-0.07
2 Anchorage	3.28	-3.24	52 Tulsa	8.10	-0.06
3 Denver-Aurora-Boulder	5.96	-3.00	53 Wilmington, DE	8.30	-0.04
4 Charlotte	5.13	-2.84	54 St. Louis	9.28	0.00
5 Bridgeport-Stamford	7.27	-2.63	55 Lexington, KY	7.39	0.03
6 Washington, DC	6.34	-2.48	56 Spokane	8.81	0.08
7 Salt Lake City	5.51	-2.46	57 New Orleans	7.96	0.13
8 Seattle	7.16	-2.22	58 Columbia, SC	7.31	0.19
9 Miami-Hialeah	9.88	-2.04	59 Fresno	7.70	0.24
10 Sacramento	7.05	-1.95	60 Tucson	8.53	0.32
11 Colorado Springs	5.56	-1.94	61 Tampa-St. Petersburg	11.94	0.33
12 Atlanta	6.19	-1.69	62 Indianapolis	8.35	0.38
13 Richmond	7.10	-1.67	63 Chattanooga	9.08	0.40
14 Minneapolis-St. Paul	6.88	-1.61	64 Jacksonville	8.29	0.41
15 Dallas-Ft. Worth	6.53	-1.47	65 Rochester	8.39	0.42
16 Austin	5.10	-1.41	66 Akron	8.92	0.43
17 Raleigh-Durham	6.25	-1.29	67 Lubbock	6.52	0.48
18 Boise	6.09	-1.27	68 Detroit	8.31	0.48
19 Des Moines	7.08	-1.21	69 Boston	8.71	0.55
20 Houston	6.01	-1.20	70 Greensboro–Winston-Salem	8.38	0.55
21 San Jose–Fremont	5.89	-1.19	71 Montgomery	8.17	0.58
22 Orlando	7.49	-1.14	72 Syracuse	8.84	0.59
23 Little Rock	6.62	-1.12	73 Baltimore	9.20	0.66
24 El Paso	5.18	-1.10	74 Cincinnati	8.89	0.69

#	City	Adjusted rate	Residual	#	City	Adjusted rate	Residual
25	Phoenix-Mesa	7.22	−1.08	75	Newport News-Norfolk	7.12	0.70
26	Kansas City	7.52	−1.07	76	Burlington	7.63	0.74
27	San Francisco-Oakland	8.47	−0.98	77	Philadelphia	9.95	0.75
28	Los Angeles-Long Beach	7.56	−0.93	78	Mobile	8.64	0.76
29	Oklahoma City	7.43	−0.92	79	Riverside-San Bernardino	8.15	0.79
30	Wichita	7.08	−0.89	80	Fort Wayne	8.63	0.80
31	Tacoma	7.51	−0.84	81	Providence-Pawtucket	9.32	0.83
32	Madison, WI	6.19	−0.75	82	Birmingham	9.26	0.87
33	Albuquerque	7.06	−0.63	83	Memphis	8.62	0.93
34	Omaha	7.58	−0.62	84	Milwaukee	8.93	1.00
35	Knoxville	7.69	−0.61	85	Portland, OR	9.54	1.14
36	Louisville	8.68	−0.60	86	Charleston, WV	10.11	1.34
37	San Diego	7.05	−0.59	87	Cleveland	9.92	1.43
38	Las Vegas	7.73	−0.57	88	Columbus, GA	8.87	1.55
39	Jackson	6.78	−0.44	89	New York City-Yonkers	11.09	1.57
40	Manchester-Nashua	7.72	−0.44	90	Chicago	9.83	1.67
41	Lincoln	6.72	−0.40	91	Pittsburgh	11.41	1.75
42	Nashville	8.01	−0.29	92	Shreveport	10.02	2.14
43	San Antonio	6.80	−0.28	93	Portland, ME	11.49	2.48
44	Ft. Lauderdale-Pompano	11.99	−0.26	94	Springfield, MA	11.04	2.50
45	Anaheim-Santa Ana	6.39	−0.22	95	Jersey City	10.83	2.53
46	Baton Rouge	6.49	−0.21	96	Flint	9.56	2.72
47	Columbus, Ohio	6.87	−0.21	97	Newark, NJ	9.71	2.77
48	Hartford-New Britain	8.86	−0.20	98	Worcester-Fitchburg	12.49	3.43
49	Corpus Christi	6.88	−0.15	99	Toledo	11.53	3.70
50	Grand Rapids	7.49	−0.11	100	Buffalo (Least Healthy)	13.14	4.23

* The residual death rate is the author's overall measure of city health. It is the difference between a metropolitan area's actual mortality rate and the mortality rate one would expect based on its median age.

SOURCE: Unadjusted rates from *Vital Statistics*; adjusted rates calculated by the author.[1] The healthiest city, i.e., with the lowest adjusted mortality rate, is Honolulu. The least healthy is Buffalo.

where people die at a faster rate, we come upon the unenlightening fact that many (like Fort Lauderdale or Tampa-St. Petersburg) seem simply to be ones with more relatively older inhabitants. For each year added to the median age of a city, the number of deaths increases by about 0.2 per 1,000 population.[2]

To allow for the fact that some cities have a younger population, we have factored out the influence of age on mortality rates by calculating what is left over (the "residual" death rate) when we remove the age factor. The interesting cities are the ones with high residuals in either direction. Miami, Bridgeport, Denver, Honolulu, Salt Lake City, Charlotte and Anchorage have *lower* death rates than one would predict from their median ages. They are the healthiest cities. But Buffalo, Worcester, Toledo, Newark and Flint have *higher* death rates than one would expect. They are the least healthy cities.

Thus Table 1-1 measures the extent to which each metropolitan area's mortality rate differs from what we might expect based on the area's median age.

So Honolulu is healthiest, based on past data. But has Honolulu's health *trend* been improving, with all the building that has gone on? Table 1-2 shows that by our measure, yes, the city is still getting healthier relative to its own past record and to other cities. Its age-adjusted death rate declined from 1986 to 1987, along with that of Columbus, Georgia; Corpus Christi; Anchorage; Omaha and 39 other metropolitan areas.

HOME/WORKPLACE, COMMUNITY, NATION

We can describe "where you live" and "where you work" in many ways. At the most intimate level, where we live is in our bedroom, in front of the television, or in the kitchen. Where we work is in our office or other work station.

Surveys reveal that Americans, even those living in very modest circumstances, express most satisfaction with their immediate surroundings—their apartments or homes.[3] People's degree of control and participation in the living environment relates closely to their degree of satisfaction with those living conditions. Those who own their houses or apartments feel a stronger sense of control and pride in their surroundings than do those who rent.

The sense of satisfaction and attachment with living space tends to decrease as one moves to larger environments and as the level of participation and control decreases. Other surveys suggest a similar theme: Americans trust local government more than state or Federal government.[4]

Within a city, neighborhoods differ. Health factors can vary substantially between upper-income and lower-income neighborhoods. The difference in death rates between New York City (11 per thousand) and

TABLE 1–2
CITY-HEALTH CHANGE, 1986–87

Metro Area	Change in Death Rate From 1986	Metro Area	Change in Death Rate From 1986
BEST TEN		**WORST TEN**	
Columbus, GA	−6.93%	Orlando	3.66%
Corpus Christi	−6.65%	Richmond	3.69%
Anchorage	−5.61%	Chattanooga	3.86%
Omaha	−5.21%	Albuquerque	4.86%
Honolulu	−5.09%	Austin	5.45%
Jersey City	−4.53%	Boise	5.79%
Burlington	−4.50%	Fort Wayne	6.40%
Ft. Lauderdale	−3.93%	Detroit	7.13%
Baton Rouge	−3.33%	Lexington, KY	7.19%
Tacoma	−3.28%	Jacksonville	9.11%

SOURCE: Derived from *Vital Statistics, op. cit.,* 1987 and 1988; change calculated and ranked by the author. The city showing the greatest reduction in the death rate is Columbus, GA. The one showing the greatest increase in the death rate is Jacksonville, FL.

Honolulu (5 per thousand) is smaller than the difference between the death rate in Central Harlem (16 per thousand, excluding AIDS deaths) and that in Greenwich Village (6 per thousand, excluding AIDS deaths).[5]

For economic and many statistical comparisons, metropolitan areas are a more useful unit of comparison than states. Everyone in a metropolitan area, both in the central city and in suburban areas, has a stake in the same downtown employers and markets. States are, however, the appropriate unit of comparison in situations where state environmental, transportation, tax or other laws (such as school financing or public-health programs) are the subject of comparison. Thus, in Chapter 8 we compare states on highway accidents because state laws regarding the minimum age for purchase of alcohol or speed limits are factors that seem to contribute to differences in auto-accident fatalities.

Regional analysis—comparisons of groups of states—is also sometimes relevant. One comparison is the East Coast vs. the West Coast. Murders are higher on the East Coast, for example, but suicides are higher on the West Coast (more than half of Americans live within 50 miles of the two coastlines).[6] Americans are migrating from east to west and from north to south. One in nine Americans now lives in California,[7] where population growth has been most rapid.

Note that western cities tend to be healthier than average; northeastern and midwestern cities tend to be less healthy than average. This observation is borne out statistically. These regional differences, however, are also significantly related to lifestyle factors as reflected in lung cancer and heart attack rates. The regional differences may have more to do with how people behave in different parts of the country than with external conditions.

HOW GOVERNMENTS AFFECT OUR HEALTH

Who is responsible for our health? Government? Yes, in part. The Federal Environmental Protection Agency (EPA) and its regional, state and local counterparts monitor air and water quality and regulate business effluent, emissions and waste disposal. The Occupational Safety and Health Act addresses worker exposure to hazardous situations; CERCLA (the Comprehensive Environmental Response Compensation and Liability Act of 1980) covers indoor air quality; Title IV of the Superfund laws regulates radon gas.[8] Sen. George Mitchell (D-Maine), Senate Majority Leader, in February 1991 reintroduced the Indoor Air Quality Act, S.455, to expand research on indoor air pollutants and develop a plan for states to follow in dealing with them.[9]

State and city environmental health varies, depending on their approach to environmental regulation. Neighborhoods also differ, as we see in our treatment of New York City in Chapter 9. Keep in mind that each level of government has a corresponding level of government service or oversight. States have their own environmental and public health agencies, and these operate through county agencies. Metro areas often have regional planning and health-care delivery committees. City governments often have neighborhood planning units or service-delivery managers, and city council members serve as neighborhood service monitors. Hospitals greatly affect the level of services for children and pregnant women, as we shall see in Chapter 7.

Also, solving one problem may create another. For example, recent concerns about conserving energy (motivated both by the cost of energy and by environmental awareness) have resulted in much more tightly constructed houses and offices. Less outdoor air is circulated in heating and cooling systems, thus trapping indoor air pollutants.[10]

ECONOMIC HEALTH

Another issue is that the *economic health* of a community can affect the health of its residents.

Surveys indicate that the most significant contributor to well-being is whether or not a person has a job (next is whether or not they are married, as we note in Chapter 5). For every additional $1,000 in per-capita income in cities we surveyed, the death rate decreases by 0.14. As we shall see in Chapter 5, within a city wealthier areas have lower mortality rates.

One reason that Los Angeles and New York have thrived over the years despite their periodic crises is their openness to immigration and entrepreneurship. More closed economies, especially those dominated by a handful of industrial companies with traditions of rigidly hierarchical management, are less hospitable to entrepreneurs—and to women.[11]

A city's economic health depends on its place in a global market as well as a local one. Western and Midwestern cities continue to have the most robust economies and continuing population growth.[12] The emergence of the European Community may help revive the East Coast (Atlantic Rim).

The test of a city's economy is its ability to provide jobs. Table 1-3 shows,

TABLE 1–3
ECONOMIC HEALTH, 1990

	Unemploy-ment	Change	Enter-prise	Average
BEST TEN				
Lincoln, NE	1	11	6	6.0
Sioux Falls	3	22	13	12.7
Columbus, OH	21	19	17	19.0
Seattle	14	19	26	19.7
Fort Wayne	56	52	72	20.0
Honolulu	3	43	22	22.7
Indianapolis	17	15	36	22.7
Norfolk–Va. Beach	31	22	20	24.3
Lexington, KY	19	40	19	26.0
Des Moines	11	27	40	26.0
WORST TEN				
Manchester	95	113	63	90.3
New York	96	102	73	90.3
Corpus Christi	108	58	107	91.0
Oklahoma City	84	91	105	93.3
Providence	90	111	85	95.3
Worcester	100	111	87	99.3
Bakersfield	111	107	82	100.0
Flint	110	85	109	101.3
Fresno	111	97	99	102.3
Springfield, MA	93	108	108	103.0

NOTES: Unemployment rates are for November 1990. Change in unemployment is between November 1988 and November 1990. The enterprise measure is based on small-business formation and growth.

SOURCES: Unemployment and changes in unemployment, derived from a special printout provided by the Bureau of Labor Statistics.[14] Enterprise data are derived from *Inc.* Magazine, March 1990.[15]

in the first column, the November 1990 unemployment ranking of some metropolitan areas. Lincoln, Nebraska, has the lowest unemployment, Stockton, California, the highest. The second column shows the change in unemployment compared with two years earlier. Baton Rouge and New Orleans (not shown) have the largest drop in unemployment; Manchester, New Hampshire, shows the largest increase.

Besides the availability of jobs, I have attempted to factor in the rate of small-business formation and growth in each metro area; these elements are the basis of community economic health, i.e., the likelihood that the level of jobs will be maintained in the long run.[13] Las Vegas is the most entrepreneurial city, Tacoma the least.

Averaging these three ranks provides an overall measure of relative economic health. Lincoln rated as the economically healthiest city in 1990; Springfield, Massachusetts, as the least healthy.

CHAPTER TWO

The Healthy Home

The 1980s saw a dramatic increase in public concern about toxic chemicals in our air, water, food and homes because they can cause allergic reactions such as fatigue or rapid weight change; puffiness in the face, hands, ankles or abdomen; or palpitations or heavy sweating unrelated to exercise.[1] The National Research Council says that 15 percent of the U.S. population is hypersensitive to chemicals in pesticides and common household products.[2]

Most toxic chemicals were developed within the last 50 years. More than 70,000 new chemical compounds have been introduced into the environment since World War II, too recently to reveal the full range of long–term effects.[3] Some exposure is unavoidable, but many *household products* available in supermarkets or hardware stores contain hazardous toxins. Many common substances qualify as indoor air pollutants—paint, dust, tobacco smoke and some household cleaning products. Other hazards like electromagnetic fields are not yet fully understood—but collectively pose worrisome health risks because they may be hard to detect or control.

This chapter covers the healthy home under six headings, in alphabetical order: energy sources, household cleaners and paper products, household electric appliances, pesticides, quality of air and water quality. Hazards relating to buildings are covered in Chapter 4 and water contamination is covered again in Chapter 6.

ENERGY SOURCES

This section addresses traditional energy–source hazards associated with electricity and gas—electrocutions, poisonous fumes and fires. Later in this chapter we examine the more recent, conflicting evidence that electric and magnetic fields created by power lines and household appliances may slow heart rates, alter brain waves or cause cancer.[4]

Electrical Hazards: Five Things to Do

Electricity is a prime home hazard because it can cause shocks and fire. Annually, 166,000 home fires are electrically caused, resulting in 900 deaths, 6,200 injuries and $935 million worth of property losses. Here is a checklist for hazard avoidance or containment:

1. *Watch for and act on signs of electrical trouble,* such as cover plates on switches and outlets that are warm to the touch, smoke or sparks emanating from switches or outlets, strange odors (like the smell of burning plastic) near the outlets or switches, periodic flickering of lights or the failure of outlets, lights or entire circuits to work.[5]

2. *Periodically check electrical wiring and cords.* Repair or replace any cords that are pinched, cracked or frayed. To prevent cords from overheating, do not place them under rugs or rest furniture on them. Do not exceed the rating for current of any cord.

3. *Avoid overloading an outlet.* Don't plug two or more appliances into the same circuit if their combined wattage exceeds 1,500 (1 watt = 1 amp current × 1 volt pressure; a typical light bulb is 100 watts or less). Air conditioners, portable heaters, broilers, washing machines or dryers, dishwashers, hot plates, full–size microwave ovens, hair dryers and toasters should be kept on separate circuits. If you blow a fuse by overloading the circuit, bring in an electrician to install more wiring, or reduce your electrical appetite.

4. *Connect third (grounding) wires that come with appliances.* They are designed to reduce the danger of your being electrocuted. Never stand on a wet or damp floor or shower or sit in a tub of water while using an electrical appliance. If a plugged–in appliance should fall into water, unplug it before trying to retrieve it, even if it is turned off. Avoid simultaneously touching an appliance and something that is grounded, like a metal water faucet.

5. *Have repairs done by a licensed electrician.* Avoid electrical tape or do–it–yourself kits from the hardware store. Replace old two–prong power outlets in the bathroom, garage, workshop and outdoors with ground–fault circuit interrupters—i.e., outlets that come with a reset button and a test button. They can detect the flow of current through unintended pathways and may be able to de–energize a faulty circuit or appliance before a fire develops.

Home Electric Safety Audit Room–by–Room Checklist and *CPSC Guide to Electrical Safety* are available for those who want to do their home survey right. Order from Consumer Product Safety Commission, Publications, Washington, DC 20207. Call (800) 638-2772 with pencil in hand.

Fires in the Home: Five Things to Do

Fires are one of the three major causes of accidental deaths in the home (the two others are falls and poisoning). Each year, more than 6,000 people die in fires, 80 percent of them in the home. Sixteen percent of all fatal fires in the U.S. begin in the kitchen, from the ignition of cooking oils, grease, clothing, towels, wax, spilled combustible liquids (alcohol and cleaning fluids) and flour.[6] When the flame or hot electric ring contacts any of these materials, combustion occurs very quickly and the resulting fire can spread rapidly. Fireplaces and wood–burning stoves can be hazardous because of the buildup of heat around the stove or fireplace and around the chimney or stovepipe. The buildup of creosote in the chimney or pipe may also lead to a fire. Quick–burning materials such as foam plastic are also a big problem.[7]

1. *Keep an ABC–rated fire extinguisher in your kitchen.* Cooking generates emissions that render smoke detectors impractical for use in the kitchen. Fire extinguishers have ratings based on the type of fires they are best suited to extinguish. The most versatile for kitchen and home use are those rated ABC. They can extinguish (A) burning paper, wood, cloth and some plastics; (B) burning grease or inflammable liquids; and (C) electrical fires. At the least, it must be rated BC to be effective.[8] It would be safest to have two fire extinguishers, one on each side of the kitchen—*in full view.* Halon-gas extinguishers are nontoxic and don't leave a messy residue, but the gas harms the ozone layer.

2. *Keep handy a fiberglass fire blanket and baking soda.* In case of fire, throw the fiberglass blanket on top of the fire. Depriving a fire of oxygen will extinguish it quickly. Baking soda is recommended for grease fires.

3. *Consider building in a sprinkler system.* Sprinklers are becoming increasingly available for the home. Fires can spread very quickly in today's houses because of the abundance of plastics in the home and small room sizes. Insulation keeps heat from fires inside the house, allowing blazes to spread more quickly.[9]

4. *Replace your smoke–alarm batteries.* To help you remember, fire– prevention officials recommend changing smoke–alarm batteries on the weekends when clocks are changed to and from daylight saving time in the spring and fall.

5. *Conduct a family fire drill at least once a year.* As a family, practice using your extinguisher (and check pressure gauge) and discuss priorities and escape routes. Post the number of the fire department and a list of procedures next to the phone.

Gas

Anything that produces high levels of heat can present safety problems. An open gas flame on a stove is a potential cause of fire; gas leaks are explosively flammable, can cause illness and they take the lives of 600 Americans every year.[10] In addition, cooking with gas generates indoor pollution, most significantly nitrogen dioxide, carbon monoxide and, to a lesser extent, nitrous oxide and aldehydes—all of which can cause or aggravate a number of ailments.[11] Poorly adjusted burners are the greatest culprits.

Nitrogen dioxide has been linked to greater risk of infectious respiratory disorders. Concentration of exposure is a bigger factor than length of exposure.[12] People suffering from respiratory diseases like asthma are more seriously affected. Even small amounts of carbon monoxide diminish the blood's oxygen level. Since low oxygen levels make the heart pump harder, heart patients, anemics and infants are extremely vulnerable to carbon monoxide.

Combustion byproducts are generally more highly concentrated in energy–efficient homes or poorly vented apartments. *The solution* to toxic combustion byproducts is a good exhaust system, which is mandatory for gas fuel; we discuss such ventilating units later in this chapter.

HOUSEHOLD CLEANERS AND PAPER PRODUCTS

Household cleaning products are among the most toxic substances encountered in our everyday environment. While deaths from fires have been declining each year, deaths from poisoning have been steadily increasing. Over 4,000 Americans die from ingesting toxic liquids or solids every year. A study of Oregon housewives found that women who stayed at home all day had a 54 percent higher death rate from cancer than women who had jobs away from the home. It suggested that this higher rate might be attributed in part to chemicals in household products.[13]

Many household cleaning products like ammonia, benzenes, phenol and cresol—and the aerosol propellants (most notoriously methylene chloride) they are often packaged with—can cause major harm, especially when misused. A significant misuse is the mixing of ammonia and chlorine bleach, producing deadly chlorine gas.[14]

Since 1977, the Consumer Product Safety Commission, under the Hazardous Substances Act, requires cleaning products to be labeled if they are corrosive, flammable, irritating, allergenic or toxic. But makers of such hazardous cleaning products are not required by law to disclose the full amount of noxious chemicals they may contain. Nor are they required to have the products approved by any regulatory agency before putting them

on the market. Three good ways to obtain safe household cleaners are to:
(1) make your own (2) buy green and (3) shop for the least toxic popular
brands.[15]

Aerosol Sprays

Most propellants contain flammable products that are toxic when inhaled;
mist particles carry the toxins to the lungs and bloodstream. So avoid
aerosol sprays. Select other sprays—or better still, liquids in a bottle.
Choose products with nontoxic, nonflammable ingredients. Use setting
lotions instead of hair spray, or shaving soap instead of shaving cream.
Aerosol deodorants can cause infections in the hair follicles under the
arms; use stick deodorants.

Bleached Paper Products

Paper products that are bleached white use chlorine, which combines with
phenol compounds from wood to produce dioxins, which the EPA once
described as the most toxic of all man–made chemicals. In 1991 key
Federal and academic experts reversed previous warnings and minimized
dioxin dangers, describing them as at worst "a weak carcinogen associated
only with high–dose exposure."[16]

Even so, tissues, towels and coffee filters made snowy white with chlorine bleaching, often are left with traces of chlorine in the paper. Oxygen–
bleached or unbleached (brown) filters avoid both potential dangers and
the chlorine taste.

Detergents

We have discussed detergents briefly. They deserve more explanation.
Synthetic detergents were invented during World War I because of a shortage of soap. They became preferred for laundry because soap reacts with
the mineral salts in "hard" water to form an insoluble curd that produces
visible oily deposits on clothes and a ring in the bathtub. Synthetic detergents prevent formation of the curd. By the early 1970s, detergents had
virtually replaced soap for clothes-washing. Chlorine is often included in
laundry detergents for bleaching—and in automatic–dishwasher detergents for removing food that has been baked on.

Most shampoos and most clothes–washing and dish–washing liquids
and powders continue to rely on detergents. The toxic character, if any, of
detergents varies with the product and depends on what additives are
included, but popular detergent brands have been used for a long time
without evidence of significant toxic effects on humans.

The major legitimate objection to detergents relates to phosphates,
which aren't inherently toxins—quite the opposite, they are essential

nutrients. In the 1970s phosphates (half from detergents) disgorged into U.S. wastewater overloaded U.S. lakes and estuaries with nutrients, choking the water surface with algae and thereby using up the oxygen in the water. So phosphates were indirectly toxic to fish. Some states banned or limited the sale of phosphate–based detergents—Indiana, Michigan, New York, and Wisconsin were among the first. Cities enacted their own bans, starting with places like Akron, Chicago and Miami. By 1983 the average phosphorus content of U.S. detergents had dropped by more than half and the proportion of phosphorus attributable to detergents fell to 35 percent in areas that didn't ban phosphate–based detergents entirely.[17]

CHEMTREC (Chemical Transportation Emergency Center), a 24–hour computerized database and emergency center, responds at any time to an emergency. Call (800) 424-9300 for assistance with chemical spills, leaks, fires or exposures. Do not use this number except in an emergency. Otherwise, call (800) 262-8200.

Floor Wax

Wood preservative is a very toxic ingredient that is absorbed through the skin and causes drowsiness, headache and nausea. Since soft liquid waxes do not hold up well and must be applied often, a house with soft–waxed floors is seldom free of toxic fumes. Alternatives include using a hard–paste wax once or twice a year with the windows open, or installing a floor covering that does not require waxing.

Furniture, Metal and Shoe Polishes: Five Alternatives

The ingredients in polishing products often include methanol, ethanes, ketones and petroleum distillates. Breathing the vapors or accidentally drinking these products can be harmful and even fatal. Long–term exposure to some solvents may cause liver or kidney problems, birth defects, central nervous system disorders and cancer.

1. *Use a paste, liquid or cream instead of aerosol waxes and polishes,* because inhalation of their toxic emissions is inevitable and they damage the ozone layer. Especially avoid polishes containing nitrobenzene, dinitrobenzene and chlorinated methanes and ethanes.
2. *Use commercially available lemon oil, or make your own nontoxic furniture polish.*
3. *Avoid shoe polish* that contains methylene chloride, trichloroethylene or nitrobenzene. Beeswax, lemon juice and oils can be used to shine shoes.[18]

4. *Avoid chemicals to clean brass or copper.* This one is a true test of your environmental commitment. Make a paste of lemon juice and salt. Or use a slice of lemon sprinkled with baking soda. Rub with a soft, clean cloth, rinse and dry.
5. *Use baking soda to remove tarnish from silver.* Dip a damp, soft cloth in the baking soda or soak tarnished silver in water with salt or baking soda along with something made of aluminum. Rub, rinse in hot water and dry.[19]

Hazardous-Waste Disposal: Five Ideas

Many household products containing toxic or harmful substances are disposed of improperly by simply pouring them down the drain or throwing them into the trash. This can cause problems with sanitation services, plumbing and septic tanks and can allow chemicals to leak into the environment.[20]

1. *Use up the can.* Find something to paint with the last bit of paint in the can, before you dispose of it. Better to have a second coat of paint on a piece of furniture than have the rest of the paint end up in our water.
2. *Give away leftover chemicals.* Give away to friends any leftover paint and paint removers, water repellent, gasoline, pool chemicals and household acids (muriatic, acetic and sulfuric). Make sure the product is in its original container and lists directions for use. Paint and paint-removal products can be donated to community organizations and theater groups. Photoprocessing chemicals can be donated to college or commercial labs.
3. *Recycle.* Local sanitation departments or recycling commissions usually have information on where to recycle specific products such as motor oil, transmission fluid, brake fluid and car batteries. Smoke detectors and gas cylinders can be returned to the manufacturer for disposal.
4. *Use community hazardous–waste services.* Many communities have household hazardous–waste collection programs. Call your local health department or environmental agency to see if one exists in your area.
5. *Mix before disposal.* Water–soluble products such as soaps and detergents can be diluted with water and poured down the drain. Other liquids that cannot be used up can be solidified and placed in the trash so as not to harm sanitation workers. To solidify a liquid, add enough absorbent material such as rags or newspapers to soak up all the liquid. Put it all into a secure plastic bag and dispose of it in the household garbage.

Spot Removers and Dry–Cleaning Chemicals

Hazardous dry–cleaning solvents including perchlorethylene or tri-chloromethane are suspected carcinogens and can damage the liver and kidneys on repeated exposure. It's best to minimize use of dry cleaning by purchasing clothes that can be washed and then using the laundry rather than the dry cleaner.

If you do use these solvents at home or bring home dry–cleaned clothing: remove the garments from their plastic wrap and be sure to air them thoroughly for at least half a day before wearing them, to allow traces of solvents to evaporate.[21]

HOUSEHOLD ELECTRICAL APPLIANCES

Many appliances are suspected of producing adverse health effects—notably cookware, microwave ovens and television sets. If you use a computer at home, see also Chapter 3 (The Healthy Workplace) for information on video display terminals.

Electrical appliances are generally considered to be safer than those that use gas. Studies also show that all-electric homes have lower concentrations of combustion byproducts *in the home* than do homes with gas appliances.[22] The problem with electricity is that generation of the power far from the homesite creates more harmful emissions. Electric appliances also cost more to operate than gas ones, but electricity costs can be reduced by installing heat pumps into the central heating system and hot-water heater. Consult a local heating and cooling contractor. "Self-cleaning" ovens may generate cancerous fumes.[23]

Electromagnetic Fields

Some people argue that electric appliances may have negative health effects because of the electromagnetic fields they generate and the power sources that feed them. The alternating current (AC) electricity used in U.S. homes and offices is produced by current that comes out of a wall outlet alternating back and forth at the extremely low frequency (ELF) of 60 cycles a second (i.e., 60 hertz). This power produces electric and magnetic fields that emit radiation. The alleged hazards relate both to the electric fields, which are produced by voltage, and to the magnetic fields, which develop as currents flow. Human skin can block electromagnetic fields and in theory the fields could produce changes inside human cells.[24]

Unlike radiation from X-rays, AC radiation is not ionizing, meaning that it does not produce chemical and molecular changes in living tissue. But a growing volume of research—even that paid for by the power industry—

suggests that cancer incidence may be linked to ELF electromagnetic fields generated by AC power and appliances that use it. *But the risk levels even in the most highly exposed populations are still low,* well below the risks to, say, asbestos workers or chain smokers. It just suggests the need for caution and additional research.[25]

The key factor in evaluating electrical devices is the source of their power and their dose. Batteries, for example, use direct current (DC) and do not emit electromagnetic fields. Electric blankets, on the other hand, come in close contact with the body, have a high electromagnetic field and are used for hours at a time.[26]

What is the dosage? The most accurate instruments for monitoring electromagnetic–field strength are expensive to purchase or rent. A few relatively inexpensive devices for measuring the most common 60–hertz (household AC) fields have become available. The lowest priced fully fledged meter I could find costs about $50 from Mentec Corp., (603) 893-8080.

Cookware Guidelines

Cookware *can* be a major health hazard. Aluminum and no-stick pots and pans seem to be safe, but copper and copper-plated tin cookware is considered dangerous by an FDA expert because the copper leaches into the food that is being cooked. Consuming enough leached copper will bring on nausea and diarrhea. Ceramic cookware can be more dangerous, because of the lead that is often used in the enamel. Cooking with ceramic cookware with inadequately sealed glaze can cause stomach cramps, constipation, insomnia and anemia. So:

1. *If you buy copper cookware, be sure it is lined.* The inside should be nickel or stainless steel.
2. *If you buy ceramic cookware, be careful of imports.* U.S., British and Japanese enameled cookware is considered safe by the FDA. But enameled cookware from China, Hong Kong, India and Mexico is not.[27]

To test for lead in your cookware:

DSK Safer Home Test Kit, 325 North Oakhurst, Beverly Hills, CA 90210 sells a kit for $32. It's in a 5-test kit from Hammacher Schlemmer, New York. *Frandon Enterprises Inc.,* P.O. Box 300321, 511 North 48th St., Seattle, WA 98103 (800) 359-9000. A kit good for over 100 tests costs $29.95 plus $3.50 shipping.

Hair Dryers, Heaters, Bedside Electric Clocks

Hair dryers require high currents and therefore generate substantial magnetic fields. Average users don't operate hair dryers long enough to pose a risk to themselves. But the hand-held dryer may be a hazard for hairdressers, who use them repeatedly each workday.

Exposure to baseboard electric heaters is not hazardous under normal circumstances, although an infant's crib should not be placed close to these heaters. Portable electric heaters, however, pose a fire, burn and electrocution hazard as well as high field intensity.

An electric clock plugged into a wall produces a magnetic field. Many people place their clock on a bedside table within a foot or two of their head. Some argue that the average eight hours' a night exposure adds up to a significant dose of electromagnetic radiation. It is simple enough to push the clock farther away or to substitute a battery-operated clock.

Microwave Ovens

Injuries, especially burns, associated with the use and *misuse* of microwave ovens have been on the rise. Microwaves heat in a different way from conventional cooking appliances, and this is rarely explained adequately in owners' manuals. Burns and scalds from liquids occur because the contents get much hotter than the package. When clear liquid is heated in glass, ceramic or smooth plastic containers, even without boiling, it can erupt violently when moved or stirred or when something is added to it.

Most alarming are reports of injuries to children using microwaves. According to the Campbell Microwave Institute in 1988, children as young as 6 years old have been allowed to use the microwave without adult supervision. When children put their eyes to the microwave door they are doing the worst possible thing in terms of exposing themselves to microwave emissions.[28]

Damage to the gasketing material around the microwave-oven door will markedly increase the level of radiation that leaks from it when it is in use. The unit should be checked every year. If it has been damaged, do not use it until it has been repaired and rechecked for radiation leakage.

Microwave Packaging and Wraps

Serious concerns have arisen regarding the food-packaging materials used for microwavable products and the interaction between their chemical compounds and the food that is cooked in them—paper trays that contain prepared meat dinners, the "heat-susceptor packaging" used with crusty foods like pizza and the plastic wraps that seal other microwaved foods. The breakdown of the packaging at a high heat level may cause a number of volatile components to become indirect food additives.[29]

The FDA doesn't regulate "microwave-safe" containers, plastic wraps or baking trays because of its housewares exemption policy, decided in the 1950s. Its jurisdiction is limited to commercial packaging.[30] FDA's limited studies so far show that the components of microwave packaging—adhesives, polymers, paper and paperboard—can migrate from the packaging to the foods that are cooked in them. Some of these components contain carcinogenic substances like benzene.[31]

So don't let plastic wrap touch food in the microwave oven, as migration of undesirable chemicals is known to occur when certain plastics are placed directly on food, especially fatty food. Until more safety data are forthcoming, the prudent thing to do is to *use glass cookware* for microwaving food, *not* the heat-susceptor microwave packages.

Television Sets

A small amount of ionizing radiation is given off as X-rays from television sets. But non-ionizing electromagnetic radiation is also given off by wiring in the unit. The electromagnetic fields are generated in the circuitry and the radiation is given off in all directions, more from the rear of most television sets or monitors than from the screen. Color monitors give off more radiation than monochrome monitors, but the total electromagnetic field depends more on the design of the unit.

Other things being equal, larger screens are associated with stronger fields. If you are concerned about these fields, stay 3 to 4 widths of the screen away from it when watching for a long period. The electromagnetic radiation also goes through wood and other building materials, so an infant or child's bed should not be placed against a wall opposite a television set in the adjoining room.

The physical hazard of television sets may be significant if a child sits close to a television for long hours. But the physical damage pales in significance next to the mental damage that is being done by these long television hours! When children graduate from television to computer terminals—whether to play video games or to do homework—the terminal should be the most recent ones, with lower levels of radiation leakage. We will discuss this in the next chapter.

PESTICIDES IN THE HOME AND GARDEN

Pesticides is a broad term for chemicals intended to control weeds (herbicides), insects (insecticides) and other pests. Exposure to commercial agricultural pesticides is difficult to avoid. But pesticide use by individuals at home is easier to avoid or deal with. For people using pesticides around the home, the most common form of exposure is through the skin. Short-term effects include shortness of breath, nausea, stomach cramps, headache and twitching muscles. Possible delayed effects of some pesticides can cause cancer and disorders of the reproductive system.

Pesticides for use around the home are regulated by the EPA. All pesticides marketed in the United States must bear an EPA-approved label that describes the proper way to handle the product. Individuals may be held legally liable for mishaps caused by misuse of these products. Be sure to read all labels carefully and follow the directions exactly.

Home Pest Control

Preventing the influx of pests is the best approach to staying free of household pests like termites, roaches, ants and fleas. You can control indoor pests without toxic substances by using a series of common-sense steps collectively referred to as integrated pest management (IPM).[32] The main idea of IPM is to eliminate the pest's habitat and disrupt its lifestyle. First, identify the pest and evaluate the extent of the problem. Learn about its life cycle, its habits, how it feeds, where it sleeps, mates and hides and when it might be most vulnerable to attack! You can then plan your course of action using nonchemical weapons.

Stopping their entry is important to your IPM strategy. For example, aphids that feed on the plants, shrubs and trees just outside your house can be eliminated with an insecticidal soap—a natural-source soap available at gardening stores. Deprive ants of their source of food and they will go elsewhere.[33] To keep ants out of your house, pour a line of cinnamon, cream of tartar, red chili pepper, salt, dried mint, sage or cucumber peels at the point of entry.

The next step might be to use nontoxic traps like roach motels. Always try other methods before resorting to indiscriminately toxic bug bombs and poisonous chemical sprays. The active ingredient in Raid is virtually as toxic as DDT and 28 times as toxic as boric acid (which is still a poison to be treated with caution). Raid is also far from selective about the creatures it kills. But boric acid, certainly a milder form of pesticide, is a powder that when used properly (spread it where roaches will walk through it) will kill many varieties of roaches.[34]

Lyme disease is a new scourge caused by tiny ticks known scientifically as Ixodes dammini. Lyme disease can be inhibited by a somewhat expensive product called Damminix—the product is a wad of cotton soaked in a chemical that is spread to the ticks by mice that use the cotton for their nests. (It works; I have used it since my wife contracted Lyme disease in our backyard.)

The No. 1 injury attributed to pets is dog bites—over a million a year are reported as serious enough to require a doctor's attention or missed work or classes.[35] To prevent dog bites, don't move to pet a dog too quickly; show it your hand first and move slowly. Back away, don't run away, from a threatening dog. Keep your own dog in an enclosed area or on a leash.

Guidance:

> *National Pesticide Telecommunications Network* (800) 858-7378, fax (806) 743-3094, is available to help you determine the relative toxicity of any commonly sold pesticide. Available 24 hours. Sponsored by EPA and Texas Tech University Health Sciences Center. Quickly and authoritatively answers pesticide-related questions regarding toxicity, health effects, residual effects and use and application. Refers callers to appropriate public and private agencies that deal with pesticide safety, environmental issues, cleanup and disposal and air and soil lab analyses.

Lawn/Garden Care and Food Hazards: Six Things to Do

1. *Control garden pests naturally.* Choose resistant plant varieties. Maintain good garden sanitation. Rotate crops. Introduce natural enemies of the pests (e.g., ladybugs). Manage the soil properly. Interplant crops. Pull weeds and use traps instead of poisons. Some pest-control materials can be made or grown.[36]
2. *Fertilize naturally.* Natural fertilizers like compost, manure, peat moss or decayed organic matter improve the productivity of the garden soil and slowly release nitrogen, phosphorous and potassium. Instead of herbicides, hand weed and mulch generously with organic material.[37]
3. *If you must use pesticides, read the directions carefully!* This will reduce the hazard to yourself and others.
4. *Wash or peel produce.* Rinsing in water will remove some of the pesticide residue on the surface. A mild solution of soap and water will help remove more. Peeling produce will remove surface residue, but it may also remove important nutrients concentrated near the surface.
5. *Buy low-pesticide or organic food.* Consumers can send a clear message to food producers and provide incentives for farmers to decrease their use of pesticides by demanding, and buying, *only* food without, or with a minimum of, pesticide residue. Buy organically grown fruits and vegetables. Buy in season and avoid the perfect-looking produce that depends on constant doses of pesticides and growth agents. Ask questions about imported produce, which often contains above-average pesticide residue and may have been treated with pesticides not legal for U.S. use.
6. *Grow your own food.*

Termite Control: Four Nontoxic Approaches

Termites are worrisome, because they can destroy your house. Subterranean termites are the worst; they nest in the soil, not inside the house.

But the chemical most commonly used to kill termites, chlordane, is a dangerous toxin. Chlorpyrios, currently the most popular termiticide, is also a potent neurotoxin that can linger in your home's air for 16 years and in the ground for 30.[38] To steer between the dangers of the termites themselves and the toxins used to kill them, here are some ideas:

1. *Inspect annually for signs of infestation.* You can inspect your own home if you have crawlspaces or unfinished basements—look for tiny holes in wood and nearby traces of wood powder. Slab-construction homes or homes with finished basements should be inspected by a professional. Never use pesticides as a preventive measure.

2. *Use nematodes against subterranean termites.* Nematodes, tiny parasitic worms, are the best nontoxic solution. Plug up all openings the termites might use to gain entry to prevent reinfestation. Limited chemical ("chemical-spot") treatment might also be used to eliminate any termites in the wood—a less toxic alternative to wholesale pesticide soaking.

3. *Use hot air, electrocution or freezing against drywood termites.* Drywood termites, found primarily in California, Texas, Florida and other Gulf Coast states, nest inside the house, usually first in attics. Look for small holes in the walls, furniture or ceilings and for oval "droppings" (resembling sawdust) anywhere near or below the holes. Severe infestations must be treated by fumigation, but new nontoxic techniques include hot air, electrocution and freezing.

4. *Use sand barriers and repair against dampwood termites.* Damp-wood termites are attracted to damp, decaying wood and are found along the West Coast. Spot treatment with pesticides and building a sand barrier at the base of the foundation are both proven methods of elimination, along with replacement of any damp wood or repair leaks that attracted termites in the first place.[39]

QUALITY OF AIR

External air and water quality are covered in Chapter 6, on the environment. Our focus in the rest of this chapter is on indoor air pollution and tap water contamination.

Air Pollution Inside the Home

People living in cities spend almost 90 percent of their time indoors, where they are exposed to toxins such as radon, pesticides, lead, asbestos, tobacco smoke and synthetic chemicals found in cleaning agents. Indoor air can be 10 to 100 times more toxic than outdoor air.[40]

Many toxins are found in building materials. Most of these chemicals lose their toxicity after a short time, but some chemicals, such as formaldehyde, can take many years. Avoid using products that contain a lot of formaldehyde—e.g., unreformaldehyde foam insulation, particle board, chipboard, wafer board, composition board and medium-density fiber board. These are often used for counter tops, kitchen and bathroom cabinets, floor underlayment, sheathing, shelving and furniture.[41]

Ventilation and Air Cleaners

Proper ventilation is especially important in the kitchen and bathroom, which contain many sources of pollutants. Installing exhaust fans in the bathroom and a kitchen range hood, vented outside, can greatly improve air quality in the home. But recirculating range hoods are often inadequate for eliminating pollutants generated in the kitchen area.[42]

Air cleaners can't remove all indoor-air problems, but will remove significant levels of dust, pollen and smoke. Filters, generally made of fiber mesh, trap particles as air passes through.[43]

Those with activated-carbon filters are even effective in removing some formaldehyde and nitrogen dioxide. Remember that all of these units require some type of yearly maintenance such as replacing filters and cleaning, and some are noisy.

In recent years, Government studies have found that harmful bacteria and molds multiply in the water tanks of humidifiers and are spewed into the air.[44]

The vented-exhaust system is the most available, the most practical and the safest system. A relatively new device called the heat recovery ventilator (HRV) can replace air in homes so that the loss of warm air is minimal. They are designed mainly for newer, energy-efficient homes and are available for the entire house or for individual rooms. See box for references.

Houseplants are an aesthetically pleasing way to reduce dangerous contaminants in the air. Spider plants and golden pothos are excellent for reducing carbon monoxide; philodendron (elephant's ear and heart leaf) can absorb large quantities of formaldehyde and carbon monoxide; and aloe vera is effective at removing low concentrations of formaldehyde.

Heat Recovery Ventilation for Housing, Superintendent of Documents, Government Printing Office, Washington, DC 20402 ($2.25).

Home Ventilation Institute, 30 W. University Drive, Arlington Heights, IL 60004.

Real Goods, John Shafer, 966-Z Mazzoni St., Ukiah, CA 95482 (800) 762-7325 or (707) 468-9292. Exhaustive catalog.

WATER QUALITY

Contaminants

Should you treat your home water? The best way to decide is to review the most likely potential contaminants, have your water analyzed and then evaluate the risks and possible benefits of treatment.

Water contaminants may be "primary" or "secondary." Primary contaminants are potentially hazardous to health. Secondary contaminants pose aesthetic or cosmetic problems that affect the taste and appearance of water but are otherwise harmless. Serious contaminants can usually be detected by taste, smell, sight or touch; but nitrates and nitrites are not detectable in this way.

Primary contaminants start with lead, the main cause for concern about toxic-metal contamination of tap water. It contributes to brain damage in children and high blood pressure among adults. It often enters drinking water through lead-soldered pipes and service lines connecting homes to water mains. It may cause a greenish stain in your sink.[45]

In May 1991 the EPA told water suppliers to treat drinking water with harmless chemicals to reduce its acidity so that less lead corrodes from pipes and solder. By 1993, all suppliers will be required to start testing tap water inside a certain number of homes for dangerous lead levels. After 1999, if tap water continues to register lead levels of more than 15 parts per billion (.015 mg/liter)—lower than the previous standard of 50 ppb—water suppliers must replace underground lead service lines. EPA rules allow 15 years for the gradual replacement of the underground lines, which means harmful lead levels could persist in some homes until 2014. But EPA deputy administrator F. Henry Habicht predicts that within the first six years, 95 percent of the benefits of the rule will be achieved.[46]

The EPA added copper to the primary contaminant list in May 1991. In high concentrations it is associated with gastro-intestinal illnesses and renal or liver failure. Copper makes water bitter, tangy or metallic-tasting and leaves blue-green stains on plumbing fixtures. The maximum permissible concentration is 1.3 mg/liter.

Nitrates (salts of nitric acid, HNO_3) and especially nitrites (salts of nitrous acid, HNO_2) are of increasing concern to the EPA, because in high concentrations they are linked to asphyxiation of formula-fed babies. These salts are byproducts of agricultural runoff but are detectable only in the lab. The EPA standard for nitrates is 10 mg/liter and in 1992 the EPA added a maximum permissible concentration of nitrites of 1 mg/liter.[47]

Secondary or cosmetic contaminants include such minerals as iron, manganese and the minerals calcium and magnesium, the salts of which make water "hard" and difficult to wash with. Most U.S. municipalities add two other chemicals, chlorine and fluoride, to their water supplies.

Iron turns water brackish (salty) or red-brown and can add a soapy taste. Residual chlorine tastes salty, corrodes pipes and blackens steel.

In 1974 the Safe Drinking Water Act empowered the Environmental Protection Agency to establish maximum contaminant levels (MCLs) for some 700 health-endangering substances found in public water supplies. As of 1990 only 30 "primary standards" had been established.[48] A 1986 amendment mandated that the EPA add 25 new MCLs every three years.

The FDA has jurisdiction over interstate sales of bottled water and presently requires bottlers to check for only 22 of the MCLs. The FDA is not bound to adopt EPA standards.

The International Bottled Water Association (IBWA), founded in 1958, is a powerful association with over 800 members including bottlers, suppliers and packagers. It has established its own MCLs for 200 contaminants and is expanding this list in 1991. Some states have adopted the IBWA's standards, which are more stringent than those of the EPA— Hawaii, Massachusetts, New Hampshire, New Jersey, Ohio, Oregon, Texas and Wyoming. California, Connecticut, Florida and New York have set water-quality standards that are more stringent than the IBWA's; but enforcement in a time of tight budgets is not always a priority.

Inorganic Contamination

Inorganic chemicals such as arsenic, asbestos, cadmium, nitrates, lead and other trace metals come from a variety of sources—industrial wastes, geologic sources, mining and agriculture are the main ones. The most hazardous of the chemicals in this category are lead and nitrates. Municipal water systems test for lead, but it can be added to your tap water as it passes through a series of pipes. Lead is found in the solder used to join the water line's copper pipe. This is especially true if the water is very acidic, alkaline, soft or hot. Since June 1988, the Federal Government has required that solder and flux be lead-free. Before this legislation, solder was typically 50 percent lead.[49] Over 90 percent of all U.S. homes and apartments have lead in their plumbing in some form.

To determine if lead is a problem in your home, have your water tested or have a plumber examine the joints of the pipes for grey-colored lead solder. Many pre-World War II homes have lead water-supply lines. If you think your supply line might contain lead, look for these characteristics: grey in color, not magnetic, scratches easily, no threads at the shut-off valve or the meter and bends when coming out of the floor or wall rather than having straight pipes or an elbow fitting. If any of these characteristics are found, invest in a new supply line.

Organic Contamination

More serious health hazards are posed by microorganisms, bacteria and viruses. The source is very often human and animal fecal matter that has entered the water system, for example through disposable diapers or many of the 20 million septic tanks that discharge into groundwater. In some areas with a high percentage of tanks per square foot, septic-tank discharge is a major cause of water pollution—Alabama, Connecticut, Florida, Georgia, Indiana, Massachusetts, Michigan, Missouri, New Hampshire, New Jersey, New York, North Carolina, Pennsylvania and Wisconsin. Organic chemicals include pesticides and herbicides like chlordane and ethylene dibromide as well as toxic substances such as vinyl chloride, benzene and carbon tetrachloride. Organic contaminants can also cause harmful effects in the liver, kidney or nervous and reproductive systems, and can also be linked to cancer.[50]

All homes serviced by wells should have their water tested periodically for bacterial contamination, usually from septic runoff. For persistent and continuing contamination, well-water purifying systems use ultraviolet radiation or ozone treatment to sanitize the water.

Other Causes of Contamination

Many contaminants relate to geography or identifiable polluters. Water contamination can be caused by uranium in the West, radium in the Midwest and Southeast and radon in Appalachia, New England and the Midwest. Industrial pollution is also a problem in many areas. The water supply's proximity to landfills, junkyards and dumps can mean it is tainted. For instance, if the water smells of gasoline, it could be tainted from one of several million underground storage tanks.

Nature itself can be a cause of pollutants. People near the sea can have high levels of chloride or sodium in their water.

An EPA survey shows that *two-thirds* of all private wells violate at least one Safe Drinking Water Act standard, with the most frequent contaminants being nitrates, fluoride, arsenic, pesticides and salt.

Testing for Contamination

Many municipal water systems and counties will test your tap water at little or no charge; contact the water utility directly or the state health department (which probably has an office in your county). By law you are entitled to see the results of water tests conducted on your municipal system. You can obtain monitor records, notices of violations of federal or state regulations and records of complaints made by other consumers.

Each state also has EPA-certified labs, lists of which can be obtained at the eight regional offices of the EPA through its Division of Drinking Water. When you inquire about a lab, be sure to find out what tests are offered, the costs and whether the lab is approved by the EPA or the Water Quality Association.

Alternatively, the Yellow Pages (for private firms look under Laboratories or Chemists) can help you find public or private labs for testing. After testing, the lab should send you printouts showing the contaminants tested, EPA "Recommended Maximum Contaminant Levels," the readings, the lab's comments on the significance of these readings and suggestions for remedies.

Federal water hotline:

EPA Safe Drinking Water Hotline (800) 426-4791. In Alaska and Washington, D.C. (202) 382-5533. EPA specialists are available from 8:30 A.M. to 4:30 P.M. ETZ, M-F.

Other resources:

Home Water Report, Jonathan O'Hall, Publisher. 502 North Main Street, Chincoteague Island, VA 23336.

National Sanitation Foundation, 3475 Plymouth Road, P.O. Box 1468, Ann Arbor, MI 48106 (313) 769-8010.

Water Quality Association, 4151 Naperville Road, Lisle, IL 60532 (708) 505-0160.

Preventing Contamination: Filtration

Pure water can be assured by filtration methods or by purchasing bottled water. "Point-of-use" sales—of bottled water and treatment devices—are now a $3.5-billion-a-year business. Over 500 manufacturers with nearly 1,000 products on the market are enjoying an annual 20 percent sales growth. Consumers are faced with many choices. The basic kinds of systems available are carbon filters, reverse osmosis, distillation and ultraviolet.

Carbon filter domestic filtration systems are available for the entire house or for individual sinks and even tabletop units. Water is passed through carbon, usually in the form of granular activated charcoal or a solid carbon block that captures contaminants. Filtration systems using activated carbon are capable of removing many contaminants such as heavy metals, chlorine, chloroform, pesticides and industrial chemicals. But they do not remove fluorides, nitrates, salts and asbestos, and are not very effective against microbial contamination. The best systems use a solid block of carbon and will not let any unfiltered water pass through it. Unfortunately, these filters can also remove minerals that may contribute to good health. Where this may be unavoidable, find alternate food sources for these lost minerals. Faucet-mounted carbon filters may run as low as $20, while higher-volume under-the-counter ones cost over $300. Carbon-filter pitchers are available for under $50. It is extremely important with the carbon-filter system to replace the filter on schedule.

Reverse osmosis is another reputable system. This is a more high-tech option that purifies water by causing it to pass through a semipermeable membrane, like plastic or cellulose, that lets in water molecules but repels pollutants. Membranes may be expensive to replace and typically cost more than carbon filters. Reverse osmosis is good at removing organic as well as inorganic contaminants like asbestos, chloride, fluoride, nitrates, pesticides, detergents and others. They are ineffective at removing high levels of calcium and magnesium. Prices for these units range from $200 to $1,000.

Distillation is a process by which water is boiled, converted to steam and then condensed. Left behind are dissolved solids, sediment and metals, including lead. Some distillers generate excessive heat and may be difficult to clean. They range in price from about $150 to $500.[51]

Ultraviolet radiation is extremely effective on microbes but little else. This device is popular because it requires no maintenance or changing of filters. The cost is about $500.

Bottled Water

The high volume and rapid growth in sales of bottled water is a sign that many Americans now distrust their public water.

Water sold in bottles is either carbonated (sparkling) or noncarbonated (still). Carbonation is simply carbon dioxide trapped in the water; natural carbonation is rare. Carbon dioxide in water also kills bacteria and relieves indigestion.

What, if anything, makes the water in bottles different from what comes from your tap? Is it really more healthful, as industry advocates encourage us to believe? One source says that as a rule of thumb, look for high minerals—calcium and magnesium contents above 50 parts per million (ppm)—and low salt, i.e., sodium levels under 35 ppm. High-mineral low-salt water is healthier than average. But the Environmental Policy Institute (EPI), a respected group in Washington, D.C. that has since merged with Friends of the Earth, has concluded that "despite the attractive packaging of bottled water, this product, in general, is not necessarily any safer or more healthful than the water that comes out of most faucets. In fact, the public water utilities supplying the same faucets are the source of more than one-third of all bottled water in the U.S."[52] For more information:

Environmental Policy Institute/Friends of the Earth, 218 D Street, S.E., Washington, DC 20003 (202) 544-2600. EPI's *Bottled Water: Sparkling Hype* was published in 1989.

H₂O: The Guide to Quality Bottled Water (Woodbridge Press, 1988); by Arthur von Wiesenberger, is useful for comparing brands.

International Bottled Water Association, 113 North Henry Street, Alexandria, VA 22314.

Saving Water: Five Things You Can Do

Many municipal water systems in growing regions such as the Southwest are hard-pressed to maintain a supply of clean water. Your health depends on conserving your water supply. Here are a few ways:

1. *Stop leaks promptly.* A dripping faucet at the rate of one drop a second uses 7 gallons a day; a steady drip can waste 5,000 gallons a month.
2. *Reduce faucet flow.* Aerate the water by installing an attachment (sold for under $10 by Seventh Generation, (800) 441-2538, or available at most hardware stores). When installing new faucets, buy the single-lever type instead of two separate controls, which require constant adjustment.
3. *Don't run water continuously for dishwashing or rinsing.* Rinse dishes in the sink right after eating; use a brush or cloth rather than the force of water to remove food; and only run the dishwasher when full and on the shortest cycle. When shaving or brushing your teeth, don't keep the water flowing. (But don't drink the first water out of the tap; wait till leached metals have had a chance to flush through.)
4. *Use plastic ice trays* that permit individual ice cubes to be removed, and keep a bottle of water in the refrigerator for drinking, rather than running tap water.
5. *Put something in your toilet tank* to reduce the number of gallons used to flush your toilet. The simplest and cheapest way is to put a bottle of water in the tank.

SUMMING UP: FOUR PRINCIPLES

Healthy living begins at home, and this chapter identified a number of health hazards that are commonplace in many homes. The review of the dangers associated with electrical appliances, energy sources, cleaning products, pesticides and air and water quality makes it clear that you should:

1. *Identify the hazards* in your house. *Read labels*, especially on bottles of fluids that promise to clean magically.
2. *Keep watch—on things that are plugged in and get hot.* Leaving anything hot and electric on when you aren't around is dangerous.
3. *Remember you are not alone when you discard things.* Your health is related to that of other people and you have a responsibility to minimize the quantity of hazardous materials you throw away.
4. *Remember you are not alone when you want something done.* If you are worried about something that you feel is harmful to your health, others probably feel the same way. Consumer groups such as the Consumer Federation of America, in Washington, D.C., applaud the proliferation of information concerning hazardous household products. The Association of Trial Lawyers is calling on its members to become whistle-blowers by bringing dangerous products to the attention of state and Federal regulatory officials.[53]

The following books, information centers and organizations may be useful, in addition to the ones already cited, in general planning for a healthier home:

Americans for Safe Food, 1501 16th St., N.W., Washington, DC 20036 (202) 332-9110. This lobbying group is a project of the Center for Science in the Public Interest.

Chemical Referral Center, operated by the Chemical Manufacturers Association (800) CMA-8200, 9-6 ETZ, M-F.

Chemical Risk: A Primer (1984), American Chemical Society, 1155 16th St., N.W., Washington, DC. (202) 872-4600.

Consumer Federation of America, 1424 16th Street, N.W., Washington, DC. (202) 387-6121.

Consumer Product Safety Commission, 5401 Westbard Ave., Bethesda, MD 20207 (800) 638-CPSC (automated telemaze). Federal agency.

Elements of Toxicology and Chemical Risk Assessment: A Handbook for Nonscientists, Attorneys and Decision Makers, Environ, Washington, D.C., 1986.

Handbook for Toxic Free Living, Group for the South Fork, P.O. Box 569, Bridgehampton, NY 11932 (526) 537-1400. $25.

Healthy House Catalog by Stuart Greenberg (Cleveland, OH: Environmental Health Watch and Housing Resource Center, 1989 with planned annual updates). Order from Environmental Health Watch, 4115 Bridge Avenue, Cleveland, OH 44113 (216) 961-7179. The catalog, priced at $19.95, is a national directory of indoor air-pollution control products, services and resources.

Home Health Products for Life, P.O. Box 3130, Virginia Beach, VA 23454 (800) 284-9123.

Home Safe Home by Paul Bierman-Lytle (New York: Nichols Publishing).

In Business Magazine, "1990 Directory of Environmental Entrepreneurs," by Nora Goldstein, March/April 1990. Listings reflect the broad spectrum of opportunities available to provide nontoxic alternatives.

Natural Resources Defense Council, 40 West 20th St., New York, NY 10011 (212) 727-2700. West Coast office: 90 New Montgomery Street, San Francisco, CA 94105 (415) 777-0220. Research and lobby group.

Pesticides Information Pamphlet (1987), American Chemical Society, 1155 16th St., N.W., Washington, DC. (202) 872-4600.

SelfCare Catalogue, 349 Healdsburg Avenue, Healdsburg, CA 95448 (800) 345-3371, 6-6 PTZ, M-Sat. Various home health-care products available.

Seventh Generation, (800) 456-1177, catalog of healthy products.

Shopping for a Better World. Council on Economic Priorities, 30 Irving Place, New York, NY 10003 (212) 420-1133; 9-5 ETZ, M-F. CEP and the book rate environmental responsibility of companies. Ask CEP for free environmental Research Report.

The Earthwise Consumer, edited by Debra Lynn Dadd, newsletter (8 issues/year, $20 per year), available from P.O. Box 1506, Mill Valley, CA 94942 (415) 383-5892. This updates her book, *Nontoxic, Natural and Earthwise*.

The Hazardous Waste Wheel, a useful guide to recognizing and disposing of hazardous household waste. It's $3.95; call (603) 436-3950.

The Healthy Home, by Linda Mason Hunter (New York: Pocket Books, 1990). An attic-to-basement guide to toxin-free living.

The Healthy House, by John Bower (Secaucus, N.J.: Lyle Stuart Books, Inc.). The book costs $17.95, from Lyle Stuart, 120 Enterprise Ave., Secaucus, NJ 07094.

Toxicology for the Citizen, Center for Environmental Toxicology, Michigan State University, East Lansing, MI, 1987. $1.

CHAPTER THREE

The Healthy Workplace

In the early 1900s, few laws protected American workers. As a result, the American workplace was more dangerous than those of most other industrialized countries. For example, in England, France and Germany miners suffered fewer than 1.5 deaths a year per thousand workers. In the United States, the figure was more than twice as high. Certain U.S. blue-collar occupations were especially hazardous, showing annual death rates from tuberculosis of more than 4 workers per thousand, while white-collar workers' death rates were under 1 per thousand.[1]

The Depression and especially the New Deal in the 1930s brought the first important steps by the Federal Government to protect worker health and safety. As Franklin D. Roosevelt took office, lawsuits were being filed against a subsidiary of Union Carbide Company over the deaths of 476 workers who were alleged in the suit to have been killed by inhalation of silica dust while drilling a tunnel in West Virginia. Company doctors had been forbidden to tell workers what their illness was; one doctor testified that he told the sick workers they suffered from "tunnelitis." Company managers knew enough about the dangers to protect themselves with face masks when they went into the tunnels; the predominantly black workers were denied such protection. With the public inflamed over this story, Frances Perkins' Department of Labor initiated many of the worker-safety programs that endure to this day.[2]

As industrial technology advanced in the post-World War II decades, public concern about environmental and occupational hazards increased. Congress passed two significant workplace health and safety laws in 1969 and 1970. The 1969 Mine Safety and Health Act sought to protect miners from job-related injury and illness. The 1970 Occupational Safety and Health Act established the Occupational Safety and Health Administration (OSHA) and the National Institute of Occupational Safety and Health (NIOSH) to protect workers' health.[3]

The OSHA regulations are the most pervasive, covering 5 million workplaces. OSHA has the authority to set job-safety and health standards for any employers in the U.S. State regulators may preempt Federal regulation only with OSHA approval. OSHA sets standards for worker safety and health, develops training programs for alerting employers and employees to these standards, has the right to inspect plants and other facilities (and question employees in private) to ensure compliance and has the authority to impose penalties for violations.[4]

But OSHA's ability to enforce the law is limited by its small staff. More than 10,000 workers still die annually from workplace accidents (see Chapter 8), according to the National Safety Council; 1.5 million suffer disabling injuries caused by workplace hazards.

Recently, such broader worker health issues as job-related stress and radiation from computer screens have emerged. This chapter examines workplace conditions and hazards, how they affect workers and what can be done to plan for a more productive and healthy workplace.

National Institute for Occupational Safety and Health (NIOSH), (800) 35-NIOSH. Sponsored by the U.S. Department of Health and Human Services. Provides information related to occupational safety.

OFFICE WORKPLACE CONCERNS

Office workplace issues are relatively new. The focus of most safety concerns has traditionally been on blue-collar work. Today, eyestrain has emerged as a legitimate workplace hazard. Other relatively less dangerous, but widely prevalent, office hazards are gaining attention.

For example, a 1989 survey by the Office Environment Index asked 1,041 office workers and 150 executives what they rated as serious health hazards. Their responses are shown in Table 3-1. Eyestrain was at the top of both lists, followed by air quality and radiation from video display terminals (VDTs).

Another survey of office managers found glare from VDTs to be considered the greatest health hazard, with 59 percent of those polled designating it an important concern.[6] Copiers and fax machines are another source of concern—their bright lights can damage the eyes of users who look at them.

Cigarette Smoke

Active smoking is well known to be hazardous to your health, causing more than 400,000 deaths a year in the U.S. and 2.5 million worldwide. The dangers of "passive smoking" have only recently been documented. The

TABLE 3–1
RATING WORKPLACE HAZARDS

	By top executives	By office workers
Eyestrain	36%	44%
Air quality	32%	27%
Radiation from VDTs	22%	27%
Exposure to AIDS	22%	10%
Exposure to hazardous materials (asbestos, etc.)	17%	12%

SOURCE: Office Environment Index.[5]

Surgeon General's Office and the National Research Council announced in the mid-1980s that hazardous compounds like nicotine and carbon monoxide in passively inhaled cigarette smoke could be linked to lung cancer and other respiratory problems. The EPA estimates that about 3,700 lung-cancer deaths can be connected to passive smoking each year.[7]

Researchers have found that secondhand smoke can cause clots to form in the arteries of the heart, leading to heart attacks and arteriosclerosis. A draft EPA-sponsored report in 1991 concluded that secondhand smoke kills 53,000 nonsmokers a year, 37,000 from heart disease.[8]

A June 1990 EPA "Guide to Workplace Smoking Policies" recommended that companies create separately ventilated smoking lounges to protect nonsmokers from carcinogenic smoke. The EPA does not yet have authority to regulate tobacco and cigarette-smoking beyond its own buildings, but it influences local smoking policies. Responding to the studies showing the dangers of secondhand smoke, many companies have initiated rules restricting smoking in work areas. The Federal Government has restricted smoking in all Federal buildings to specially designated smoking areas. More than half of the states have laws restricting smoking in public and in workplaces, and many city and county governments have further limitations on purchase of cigarettes (for example, many communities ban selling cigarettes in vending machines) and on smoking in public places.[9]

Action on Smoking and Health, 2013 H Street, N.W., Washington, DC 20006. This is a national nonprofit organization concerned with the problems of smoking and the rights of nonsmokers.

Other Toxic-Air Hazards

Some small, but potentially significant, toxic hazards lurk in unlikely places in the office. Liquid Paper correcting fluid, used in many offices to "white out" typing mistakes, as originally formulated contained toxic chemicals such as trichloro-ethylene. The Gillette Company agreed to remove the cancer-causing elements from the product. California's Proposition 65, a voter initiative aimed at removing unnecessary toxic risks from offices, requires businesses to place warnings on products that contain toxic chemicals.[10]

Older copying machines that used chemical toners posed a significant hazard, but the new dry copiers are less worrisome. The chemically treated paper used in many fax machines is a potential hazard. A more likely source of toxic emissions in the workplace air is cleaning fluids used to clean floors and walls.

Occupational Safety and Health Guidelines for Chemical Hazards is published by NIOSH and OSHA. It lists certain hazardous chemicals, describing each one's hazards, exposure limits, medical and first-aid procedures, monitoring procedures, protection and waste-removal and disposal procedures. Contact the Publications Dissemination Section of NIOSH in Cincinnati, OH (513) 533-8287. Ask for DHHS (NIOSH) Publication No. 81-123. Or write to Superintendent of Documents, U.S. Government Printing Office, Washington, DC 20402.

Lighting

Inadequate or inappropriate lighting in the workplace can increase eyestrain and has been linked to stress and sluggishness. Some claim such lighting can interfere with calcium absorption and can lead to fragile bones, especially among the elderly.

Fluorescent lighting is widely used in public buildings and offices, and has to a large extent replaced the more expensive incandescent bulbs, which more closely simulate natural sunlight. Fluorescent lighting is far more energy-efficient and less expensive—fluorescent bulbs operate with one-sixth the electricity.

But standard fluorescent lights are also said to be the most "nutrient-deficient" artificial lighting.[11] The glare and flickering of fluorescent lighting can cause eyestrain and headaches. Also, a 10-watt compact fluorescent (CF) light bulb produces a magnetic field 20 or more times stronger than that of a 60-watt incandescent bulb. All fluorescent lights (compact and regular) also contain at least a tiny amount of mercury, and some CFs also contain radioactive material.[12] For all of these reasons, those concerned about healthy workplaces oppose such fluorescent lights.

But times are changing. The alleged adverse affects of fluorescent lighting can be reduced if the bulbs that are used more closely simulate full-spectrum natural light and sunlight. Although some experts are not convinced of the difference, under full-spectrum fluorescent lighting (defined as the light emitted by a certain metal at 5,000 degrees Kelvin), workplace productivity has been found to increase while absenteeism dropped.[13] CFs screw into incandescent sockets and some brands have a much wider spectrum of light (2,700 degrees Kelvin) than the old fluorescent tubes or the old incandescent lights.

Noise Pollution

The quality of office acoustics has been found to affect the performance of workers. Studies show that office productivity can be cut by 40 percent if office noise is excessive (60 decibels); keyboard errors, for example, were found to increase by 30 percent. Phones, typewriters, impact printers and copy machines tend to be the greatest contributors to noise pollution in the office. Their effects can be limited by placing acoustic hoods on noisy office machines, by absorbing the noise with acoustic materials on floors, ceilings and walls, or by masking the noise with soothing background sounds.[14]

Video Display Terminals (VDTs)

The expanding role of workplace computers has raised concerns about radiation from video display terminals (VDTs, computer screens). The radiation pattern of a computer is similar to that of a television. The major difference in the hazards is that the computer operator usually sits much closer to the device, so the field is stronger. Shielding computers fully can add as much as $3,000 to the cost of each terminal. Very few computers in the U.S. are shielded to that extent, but many computer manufacturers are producing low-emission monitors that comply with Swedish guidelines; most expect to charge a premium of only $50 to $100.[15]

Until 1982, personal and office computers produced such high levels of radiation that they were capable of interfering with operations in air-traffic control in many airports. The Federal Communications Commission issued regulations restricting both types of radiation a computer could emit (what it calls Radio Frequency Interference and Electromagnetic Interference), so newer computer models have lower levels of radiation leakage.

Eager to do something (especially something that costs government little) about possible hazards, some legislators have imposed modest regulations concerning the use of VDTs in the workplace. Since December 1990, for example, San Francisco requires that employers of 15 or more

VDT operators provide adjustable chairs and screens, detached keyboards and proper lighting.[16]

Recently, optometrists have developed a protective film to coat spectacles to keep out ultra-violet rays. They argue that the film is protection against both sun and VDT emissions. But computers and indoor lights don't give off significant amounts of ultra-violet rays. The film may be of some use against the sun, the strongest source of ultra-violet rays.[17]

Three Steps to Take About VDTs

1. *Use a detachable keyboard* and keep it at least 30 inches away from the disk drives and computer monitor; this will reduce the radiation.
2. *Buy low-emission monitors* when the office replaces its monitors.
3. *Measure the levels of low-level electromagnetic radiation in the office.* A small office could purchase a meter of the kind described in Chapter 2. A large office might prefer to turn the matter over to a professional engineer or an environmental consultant to measure the strength of electromagnetic fields and make recommendations.

GENERAL WORKPLACE CONCERNS

Cumulative-Trauma and Repetitive-Motion Disorders

It has long been known that jobs involving physical activity entail risk of injury. A newly prominent danger results from repeating a single physical task or motion, as on an assembly line. Such jobs can create a condition called cumulative-trauma or repetitive-motion disorder.

This disorder has become the most frequent occupational complaint. The Bureau of Labor Statistics says that cumulative-trauma disorders accounted for 48 percent of the 240,900 workplace illnesses in 1988, compared to 18 percent of 126,100 illnesses in 1981.[18]

Jobs in car assembly, poultry processing and meat packing, involve heavy physical work and are typical occupations with a high incidence of cumulative trauma. Automation has reduced the amount of heavy lifting involved in these jobs, but has required faster-paced and more repetitive tasks.[19]

But cases of repetitive-motion disorders are spreading from physical, blue-collar jobs to jobs that involve "white-collar work with blue-collar rhythms and discipline," particularly data-entry workers. Supermarket checkers and cashiers have also experienced these disorders. The ailments encountered as a result of repetitive-motion jobs include: ganglionic cysts, tendonitis, bursitis, carpal-tunnel syndrome and other inflammations and problems of the hands, arms and shoulders. Carpal-tunnel syndrome (CTS) affects the vital median nerve that runs down the arm, through the wrist and into the thumb and index and middle fingers. CTS is recognized by burning, tingling and numbness in your hand and wrist. Get medical advice as soon as possible, because irritating the tendons over time can cause serious damage to the nerve.[20]

Four Remedies for CTS Symptoms

Some people are being misdiagnosed for CTS when a few self-help measures could alleviate the pain, says Dr. Vern Anderson of NIOSH. Here are some remedies:

1. *Adjust your chair or desk height* so that the middle row of the keyboard is at or below elbow height.
2. *Try foam wrist rests*, which help the wrists maintain a natural, comfortable position.
3. *Try a wrist support* available for $22 (specify left or right hand) from the SelfCare Catalog (800) 345-3371.
4. *Take regular relaxation breaks.* Stand up and walk around and then resume work.[21]

Stress

In addition to workplace conditions, the demands and pressures found in many businesses can lead to job-related stress. While not having a job is generally more stressful than having one, job-related stress creates health concerns for many workers and has been linked to such severe health conditions as high blood pressure and heart attacks. The most stressful jobs are those where the demand placed on workers is high *and* which allow little latitude for decision-making. People in such jobs often have two-to-four times the risk of illness (in addition to other isolated risk factors) than those in other low-strain jobs.

Some examples of "high-strain" jobs are assembly-line work, waiting on tables, and certain office jobs. Characteristics of this type of occupation are rigid hours and procedures, high risk of layoffs, limited learning of new skills, little room for innovation and difficulty in getting time off for personal needs. The lower levels of the job ladder tend to have more high-strain jobs, and thus more job-related illnesses.[22]

People employed in these high-strain jobs tend to have a higher heart-attack rate and often experience depression and other psychological disorders; speculation is that stress interferes with the body's nerves, hormones, or immune system. Workers with high-stress jobs have been found to have a risk of high blood pressure about three times greater than those who did not suffer from job strain.[23]

Stress-related headaches and back pains are the two leading causes of lost work time in the United States. Many drug-free treatments are on the market which help to release tension and pain related to stress.

OCCUPATIONAL HAZARDS

The conditions found in many office and work areas, such as VDT radiation, poor lighting and ventilation, and stress are common hazards, but they generally do not lead to fatal or crippling health concerns. Many businesses and industries have fatal dangers. Those most threatened in these high-risk industries are workers in nuclear-power and chemical plants.

Occupational Illness and Injury

In 1988, the Bureau of Labor Statistics reported an injury and illness rate of 8.6 per 100 full-time workers—a total of 6.4 million job-related injuries and illnesses.[24] Occupational *injuries* are any that occur from an accident in the workplace and result in death, loss of consciousness, restriction of mobility, medical treatment beyond first aid, or that result in transfer to another job. Job-related *illnesses* are those that are acute or chronic, with symptoms that are relatively clearly related to the workplace.

Musculoskeletal disorders are the leading cause of injury or disability among workers in the United States. These injuries—back problems, inflamed joints, ankle, knee and shoulder problems being the most common—exceed any other health disorder, as measured by earnings lost and worker compensation payments. The National Safety Council has estimated that of two million workers sustaining job-related disabling injuries, 70,000 suffered permanent impairments such as amputations, fractures, eye loss, irreversible hearing loss lacerations and death.[25]

According to NIOSH reports, some of the most significant occupational illnesses are those that involve lung and heart diseases, cancers and disorders of the nervous system. In addition, skin conditions and certain psychological disorders are major issues in job health. Exposure to toxic substances in the workplace can often cause problems in the reproductive system, such as spontaneous abortions, birth defects, sterility and impotence.

Neurotoxic chemicals can cause such effects on the nervous system as lack of coordination, tremors, impaired sight, hearing and touch, loss of alertness and lapses in judgment. These job-related conditions can impair an individual's ability to react to hazardous situations. NIOSH is attempting to develop new methods of detecting nerve degeneration induced by neurotoxic chemicals in the workplace. Skin disorders account for at least 40 percent of all occupational diseases, but even these figures might be deflated as a result of under-reporting. The skin and the lungs are the areas most susceptible to dangerous fumes and chemicals.[26]

During the 1972-79 period, OSHA made more than 12,000 inspections of chemical companies and ended up citing over 110,000 violations of its regulations. Roughly 84 percent of those citations were for safety, while 13 percent were for health. Workers can get involved in the inspection process through employee complaints, which often result in general inspections, and by accompanying the OSHA inspector during the visit.[27]

Obstacles to the Healthy Workplace

Surveys indicate that safety rates No. 1 among worker concerns, above such issues as salary, benefits or day care. But we have observed already that more than 10,000 workers still die annually from workplace accidents. If safety is such a great concern, why is this happening?

- Some work is inherently risky. Steeplejacks, office-window washers, riveters and police officers are like racing drivers and jockeys—some risk of bodily harm is inevitably connected with their work.
- States are taking over much of the regulation of workplace standards, but few are very active in enforcement and prosecution.
- Many companies fail to report occupational hazards. Illnesses and injuries incurred in the workplace may be wrongly blamed on outside factors such as the personal health and habits of the workers.[28]
- Many workers choose to ignore or refuse to report serious dangers because they are afraid of losing their jobs. Despite several Federal statutes designed to protect employees who express concerns about health and safety violations in the workplace, many employees in fact receive no such protection. The Employee Health and Safety Whistle-Blower Protection Act is designed to protect the free-speech rights of employees who express concern for safety and health standards in the workplace. The aim is to eliminate the incidence of workers being blacklisted, harassed, demoted or fired for "blowing the whistle" on the employer.[29]
- Reduction of workplace hazards is further impeded by what seems to be a double standard. The accepted level for toxic lead fumes is 33 times greater in the workplace than in the outside air. While most commercial products have been tested, the National Academy of Sciences found that 60 percent of the chemicals found in the workplace have not been tested. Former NIOSH safety director John Moran says: "Injury, illness and death in the workplace [are] still socially acceptable."[30]
- OSHA is underfunded. The EPA's budget is over 21 times greater than OSHA's.

• Industry lobbying against stricter standards is constant, because safety can be expensive. In 1987, a bill entitled "The High Risk Occupational Disease Notification and Prevention Act" was passed in the House of Representatives. It sought to speed up the notification process of OSHA's "Hazard Communication Standards" and among other provisions required companies to give workers access to their personal medical records. The bill was killed by filibuster in the Senate.[31]

CHAPTER FOUR

The Healthy Building/Environment

The preceding chapters have addressed health concerns in the home and workplace, citing potentially hazardous products or conditions. But many hazards are found in the building materials and structures themselves. This chapter examines ways to avoid or remedy such conditions and considers alternative visions of the healthy building.

BUILDING MATERIALS AND STRUCTURES

Asbestos, insulation, paint, roofing and floor coverings are common building materials; they all can have adverse health effects. The problems range from rashes and allergic reactions to respiratory problems or cancer. In most cases, the concentrations of the toxins decrease as the materials age. But according to the EPA, indoor air pollutants—most of them from building materials—now outrank outdoor air pollutants as a cause of cancer.[1]

Asbestos

"Asbestos" refers to a family of relatively indestructible, flexible mineral fibers that are heat resistant and chemically stable. It is found in floor and ceiling tiles, cement shingles, water pipes and many other familiar building products.

Starting in the 1930s, asbestos was viewed as a wondrous insulator, fireproofer and textile. As of 1979 more than half of the high-rise buildings in the U.S. contained some form of asbestos. Knowledge of the hazards of carcinogenic elements began to emerge in the 1960s, and the use of asbestos began to drop significantly in the 1970s even before the EPA intervened.

Scientists found that asbestos can crumble into dust and tiny particles, especially when its fibers are not firmly bonded within another material, and that in this form, asbestos is easily released into the air, where it is swallowed, inhaled or becomes attached to clothing. Epidemiological studies show that any exposure to loose asbestos is risky; smokers are at greater risk than nonsmokers.[2] Tightly bonded asbestos is considered to be relatively safe unless disturbed.

Exposure to asbestos can increase the risk of contracting four serious diseases that affect the lungs and digestive tract: lung cancer; mesothelioma, a cancer of the lining of the lung or abdomen (which is almost always caused by asbestos); gastro-intestinal cancer, and asbestosis, a condition that results from chronic occupational exposure to airborne asbestos fibers. Except for the last, these diseases usually develop 20 or more years after the initial exposure.[3] The effects of low levels of exposure are not so clear and are the subject of much debate; some argue there is no safe threshold.

Although the EPA banned all asbestos production in the 1980s, asbestos can be found in older homes as insulation, fireproofing or old flooring. Asbestos, in fact, was *required* as fire protection in specific building areas until 1976. The Asbestos Hazard Emergency Response Act passed by Congress in 1986 required that all public and private school buildings be inspected for asbestos. If any was found in deteriorating condition, the school was required to delineate plans to remedy the situation. A major concern is asbestos removal; because of required safety precautions, removal can cost *ten times* what it cost to spray the asbestos on during the 1960s.[4]

Optimistic scientists—taking a position that is closer to the view of the asbestos industry—minimize the asbestos hazard, arguing that only asbestos workers handling the coarse amphibole asbestos, the kind used in office buildings, suffer from such illnesses as mesothelioma.[5]

Pessimistic scientists—taking what could be described as an anti-industry view—argue that exposure to even low levels of chrysotile is as hazardous as any other form of asbestos. They cite studies that have shown that chrysotile causes cancer in animals and can carry many of the same risks in humans inhaling the substance. Studies of sheet-metal workers and of firefighters (see Chapter 3) and a study of families of asbestos workers have all found higher-than-normal rates of asbestos-related illness, particularly precursors of cancer and mesothelioma.[6]

Ironically, the pessimists are often the first to oppose removal because workers and the public may be endangered if asbestos is disturbed. The risk of asbestos exposure in a nonoccupational setting is often strongest when the asbestos is being removed. Removal may be warranted when asbestos is lining an air duct or is in a place where it will be constantly disturbed. But the removal process, especially when done improperly, can greatly increase the amount of airborne asbestos. A growing international consensus is emerging that the needless removal of asbestos is actually causing greater risks than it is preventing.[7]

Few, therefore, disagree with current EPA policy that (1) undisturbed asbestos in schools should not be removed, (2) exposed asbestos should be enclosed so as to eliminate its vulnerability to damage, and (3) damaged asbestos should be removed from school buildings only by government-certified workers. Congressional hearings have reviewed EPA's asbestos policy and the EPA itself has convened a special panel to review evidence of the relative health risks.[8]

For more information:

Asbestos in the Home, a 12-page publication available from Publication Request, Consumer Product Safety Commission, Washington, DC 20207. Call (800) 638-CPSC for advice.

Environmental Health Watch, 4115 Bridge Avenue, Cleveland, OH 44113 (216) 961-4646. Educates the public about the health effects of such hazards as asbestos, lead and formaldehyde.

EPA Asbestos Information Hotline (800) 835-6700.

NIOSH Hotline, for asbestos in the workplace (800) 35-NIOSH.

Insulation (Formaldehyde)

Too much insulation can restrict fresh air and proper circulation, preventing harmful pollutants from leaving your home. However, a well-sealed house (i.e., foil-backed drywall, sealing all electric boxes, windows, doors and other openings) will prevent insulation from contaminating the inside air.[9] Home insulation materials often contain large amounts of chlorofluorocarbons (CFCs), the same kind that are used in aerosol cans and make their way into the atmosphere where they destroy the vital ozone layer.[10]

Formaldehyde is a strong-smelling liquid used as an adhesive. Its fumes, even in small amounts, can cause respiratory problems, dizziness, lethargy, menstrual problems, eye and throat irritations and rashes. Products containing formaldehyde release low levels of fumes over several years, and continued exposure to the toxic gas can lead to disorders of the central nervous system and cancer. The National Research Council estimates that one in ten Americans are hypersensitive to formaldehyde. In 1987 the EPA upgraded the classification of formaldehyde from a "possible" to a "probable" carcinogen. It causes nasal/bronchial cancer in laboratory animals and may cause cancer of the liver, lungs and pharynx in high exposures. Formaldehyde is believed to cause bronchial asthma and can produce allergic dermatitis.[11]

Urea-formaldehyde foam insulation (UFFI) is dangerous because of its formaldehyde content. In August 1982 the Consumer Product Safety Commission (CPSC) banned the use of UFFI in schools and residences. The ban was overturned a year later in the courts, but the CPSC continues to warn consumers about the health risks associated with this insulation. UFFI is found in about 500,000 American homes, mostly from installation in the 1970s.[12]

Fiberglass and blown-in cellulose are two alternatives to UFFI. The latter is cheaper and safer; fiberglass particles are easily inhaled and can have adverse effects on health.

Formaldehyde information sources:

American Lung Association, 1740 Broadway, New York, NY 10019 (212) 315-8700. Provides publications on issues such as formaldehyde, radon and air pollution. Ask for Ronald White.

The Consumer Product Safety Commission is the place to call if you suspect that your home is insulated with UFFI; phone (800) 638-CPSC for information about detection and removal.

Paint and Paint Removers

Paint may contain more than 300 toxic chemicals and 150 carcinogens. Oil-based paints contain such chemicals as benzene, methanol and ethane. These chemicals are carcinogenic and can cause liver and kidney damage, dizziness, headache, fatigue and loss of coordination. Symptoms such as irritability, insomnia, rapid heartbeat, headaches, low-grade fever and leg cramps are commonly caused by mercury poisoning from paint and paint fumes.[13]

Although oil-based paints and varnishes provide a harder, more durable and more vapor-proof finish, they are very toxic and can take months to be completely dry and odorless. Latex is the best option. In 1990, the EPA banned the use of mercury in latex interior paints.[14] Even so, latex paint can cause symptoms such as nervous stimulation, depression, vomiting and kidney damage.

The alternatives are certain hypo-allergenic and nontoxic paints, which can be relatively costly. They include old-fashioned, limestone-based whitewash or casein-based "milk paint." Milk paint is the commercial paint with the least odor, but it has a tendency to mold in damp locations like kitchens and bathrooms.[15]

Here are five steps for avoiding both the expense of nontoxic paints and most of the toxic and odor problems of regular paints:

1. Paint during a warm, dry season.
2. Paint with water-based latex paint wherever possible; use oil-based paints or varnishes sparingly.

3. Be sure areas being painted are fully ventilated.
4. After painting, "bake" the painted areas by turning on a heat source such as a high-watt light for a week; close all doors and windows and vacate the rooms.
5. Have a professional do your painting.[16]

Doors and Windows

Metal doors and door frames and windows, though not always aesthetically pleasing, are often safer alternatives to wooden ones, which tend to use a lot of potentially toxic glue during construction. Sealants can be effective in reducing the amount of noxious fumes emitted from preservatives in wooden window frames.[17]

Standard single-pane or old-style double-pane windows found in most homes leak heat and energy. New windows have the insulating capacities of fiberglass-insulated walls and can insulate four to eight times better than single-pane glass and twice as well as double-pane windows.[18] The so-called low-E (emissivity) windows are the best buy.

Flooring

Ceramic tiles, brick and concrete are often the best type of flooring for people who are sensitive to carpet dust and gases. Hardwood floors are also available with nontoxic wood finishes. The best types of hardwood flooring to install are the pre-finished hardwood floor tiles that have a baked-on finish.

Tile, concrete, brick or stone are excellent for those with serious sensitivities, provided they are installed with nontoxic adhesives. But because they don't yield to the feet they can be hard on the joints. Wood and hard vinyl are the next best options and should not present problems, except for hypersensitive individuals. Avoid the soft, pliable sheet-linoleum and vinyl tiles. They contain a volatile plasticizer to keep them flexible, and can emit carcinogenic fumes. Instead, look for hard vinyl, which breaks when you bend it. *Consumer Reports* says vinyl-asbestos with a "no-wax" surface is the best choice from an odor standpoint.

Roofing

Fire-retardant plywood, commonly used in roofing, has been found to decompose after a few years, causing leaky and unsafe roofs requiring expensive repair work. Introduced in the early 1980s, it has been used in millions of homes, and many suits have been filed against makers and suppliers. Repairs and replacement are very costly, but many developers have begun replacing the roofing with new plywood.[19]

Tar is the most dangerous of all roofing materials. It is especially noxious during installation and continues to emit fumes long after it is in place, especially in warmer climates. Most other types of roofing are acceptable; best are slate, tile or metal. If you already have a tar roof that needs retarring, try asphalt-free "rubber" roofs. These rubber roofs, made of sheets of synthetic rubber or plastic that are heated, nailed or glued into place, are extremely durable. Installation costs are two to three times greater than for tar roofs, but the rubber roof can last up to five times longer.[20]

Other Hazards

Termite treatments for wood framing, needed in many parts of the country, are toxic. They may be avoided by using steel framing—often more expensive than wood framing, but usually not more expensive than the cost of preventing termites.

Shattering glass can cause serious injuries. Three types of safety glass have been developed—tempered, laminated and plastic—all of which break into small pieces on impact.

National Glass Association, 8200 Greensboro Drive, #302, McLean, VA 22102 (703) 442-4890.

SOURCES OF DUST AND TOXIC SUBSTANCES

Carpeting

Synthetic carpeting contains up to 100 volatile chemicals, including formaldehyde, and as the carpet ages it creates synthetic dust. This dust can enter the heating system and produce toxic gases. Most carpets, even natural-fiber, wool or cotton, can be full of insecticides, preservatives or other chemicals. In recent years scores of complaints have been received by the Consumer Product Safety Commission regarding carpeting. Most were about eye and throat irritation, but some were of dizziness and flu symptoms believed to be related to office carpeting. One theory is that these conditions stem from storing carpets in warehouses for long periods without proper ventilation. The EPA has not yet found any particular offending chemical, but suspects the adhesives used to secure carpeting to the floor.[21]

Natural carpet sealants and cleaners protect carpets and keep them water-resistant, while also remaining nontoxic. Wall-to-wall carpeting is not recommended; area rugs, which can be washed regularly, are preferable. See "Flooring" for more alternatives to carpeting.

American College of Allergy and Immunology (800) 842-7777, 24 hours. Sends information on specific allergies and refers callers to board-certified doctors listed in each state.

Carbon Monoxide and Other Gases and Respirable Particles

Common noxious gases like carbon monoxide and nitrogen dioxide, and vapors with respirable particles, can be found in homes and office buildings. They are believed to cause bronchial constriction, burning eyes, headaches and general respiratory difficulties. In addition to car exhausts and tobacco smoke, fumes can emanate from unvented combustion appliances such as kerosene and gas heaters, leaking chimneys and furnaces, down-drafting from wood stoves and fireplaces and improperly adjusted gas stoves. Carbon monoxide and nitrogen dioxide are very dangerous at high levels and can cause allergic reactions in many people, even in smaller amounts. Carbon monoxide can be lethal even in small concentrations because it accumulates on hemoglobin and interferes with oxygenation of blood and tissue. Respirable airborne particles may be invisible and can be found in a variety of sources such as dust, carpet and clothing fibers and soot from improperly vented heaters and stoves.[22]

To limit possible emission of dangerous gases or particles, gas appliances should be adjusted to the manufacturer's specifications, and any gas or kerosene space heaters or wall or floor furnaces that don't vent outside should be replaced by units that do. Cars left running in a garage attached to a home, even with the garage door open, can release harmful and potentially fatal fumes that could be drawn into the house.[23]

Formaldehyde

Besides being used in insulation, formaldehyde can be found in carpets, draperies, particleboard, plywood, wood paneling and fiberboard. Man-made or pressed-wood products emit high levels of formaldehyde gas, as do the adhesives used to bind them. Other sources include tobacco smoke, glue and certain textiles.[24] Kitchen cabinets are a source of formaldehyde gas. Cabinets that are up to ten years old probably contain particleboard covered with a wood, paper or vinyl coating. Much of the formaldehyde will build up on the inside of the cabinet, as the doors are generally left closed, but the cabinets can be sealed with foil vapor barriers and tapes lining the cabinets, or the cabinet doors can be sealed with a nontoxic wood finish. To avoid these fumes, use exterior-grade pressed wood products or solid wood whenever possible. As with most other forms of indoor air pollutants, thorough ventilation will limit buildup of the gas and over time these materials will emit less and less formaldehyde.

Lead

Another harmful substance found in or around home, office and, unfortunately, school buildings, is lead. Lead, widely used in the U.S., is toxic and can accumulate in the body. Several studies have shown that exposure to lead can produce the symptoms of poor appetite, fatigue, hypertension and diminished mental capacity. Prolonged exposure can cause permanent and irreversible damage to the brain and nervous system, especially in children. The EPA reported in 1986 that about 250,000 children had suffered small but measurable losses in IQ from exposure to lead poisoning from water, and the agency estimates that 20 percent of all Americans drink water contaminated with unsafe levels of lead. Although stringent Federal rules about lead in school water were passed in 1986, the rules have not been effectively enforced either by the EPA or by state authorities.[25]

Lead can enter the air, as well as food and dust, in the home or office in several ways, including car exhausts and lead-based paint. The EPA has sought to cut the amount of lead in drinking water, where it exists as a corrosive byproduct from the pipes and solder. Recently, Federal and state laws have banned lead plumbing in drinking-water systems. Grounding electrical equipment to water pipes can increase the corrosive process in the pipes and raise lead levels in the water. Water coolers have been found to release lead into drinking water, and Federal law requires only that water be tested in water towers, reservoirs and other places where public water is stored. Lead-based paint can be found in millions of homes on interior surfaces and is a major hazard for children, as the paint chips or dust can be easily ingested. The greatest hazard of lead poisoning comes from inhaling the paint dust that flies in when opening and closing a window.[26]

Use of lead paint in houses is banned, but it is still used commercially. Children living in deteriorating housing built before 1950 are at high risk for excessive lead exposure. In addition, poor, black children in urban areas are disproportionately affected by lead poisoning. In April 1991, the Appellate Division of the New York State Supreme Court, affirming a lower-court decision, upheld a law passed by the New York City Council in 1982 that requires the city to inspect for and remove lead paint from all multiple-dwellings.[27]

The Centers for Disease Control previously conducted lead-screening programs, but in a tight Federal budgetary environment it ended them; lead screening is now in the hands of the states. Children should be tested for lead by the age of 5; lead poisoning is entirely preventable. Federal officials say that only one-third of the poor children in the country are tested for lead poisoning, even though such testing is required by a 1989 law.[28]

During home and office renovation, replaster or drywall over lead-based paint or cover it with wallpaper. If stripping lead-based paint from moldings or woodwork, do not sand or burn it off; use a chemical stripper with thorough ventilation or, even better, remove the pieces and have them stripped off-site.[29]

Radon

Radon, a byproduct of naturally decaying uranium found beneath the surface of the earth, is a very radioactive gas. It is invisible, odorless, tasteless *and* carcinogenic. Typically, it can seep into the basements of homes and buildings through cracks or holes in the foundation, crawl spaces, loose-fitting pipes, sumps and floor drains and it can circulate through the air when the inert radon gas breaks down into radioactive isotopes. It can emanate from all types of soil and rock, water and nuclear wastes, dispersing easily into the air. Common "hotspots" of radon concentration are found in geologic deposits of granite, shale and phosphate and in rock formations and soil containing uranium. It can pass through solid materials and can permeate buildings. Radon becomes concentrated only when it enters a confined space, such as a home. In poorly ventilated living or working areas, radon may be inhaled into the lungs, where it can damage the genetic material or cause cancerous tumors in tissue and the cells of the bronchial lining. While exposure to radon shows no immediate symptoms, it accounts for about 10 percent of lung-cancer deaths.[30]

In 1988, EPA officials and the Surgeon General informed the public that in their view 21,000 cases of lung cancer per year can be attributed to radon. Smokers are especially susceptible to radon-induced lung cancer. The EPA estimated that radon can be found at levels above EPA standards in 8 million U.S. homes and it said that radon is the most hazardous of all EPA-regulated pollutants. Congress has passed legislation setting desired maximum levels of radon, but the EPA claims there is no *safe* level of radon exposure. The EPA says radon is the second largest cause of lung cancer in the U.S. after cigarette smoking.[31]

Critics of the EPA have responded that its test results overstate the true risks of radon, because the readings are usually taken in basements. They contend that this is inappropriate since the basement is usually poorly ventilated, greatly inflating radon readings, and that few people actually live in the basement. Experts are still arguing over the extent of the cancer risk posed by radon. Meanwhile, in February 1991 the EPA retreated somewhat from its 1988 position; it reduced its estimate of radon-caused deaths to 16,000.[32]

Still, the EPA has long advised homeowners to test for radon, yet only 5 percent of them have done so. Utility companies sometimes provide free radon testing and many states have taken action in radon testing and in funding home repairs to remove radon. Radon detectors are sold in many hardware stores and even some supermarkets as charcoal-absorbent canisters and alpha-track detectors. The charcoal-absorbent canisters are short-term devices that can provide radon readings after three to seven days of exposure. The long-term tester, the alpha-track detector, provides an average reading after an exposure period of three months to a year. Both are sent to a testing agency for analysis and cost approximately $25, including lab analysis.[33]

Radon levels are higher during the colder seasons, when houses are closed up tightly. Be careful which testing company you use. Buyers Up, a Ralph Nader group, warns that some radon-testing labs are unreliable, and that some frauds have occurred.

U.S. Consumer Product Safety Commission, 5401 Westbard Ave., Bethesda, MD 20207 (800) 638-2772.

U.S. Environmental Protection Agency (EPA), Radon Division, Office of Radiation Protection Programs, Washington, DC 20460 (202) 544-1404. Radon Test Information Hotline: (800) 767-7236. Sells *A Citizen's Guide to Radon* (Publication OPA-86-004) and gives away *Radon Reduction Methods* (suggests fair prices). Some states with toll-free radon hotlines are: Maryland (800) 872-3666, Minnesota (800) 652-9747, New Jersey (800) 648-0394, New York (800) 458-1158, Ohio (800) 523-4439, Pennsylvania (800) 23-RADON, Virginia (800) 468-0138.

The best way to *reduce* radon levels is to ventilate your basement and other areas where radon may enter, to keep it from accumulating. In addition, seal all possible areas where radon could enter the home, such as cracks in the basement floor and walls; cover drainage pipes; reduce dust in the air and lower the indoor air pressure through venting systems.

Indoor Pollution: State Laws

States can be rated for their indoor pollution concern, based on the strength of their programs and legislation to eliminate indoor pollution. Indicators for indoor pollution policies are anti-smoking laws, radon programs (funding and testing available to residents, radon education, percentage of homes tested and number of excessive radon levels), number of children tested for lead poisoning, banning the use of lead in drinking water and household hazardous waste programs. The states showing high concern are New Jersey (highest), Florida, New Hampshire, and New York. The state with the lowest concern is Mississippi.[34]

BEYOND HAZARDS: THE HEALTHY LIVING ENVIRONMENT

Healthy Placement: *Feng Shui*

Beyond avoiding direct hazards in the home and working areas, design and architecture can contribute to establishing a healthy living and working environment. Some old and new approaches offer food for thought in the planning and development of buildings and communities.

Feng shui (pronounced fung shway), the Chinese art of designing a harmonious environment, is a 2,000-year-old approach to the physical environment that weaves together Buddhist and Taoist rules to guide the placing of a single flower or the design of large cities. *Feng shui*, literally "wind and water," pursues the most harmonious and auspicious place to live and work, giving people ways to improve their lives by changing and balancing their surroundings.

A basic principle of *feng shui* is to seek the *ch'i* (harmonious, meandering, irregular) forces and deflect the *sha* (vicious, direct) forces. Thus a path to the front of a house should not be straight. If a path is straight, front steps (at very least) are needed to deflect *sha*. A house should be above, not below, a road. Dead trees around a house should be cut down. Shrubs shield a house from bad energy flow.

Indoors, stairways should be curved or they drain energy from the upper floors. Any wall blocking the view into a room should have a deflector in front of it—a mirror, aquarium or screen. A room lacking life needs plants. Doors should not have spaces behind them; beds should have their headboards to the wall and should not face or be next to the door (the "mouth of *ch'i*"). Chairs should neither face nor have their backs to windows or doors.

Feng shui is enjoying revived interest among architects, interior designers, gardeners and homeowners in America. Woodstock, N.Y. builder Curry Rinzler used *feng shui* to locate the optimal position of a new house on the top of a mountain. The house, called "dragon's eye," is situated not at the very top but closer to where the eye of a dragon would be in relation to the whole head. Below the house, a long stretch of cleared area opens up the vista of the surrounding mountains in true *feng shui* tradition. "When I looked at the property," says Rinzler, "it fitted exactly into the *feng shui* scheme." The house was sold to a rock star in 1990.

Feng Shui: The Art of Placement and *Interior Design with Feng Shui*, by Sarah Rossbach (New York: E.P. Dutton, 1983).

Feng Shui: The Chinese Art of Designing a Harmonious Environment, by Derek Walters (New York: Simon & Schuster, A Fireside Book, 1988).

Yun Lin Temple, 2959 Russell St., Berkeley, CA 94705 (415) 841-2347. Prof. Thomas Yun Lin is a revered lecturer on *feng shui*.

Bau-Biologie

Another philosophy that deals with the living and working environment is the German philosophy Bau-Biologie, pronounced "bow (as in bow-wow) biology." Literally translated as "Building Biology," Bau-Biologie looks beyond locating toxic and hazardous building materials and products. It seeks to take these practical concerns and place them in a broader theoretical context that draws on ecology, biology, medicine and engineering to develop a *healthy environment*. Proponents of Bau-Biologie wish to:

- Take control of design and construction of buildings away from "experts" and give it to actual users, because serving only the interests of the experts decreases the chances of achieving a harmonious balance for the living and working environment.
- Subordinate technology to nature, life and culture; subordinate profit and performance to health concerns.
- Reach out not just to professional architects and builders but to anyone who wants to build a healthy, nontoxic home.[35]

Bau-Biologie uses a concept of harmony that can also be found in *feng shui*. The basic concerns in Bau-Biologie involve finding a proper site and design and then using proper building materials or products, ventilation, lighting and interior design to provide an energy-efficient and healthy living or working environment.[36]

Foundation for Timeless Architecture, Henry MacLean, P.O. Box 513, Boston, MA 02258 (617) 964-6384. Dedicated to the revival in architectural practice of global worldwide traditions.

Nacul Products and Resources, Roc Ahrensdorf, 592 Main Street, Amherst, MA 01002 (413) 256-8025. The Nacul Architecture Center consults regarding purchase of nontoxic building construction and household products.

The International Institute for Bau-Biologie & Ecology, Inc., Clearwater, FL 34615 (813) 461-4371.

Community or Social Architecture

"Community architecture" began in London in the 1970s and grew in the 1980s when community riots—such as those on the Broadwater Farm estate in 1985—showed that something was wrong with some of the area's built environment. The movement seeks to improve living and working conditions through increasing involvement and control by the people over their environment.[37]

The movement has undertaken many projects to build appropriate communities, such as technical-aid centers for community leaders (starting in the 1970s); self-build housing programs (one in Lewisham was completed in 1981); public-sector rehabilitation involving tenants (Lea View House, London, 1983) and occupant-managed settlement (Lightmoor, Shropshire, 1984). A U.S. example is resident-managed housing for the homeless in Seattle.[38]

The founding principle of community architecture is that "the environment works better if the people who live, work and play in it are actively involved in its creation and management. Like Bau-Biologie, it opposes leaving community development in the hands of bureaucrats and professionals and instead argues for:

- Involving members of the community in a "creative partnership" among professionals, politicians and citizens in the planning and development of housing and working environments.
- Easily managed and maintained, energy-efficient structures to improve the local quality of life.
- Small-scale building and production, "user-friendly" technology, recycling, conservationism and housing individuality epitomized by the handmade house.[39]

The National Civic League, 1445 Market Street, #300, Denver, CO 80202 (800) 223-6004. Some issues of the League's *National Civic Review*, in its 81st year in 1991, include a section on "Healthy Communities" (contact David Lampe, Editor, at the League) and the League is preparing a *Guide to the Healthy Community*.

The following organizations are among those that provide information about model building codes, standards and housing maintenance.

American National Standards Institute (ANSI), 1430 Broadway, New York, NY 10018 (212) 354-3300.

American Society of Heating, Refrigerating and Air Conditioning Engineers (ASHRAE), 1791 Tullie Circle, NE, Atlanta, GA, 30329 (404) 636-8400.

American Society of Mechanical Engineers (ASME), 1825 K Street, NW, Washington, DC 20006 (202) 785-3756.

American Society for Testing and Materials (ASTM), 1916 Grace Street, Philadelphia 19103 (215) 299-5400.

Council of American Building Officials (CABO), 5203 Leesburg Pike, Suite 708, Falls Church, VA 22041 (703) 931-4533.

Housing Resource Center, 1820 W. 48th Street, Cleveland, OH 44102 (216) 281-4663. Provides practical home-maintenance, repair and improvement information.

International Conference of Building Officials (ICBO), 5360 South Workman Mill Road, Whittier, CA 90601 (213) 699-0541.

National Association of Home Builders, 15th and M Streets, NW, Washington, DC 20005 (800) 368-5242, ext. 300.

National Conference of State Building Codes and Standards (NCSBCS), 505 Huntmar Park Drive, Suite 210, Herndon, VA 22070 (703) 437-0100.

National Fire Protection Association (NFPA), Batterymarch Park, Quincy, MA 02269 (617) 770-3000, (800) 344-3555. Prepares fire-prevention standards. For example, Standard 89M covers heat-producing appliances.

CHAPTER FIVE

Mortality Rates

In 1987, the total number of American deaths from all causes was 2.1 million, 18,000 more than the previous year. It was the largest number of U.S. deaths ever recorded, reflecting the country's population growth and the increasing number of elderly people.[1]

U.S. LIFE EXPECTANCY

But the death *rate* for 1987, at 872.4 deaths per 100,000 population, was slightly *lower* than the 873.2 per 100,000 in 1986. This reflected the continued growth of the American life span. Over the last three decades it has lengthened from 69.7 years in 1960 to 75.0 in 1987 and an all-time high of 75.4 years in 1989. In the 19th century, citizens of industrialized countries could expect to live only 40 years.[2]

U.S. life expectancy is projected to increase to 76.7 years by 2000, but with the growing incidence of AIDS, which kills most of its victims at a young age, these forecasts may prove to be somewhat optimistic. If we don't count the deaths that occur immediately after childbirth, only 12.4 percent of all deaths now occur before the age of 50.[3]

Despite its wealth, the United States ranks below 15 other countries in life expectancy. Japan heads the list shown in Table 5-1, which averages the numbers for men and women (women tend to have higher life expectancies); life expectancy in Japan was extended dramatically, by a full year, from 1989 to 1990.[4]

U.S. life expectancy has been increasing at a much slower rate than in Japan. In 1955, U.S. men had a life expectancy of 66.7 years, more than three years longer than Japanese men's 63.6 years. By 1986, an American baby boy could look forward to 71.3 years of life, compared to a Japanese

TABLE 5–1
LIFE EXPECTANCIES, HIGHEST 16 COUNTRIES

Rank	Country	Life expectancy at birth (years)	Rank	Country	Life expectancy at birth (years)
1	Japan	79.0	10	Germany	
2	Switzerland	78.0		(west only)	75.9
3	Sweden	77.4	10	France	75.9
4	Spain	77.3	12	Cuba	75.7
5	Canada	77.2	13	Austria	75.6
5	Netherlands	77.2	14	Belgium	75.5
5	Greece	77.2	14	Denmark	75.5
8	Italy	76.8	16	United States	75.4
9	Australia	76.2			

SOURCE: U.S. Bureau of the Census, *Statistical Abstract of the U.S., 1990*, 110th ed., Table 1440, pp. 835–836.

boy's 75.2 years—nearly four years longer for the Japanese baby, a relative gain of seven years.[5]

Americans thus far have been unwilling to adopt the diet and other lifestyle factors that would permit them to live as long as the more disciplined Japanese, Swiss and Swedes. But the difference looks even more stark when we consider that the United States is behind *other* countries noted for their heavy consumption of cigarettes and alcohol; one explanation may be the greater availability of health-care services for the poor in these other countries.

Also, while Americans are living longer, they are also sick more often, and longer. Women lose more time to illness than men.[6] It would be desirable for the government to develop data that could incorporate into the traditional mortality-rate yardstick of health a "disability standard" reflecting not just survival but freedom from chronic disease and disability.

WHAT AMERICANS DIE OF

The two leading killers of Americans are cardiovascular diseases and cancer. They accounted for two-thirds of U.S. deaths. Cardiovascular diseases (mostly heart disease, then strokes, with some less-common vascular diseases) caused 46 percent of deaths in 1986 and 1987, while cancer caused 22 percent.[7] Although heart disease has been declining in recent years, cancer continues to increase.

Heart disease deaths (including deaths from related artery diseases) increased 167 percent from 1900 to 1970, from 148 deaths per 100,000 population to 394. But since 1970, deaths from this cause have *decreased*, to 312 per 100,000 in 1988.[8] Heart disease is linked to smoking, intake of high levels of saturated fat and alcohol and lack of exercise. Consumption of saturated fat began declining in the late 1980s, in response to warnings from the Surgeon General; smoking had begun to decline earlier.

Cancer deaths, however, have been *increasing steadily*, from 68 per 100,000 in 1900 to 199 in 1988. Of the 985,000 new cases of cancer in 1988 (five-year average survival rate 49 percent), 152,000 were lung cancers (survival rate 13 percent), 152,000 were breast cancers (survival rate 74 percent) and 105,000 were colon cancers (survival rate 54 percent).[9] These diseases are linked to smoking, alcohol and toxic chemicals in air, food and water, as well as to the greater longevity that results from successful treatment of other diseases.

The third- and fourth-leading causes of death in the U.S. are strokes (included among the cardiovascular diseases along with heart disease) and accidents. Automobile accidents (see Chapter 8) are the most common form of U.S. accidents, with workplace and home accidents (see Chapters 3 and 8) contributing substantial numbers.

Certain diseases are on the increase. AIDS is one, so far striking mainly homosexuals and intravenous drug users. The death rate from AIDS among men in some parts of New York City is double the death rate from all causes in Anchorage. Alzheimer's disease is another—between 1979 and 1987, the incidence of the disease rose more than tenfold, from under 900 to over 11,000 cases. Some observers attribute the increase in reported incidence of Alzheimer's to increased awareness of the disease; instead of describing the cause of death as "senility," a doctor may now be more specific.[10]

STATES WITH HIGH MORTALITY RATES

The age-adjusted mortality or death rate is a crude overall measure of the health of a community. A mortality rate is simply the rate at which people are dying. As we saw in Chapter 1, we should look at unadjusted death rates cautiously because they are affected by the age composition of the community. The age-adjusted death rate (see Table 1-1) takes age composition into consideration.

State mortality rates vary substantially, because of differences in lifestyles and environment. The Centers for Disease Control collected information on state death rates from "chronic" and "largely preventable" diseases—coronary heart disease and stroke, chronic obstructive pulmonary disease, lung cancer, breast cancer and colorectal cancer and cirrhosis and diabetes. Death rates from these diseases in 1986 ranged from a low of

326.8 deaths per 100,000 in Hawaii to 517.6 deaths per 100,000 population in Michigan. The ten "best" and "worst" are shown in Table 5-2.

The mortality data of some of the "worst" states clearly show the human cost of industrial activity and coal mining. They are also interesting in the context of pesticide-intensive farming. Several states with the highest mortality rates (New York, Delaware, Indiana) have been the slowest to show interest in reducing use of toxic chemicals in the growing of food.[12] Use of toxins on farms is especially bad for the farmers, but also affects the urban dwellers who consume the food.

In the remainder of this chapter we review the major categories of mortality and the rankings of cities in each category. We leave discussion of infant mortality to Chapter 7 and accidents to Chapter 8.

CARDIOVASCULAR DISEASES

Cardiovascular diseases include high blood pressure, leading to strokes, and hardening of the arteries, leading to heart attacks. *The average American is estimated to have a one-in-three probability of a significant cardiovascular "event" (heart attack or stroke) by the age of 60.*[13]

Comparative data on heart-attack death rates by metro area is shown in Table 5-3. The residual mortality rate for these diseases was explained in Chapter 1. It adjusts the crude mortality rate to allow for the fact that the median age of residents of cities varies. We do this by calculating what is left over (the "residual" death rate) when we remove the age factor, showing

TABLE 5–2
DEATH RATES, CHRONIC/PREVENTABLE DISEASES

State	Death Rate, 1986*	State	Death Rate, 1986*
BEST TEN		**WORST TEN**	
Hawaii	326.8	Illinois	487.9
North Dakota	361.1	Indiana	490.6
Utah	361.7	Rhode Island	491.0
New Mexico	382.0	South Carolina	493.2
Texas	387.6	Delaware	494.2
Minnesota	388.4	Kentucky	497.2
Idaho	394.9	Ohio	501.2
Arizona	396.2	New York	508.5
Nebraska	398.3	West Virginia	512.5
Colorado	400.3	Michigan	517.6

* Rates are per 100,000 population.

SOURCE: Centers for Disease Control, *Morbidity and Mortality Weekly Report,* January 19, 1990.[11]

TABLE 5–3
FATAL HEART ATTACKS

Metropolitan Area	Residual IHD Death Rate	Metropolitan Area	Residual IHD Death Rate
BEST TEN		**WORST TEN**	
Washington, DC	−1.14	Pittsburgh	0.71
Honolulu	−1.11	Jersey City	0.76
Seattle	−0.94	Shreveport	0.80
Denver–Aurora–Boulder	−0.90	Worcester–Fitchburg	0.88
Albuquerque	−0.84	Cleveland	0.89
Des Moines	−0.83	Newark, NJ	0.97
Anchorage	−0.81	Flint	1.11
Salt Lake City	−0.77	New York–Yonkers	1.18
Las Vegas	−0.77	Toledo	1.27
Atlanta	−0.71	Buffalo	2.14

NOTE: Fatal heart attacks, known medically as deaths from ischemic heart disease (IHD), constitute the major category of heart disease deaths, which in turn constitute the major category of cardiovascular disease.

SOURCE: Unadjusted rates from *Vital Statistics of the U.S., loc. cit.*, 1987; residual, age-adjusted rates calculated by the author (see Table 1–1 for explanation of procedure).

the extent to which each metropolitan area's mortality rate is lower or higher than would be expected based on the area's median age.

Cities with high levels of cardiovascular diseases are likely to have: (1) a high level of stress, (2) a high consumption level of fat, especially red meat, or (3) inadequate recreational facilities and a lack of interest in exercise.

Stress as a cause of heart attacks could be an especially serious problem in a community that is in economic decline, losing jobs and people. The metropolitan areas with the lowest heart-attack rates in Table 5-3—like Washington, D.C., Honolulu and Seattle—have been growing in recent years. The areas with the highest heart-attack rates—like Buffalo, Toledo, New York and Flint—have been suffering job losses.

Those who are left behind could be dying in larger numbers because of stress—worries about paying the rent, a feeling of failure, a loss of a sense of purpose—a collective version of the loss of a will to live. The health effects of stress are aggravated by a lack of exercise, which could also follow from economic decline.

According to the Centers for Disease Control, the six most important factors that lead to heart attacks are, in decreasing order: sedentary lifestyle (importance rating of 58), high serum cholesterol, which is related both to fat consumption and heredity (31), smoking (25), overweight (22), hypertension/stress (17) and diabetes (5). The leading preventable cause of heart attacks is lack of exercise.[14]

Sedentary people are twice as likely to die from a heart attack as people who are physically active. A person escapes from the label of "sedentary" by (1) doing any purposeful physical activity or regular exercise as often as three times a week, and (2) doing it for at least 20 minutes at a time. By this definition, of those surveyed in 37 states, *58 percent* of respondents described themselves as being sedentary![15] Of the states examined, New York had the highest percentage of inactive people, *74 percent*, while Washington had the lowest, 45 percent.

People who exercise moderately but regularly live the longest and are the least likely to suffer from heart attacks. Exercise also reduces the incidence or seriousness of hyperlipidemia, obesity, noninsulin-dependent diabetes mellitus, osteoporosis, psychological impairment, colon cancer, stroke and back injury. Many states promote physical-activity programs; see Chapter 7.[16]

So your health is affected by your economic and recreational environment. A community like New York City—with a high heart-attack rate and a high percentage of sedentary people—that responds to an economic downturn by cutting its parks and recreation budget virtually in half (as New York is doing in 1991) is compounding what might be called a Loss-of-Heart Syndrome (LOHS).

CANCER RATES

As described in Chapters 2-4, cancer incidence is commonly related to pollutants in air, water and food. Other diseases that are exacerbated by air pollution include multiple sclerosis, emphysema and pneumonia. After adjustment for median age, Denver, Salt Lake City and Honolulu have the lowest death rates from cancer (see Table 5-4). Buffalo, Worcester and Portland, Maine have the highest cancer rates.

Cancer deaths among people 55 and older are climbing rapidly not only in the United States, but also in Japan and many European nations.[17] While rates of some cancers have been dropping, the overall cancer mortality rate has soared in the last 20 years. Though lung and stomach cancer in men have decreased, other cancers such as brain tumors and cancer of the breast, kidney, skin, lymphatic system and bone marrow have dramatically increased. But it is unclear whether these increases reflect new carcinogens in our environment or whether they reflect better diagnoses (previously many cancers may have gone undetected and untreated).

People in certain professions may be more vulnerable to certain cancers. For instance, it has been suggested that farmers are more at risk for cancers of the blood and lymph systems, namely leukemia, non-Hodgkin's lymphoma and multiple myeloma,[18] which have been associated with agricultural chemicals.

But other, more common, types of cancers are not linked to chemicals. Nonmelanoma skin cancer, the most common form of cancer in whites in

TABLE 5—4
CANCER DEATHS

	Residual Cancer Deathrate		Residual Cancer Deathrate
BEST TEN		WORST TEN	
Denver–Aurora–Boulder	−0.80	Springfield, MA	0.53
Salt Lake City	−0.78	Pittsburgh	0.54
Honolulu	−0.78	Shreveport	0.58
Miami–Hialeah	−0.65	Flint	0.62
Charlotte, NC	−0.65	Newark	0.70
Anchorage	−0.64	Charleston, WV	0.72
Colorado Springs	−0.57	Toledo	0.74
Washington	−0.46	Portland, ME	0.82
Bridgeport–Stamford	−0.45	Worcester–Fitchburg	0.87
Atlanta	−0.45	Buffalo	0.98

SOURCE: Unadjusted rates from *Vital Statistics of the U.S.*, for 1987; (which was the latest year for which data were available when the author's research was done in 1990); adjusted rates calculated by the author (see Table 1–1 notes).

the U.S., is increasing at an annual rate of 3 percent a year and is directly related to exposure to ultraviolet-B radiation from the sun. Exposure to the sun causes even more widespread ailments such as facial blemishes, varicose veins, wrinkled skin and oral lesions.[19]

The more lethal form of skin cancer, melanoma, increased 57 percent, or about 4 percent annually, between 1973 and 1985 for white Americans. Among blacks, who are much less at risk of this cancer, the rate has been decreasing. Future ozone depletion in the earth's stratosphere will lead to greater increases in both melanoma and nonmelanoma skin cancer, since the ozone layer reduces the harmfulness of the sun's ultraviolet-B rays. Children, whose cells are multiplying as they grow and have more sensitive skin, are especially vulnerable to getting skin cancer from radiation.

HOMICIDES AND ROBBERIES

With homicides involving partners or family members, the victims are slightly more likely to be female (52 percent) while the killers are predominantly male (74 percent). The rates for violent assault between partners or family members show an even more pronounced tendency for victims to be females (73 percent) and the assaulters male (80 percent).[20]

Table 5-5 shows that the lowest homicide rate in 1989 was in Boise (0.5

> *Cancer Information Service* (800) 422-6237, (800) 524-1234 (Hawaii), 8:30-10 ETZ, M-F. Offers counseling and information on cancer treatment, diagnosis, clinical trials, rehabilitation, home care, financial aid, prevention information and a physician-referral service.
>
> *National Foundation for Cancer Research* (800) 321-CURE, 9-5 ETZ, M-F. Conducts scientific research on various types of cancer and provides referrals to other cancer organizations.
>
> *Y-ME Breast Cancer Support Group* (800) 221-2141, (312) 799-8228 (Illinois), 9-5 CTZ, M-F. Offers counseling with other cancer patients. Provides medical information on treatments for cancer, such as chemotherapy.

per 100,000 residents). The highest rate was in New Orleans (24.7 per 100,000), New York–Yonkers (22.7) and Miami–Hialeah (21.8). An important advantage of homicide rates as a measure of violence is that deaths tend to be fully investigated, and therefore are better reported, than less serious forms of assault.

Early data on 1990 homicide rates showed that they rose 16 percent in middle-sized cities (500,000-1 million population), twice as much as for cities of 1 million or more. This continues a trend throughout the latter half of the 1980s, during which homicide rates increased sharply in some middle-sized U.S. cities. In 1990, homicide rates for Memphis and St. Louis exceeded that for New York City. Drug rings have moved to smaller cities where costs of doing business are lower.[22]

Robberies are a better indicator of the likelihood of being killed by a

TABLE 5–5
HOMICIDE RATES, 1989

Metro Area	Homicides per 100,000	Metro Area	Homicides per 100,000
BEST TEN		**WORST TEN**	
Boise	0.5	Washington	17.0
Lincoln, NE	1.9	Dallas–Garland–Ft. Worth	17.3
Rochester, NY	2.0	Houston	17.4
Syracuse	2.6	Detroit	17.5
Spokane	2.7	Los Angeles–Long Beach	18.0
Grand Rapids	3.1	Jacksonville, FL	19.2
Pittsburgh	3.2	Shreveport	19.6
Manchester	3.4	Miami–Hialeah	21.8
Salt Lake City	3.4	New York–Yonkers	22.7
Springfield, MO	3.4	New Orleans	24.7

SOURCE: FBI.[21]

stranger than the overall homicide rate, since robbery is a stranger-to-stranger crime and a (small) percentage of them end in homicide (see Table 5-6). The lowest robbery rate was in Boise, the highest in Miami.

TABLE 5–6
ROBBERIES, 1989

Metropolitan Area	Robberies per 100,000	Metropolitan Area	Robberies per 100,000
BEST TEN		**WORST TEN**	
Boise	24.6	Baltimore	445.0
Lincoln	48.9	Dallas–Garland–Ft. Worth	452.9
Burlington, VT	50.8	Jacksonville, FL	460.6
Portland, ME	57.6	New Orleans	549.8
Madison, WI	64.0	Jersey City	551.1
Manchester	68.1	Newark, NJ	551.7
Salt Lake City	77.8	Chicago	561.9
Springfield, MO	85.9	Los Angeles–Long Beach	616.4
Syracuse	87.9	New York–Yonkers	1,107.8
Colorado Springs	94.0	Miami–Hialeah	1,108.2

SOURCE: FBI.[23]

SUICIDES

The murder rate in America is high, but more people kill themselves than kill others. Suicides are widely viewed as a mental-health problem. Yet the pattern of high suicide rates suggests that the causes are complicated and that those who commit suicide are not necessarily mentally unbalanced. The highest suicide rates tend to be in retirement communities like Phoenix and Tampa, and in the Rockies and the West, where life is commonly thought of as being less stressful, with a lower population density and with strong economies. Thus, Las Vegas, Tucson, Boise and Albuquerque all have suicide rates above 20 per 100,000 residents (see Table 5-7).

Having followed these numbers with care for more than 20 years, I see a connection between high suicide rates and rapid community growth. People go to these cities of opportunity with high expectations and their expectations are not always met. Las Vegas is a prime example, at the highest end of the suicide list. Most people go there to gamble or divorce, or both. The odds are against them. Those who are disappointed may take it out on themselves.

Retirement communities also by their nature attract elderly people who are looking for a paradise in their golden years and who may end up missing home. Elderly people may also face incurable diseases or the death

TABLE 5–7
SUICIDE RATES

	Suicide Deaths per 100,000		Suicide Deaths per 100,000
BEST TEN		**WORST TEN**	
New York–Yonkers	4.2	Riverside–San Bernardino	17.2
Montgomery	6.4	Portland, OR	17.7
Charlotte, NC	6.6	Tampa–St. Petersburg	17.7
Jackson, MS	6.8	Colorado Springs	18.1
Dayton	6.9	Phoenix–Mesa	18.4
Bridgeport–Stamford	7.6	Tacoma	19.1
Syracuse	8.2	Albuquerque	20.3
Newark, NJ	8.5	Boise	21.3
Lincoln, NE	8.6	Tucson	23.0
El Paso	8.7	Las Vegas	26.2
Raleigh-Durham	8.7		

SOURCE: *Vital Statistics of the U.S., 1987.*[24]

of a spouse or other close person, and may choose death rather than a long period of suffering and accumulation of medical bills.

Low suicide rates prevail in the East, Midwest and Deep South. New York City has the lowest suicide rate in the country, perhaps because people are too busy fighting for survival to consider taking their own lives. Two other possible explanations are: (1) New Yorkers don't blame themselves for their shortcomings when so many other possible explanations of why things go wrong are all around them, like government and other people, and (2) New York attracts and retains risk-oriented people in the entrepreneurial economy and such people always keep hoping for better times. The rootedness of the communities in these areas may be another factor, as well as the more realistic expectations of people who live in these cities and the strength of religious institutions. A strongly rooted community will have support groups to help depressed people.[25]

Suicide rates are increasing and in the last two decades the teen suicide rate has nearly doubled. The rate remains highest among older people, but between 1969 and 1987, the rate of suicides among 14-to-19-year-olds rose from 5.7 per 100,000 to 10.2. One-fourth of adolescent boys and 42 percent of adolescent girls said in 1987 that they had seriously considered committing suicide. Just under half of those who had considered it—11 percent of the boys and 18 percent of the girls—reported having attempted suicide.[26]

Suicide is currently the eighth leading cause of death, but quite likely would rank higher if reporting procedures permitted dual classification of suicidal accidents—many fatal car accidents, for example, have all the earmarks of suicides, yet are not reported as such. Among college students, suicide ranks as the second leading cause of death, after auto accidents— but suicides and auto accidents are often linked, and both are related to alcohol and drug use.

Suicide is unique among causes of death because it is an outcome desired by the victim. Men are *three times more likely than women to kill themselves,* but *women make three times as many attempts!* Whites commit suicide more than nonwhites. *Divorced men are three times more likely to kill themselves* than married men. Other factors identified with suicide include alcoholism, homosexuality (especially since and in relation to the appearance of AIDS, discussed next) and a family history of suicide.

SEXUALLY TRANSMITTED DISEASES

Acquired Immune-Deficiency Syndrome (AIDS) is the most deadly of the diseases that are primarily transmitted through sexual intercourse. In the United States it takes its toll primarily among homosexuals, whereas elsewhere in the world the AIDS virus is spreading rapidly among hetero- sexuals as well. AIDS is fast becoming a major contributor to the U.S. mortality rate, accounting for 100,000 deaths since 1981, with another 350,000 deaths expected by 1992. As many as 1.5 million Americans may be carrying the AIDS virus; most of them are undiagnosed and untreated. Much progress has been made in life-prolonging drugs, but AIDS is still eventually fatal.

In 1987 the AIDS virus—Human Immunodeficiency Virus infection (HIV)—was the 15th leading cause of death in the United States. This was the first year that AIDS was given a code number for state reports and ranked as a cause of death. Of the 15 leading causes of death, the greatest difference in the mortality rate between men and women was for HIV infection by a ratio of 9 to 1 (13,886 deaths of men versus 1,577 deaths of women from AIDS in 1988).[27]

AIDS cases may be underreported because the actual cause of death may be listed by a doctor or hospital (sometimes out of deference to the wishes of the victim's family) as a particular pneumonia, cancer, or other disease, rather than the HIV virus that destroyed the victim's immune system. In 1989 seven states reported 700 or more AIDS cases. While more than half of the cases in 1981–82 were in New York State, in 1989 more cases were reported in California than New York (see Table 5-8), with San Francisco being the most afflicted city in California.

New York City has more AIDS cases than any other city in the world, with more than 16,000 deaths by 1989. AIDS ranks as the third leading cause of death in the city, behind heart disease and cancer but ahead of auto accidents. AIDS cases are concentrated heavily in certain neighborhoods. (See Table 5-9.)

TABLE 5–8
REPORTED AIDS CASES BY STATE, 1989

State	Cases	Percent
California	3,645	19.1
New York	3,350	17.5
Florida	1,781	9.3
New Jersey	1,386	7.3
Texas	1,278	6.7

NOTE: The data are provisional. The five states included are those with 700 or more AIDS cases reported from January through July 1989.

SOURCE: U.S. Centers for Disease Control (Atlanta, GA), unpublished data report in U.S. Bureau of the Census, *Statistical Abstract of the U.S., 1990*, Table 187, p. 117.

For the two neighborhoods where AIDS has struck most acutely—Chelsea-Clinton and Greenwich Village—the probable explanation is that these are the two most popular neighborhoods for homosexual males, one of the groups most at risk for AIDS, to live. The high ratio of male to female deaths points to this interpretation. In the other neighborhoods, intravenous drug use is a more likely explanation because females are a higher proportion of the victims; sharing needles is another major risk factor for AIDS.

TABLE 5–9
AIDS DEATH RATES IN NEW YORK CITY NEIGHBORHOODS
Deaths per 100,000 Residents

Neighborhood	Men	Women
Chelsea & Clinton	404	18
Greenwich Village	371	5
Central Harlem	196	55
Midtown	213	21
Lower East Side	194	38
East Harlem	176	49
Brownsville	136	75
Bedford-Stuyvesant	153	56
Concourse/Highbridge	161	41
Melrose/Mott Haven	152	49
Upper West Side	188	11

NOTE: The neighborhoods were ranked according to *total* AIDS deaths per 100,000 residents in 1988.

SOURCE: New York City Bureau of Health Statistics and Analysis, *New York City Community District Vital Statistics Data Book, 1988*.

As measured by years of productive life lost (i.e., working years up to age 65), AIDS is the No. 1 cause of death in New York City and is one of the most devastating and costly causes of death in the country. Of the 19,000 reported AIDS deaths in 1989, 56 percent of the victims were white and non-Hispanic and 88 percent were under 50 (46 percent were in their 30s, 22 percent in their 40s and 20 percent under 30).[28]

Besides AIDS, other sexually transmitted diseases are on the increase and are taking their toll, although not in the same numbers as AIDS (many may, unlike AIDS victims, be cured with antibiotics). The Hepatitis B virus can be fatal and is sexually transmitted as well as through sharing needles by drug users. Most at risk are those who change sexual partners frequently.

THE CASE FOR MONOGAMY

The spread of hazardous sexual diseases is an argument by itself for monogamous relationships. But independent of such threats, marriage extends the life of both partners, but especially men—unmarried middle-aged men are twice as likely to die as those who have wives. The men most at risk are those who were previously married (as with all statistics, reverse causation is possible—i.e., sickly singles can't find spouses). The exceptions appear to be among certain groups such as those of Japanese ancestry in Hawaii; possibly it is because they have strong inter-generational social ties, independent of marriage.[29]

Women's liberation has led to more women taking on some of the same hazardous jobs as men, but it's also possible that (1) by taking on higher-level positions in management, working women have increased their control over their work and have reduced their stress, and (2) fewer pregnancies mean fewer deaths from childbirth. In any case, U.S. women still can expect to outlive men by 6.9 years.[30]

BLACK VS. WHITE MORTALITY RATES

The difference in U.S. mortality rates between blacks and whites is shocking. In 1981, the life expectancy for whites was 74.8 years, for blacks, 68.9 years, a gap of 5.9 years. In 1988, whites were expected to live to 75.6 years, blacks only to 69.2 years, a gap of 6.4 years.[31] So the gap between the life expectancies of whites and blacks has been widening. Blacks have higher rates than the white population for most of the leading causes of death.

The largest difference continues to be in the area of homicide, where the rate for blacks is *six times* that for whites. Homicide is most likely at younger ages; young black men are much more at risk than whites. Homicide is the leading cause of death for black males between the ages of 15 and 24.[32] One reason is the failure of social support systems for black families—only 38.6 percent of black children lived with both parents in 1988, a tragic 67 percent decline from 1960. Significantly more than half of all black children live in female-headed households, a consequence in part of welfare laws that historically have barred aid to poor families in which the father lives at home.

The homicide rate among black males aged 15–24 rose two-thirds from 1984 to 1988, nearly entirely because of increased use of guns. Of the more than 20,000 young black males who died between 1978 and 1987, homicides claimed the lives of about 40 percent, and about 80 percent of the homicides involved guns. Homicide can result from domestic violence, child abuse, rape and fighting among acquaintances. More than half of all homicide victims are killed by people known to them. Factors contributing to the rising numbers of homicides are easy access to firearms, alcohol and substance abuse, drug-trafficking, poverty, racial discrimination and acceptance of violent behavior.[33]

Academic underachievement among blacks in one effect of childhood neglect, and this in turn perpetuates a cycle of poverty. Although blacks are graduating from high school in much greater numbers than used to be the case, many employers now insist on two or four years of college. Blacks are just not going on to college at anywhere near the rate of the rest of the population of high school graduates. Of young black men in their 20s, nearly one in four (23 percent) is in prison or on probation or parole. While blacks account for only 6 percent of the U.S. population, they are 46 percent of state prison inmates.

Blacks live disproportionately in the inner cities and rely on crowded public hospitals for their medical care. This accounts for some of their higher mortality rates. For example, asthma deaths have been rising steadily, with the highest rate among black male children. Asthma attacks an estimated 9.9 million Americans—mostly children, blacks and the poor.[34] Asthma hospitalization rates and mortality are more than twice as high among blacks as whites. The two most plausible explanations of these figures are that the unhealthy urban air causes asthma problems (New York City and Chicago alone account for 21.1 percent of deaths from asthma) and inner-city children do not receive the instruction in or access to inhalers that would prevent serious asthma attacks. Poor children in New York City and other urban areas suffer from such attacks to a significantly higher degree than the rest of the population.

CHAPTER SIX

The Environment

Conditions in our community can greatly affect our health—for example, through the quality of the air we breathe, the water we drink and the stress we are subjected to. In recent years, Americans have grown increasingly aware of practices that can put entire populations at risk. One authoritative survey pointed to hazardous waste as the greatest environmental concern, with more than 60 percent of respondents considering it "very serious" (see Table 6-1).

TABLE 6–1
TOP ENVIRONMENTAL CONCERNS OF AMERICANS

1. Active hazardous waste sites	62%
2. Abandoned hazardous waste sites	61%
3. Workers exposed to toxic chemicals	60%
4. Industrial water pollution	58%
4. Nuclear accident radiation	58%
4. Radioactive waste	58%
7. Underground storage tank leakage	55%
8. Pesticide residues harming farmers	54%
9. Pesticide residues harming consumers	52%
10. Industrial accident pollution	51%

SOURCE: Roper Poll, 1988.[1]

Many of the situations the public considered most serious in that 1988 survey involve corporate pollution—industrial hazardous wastes, water quality and the exposure of workers to chemicals. Situations over which the public has more control, such as indoor air pollution, radon and microwave-oven radiation, were considered much less serious. Such global issues as acid rain, destruction of the ozone layer and the greenhouse effect, the latter two of which were only theoretical worries in 1988, were near the middle or bottom of the list.

Release of wastes into the ground, air and water affect our communities and environment at every level. In this chapter we analyze the ways these problems affect the healthfulness of where we live and work. A general environmental resource is:

Environmental Protection Agency (EPA) (800) 424-4000 (Ex D.C.). Available 10:00-3:00 ETZ, M-F. Provides referrals to state and local agencies on environmental issues such as air pollution and gas in ground.

STATE AND LOCAL CONTROL OF INDUSTRIAL WASTE

Some of the most toxic substances are released by the petrochemical industry and as byproducts of industrial processes such as the manufacture of alloys and paints, and aluminum processing. Companies also use toxic substances as solvents, cleaners and fuels—a large portion of hazardous waste is liquid. Some waste causes respiratory problems and cancers, other waste is immediately fatal if inhaled or ingested. Some toxic substances emitted in industrial processes can deplete the ozone layer.[2]

Underground storage tanks are commonly used to store the radioactive byproducts of plutonium and uranium. Disposal of radioactive wastes can become a major preoccupation for people near nuclear power facilities and weapons plants.[3]

The Danger of Explosions

These toxic substances can also be flammable or explosive. This aggravates the risk of chemical and radioactive wastes because if organic chemicals were to seep into storage tanks, some fear it could result in giant explosions.

Many towns with toxic-chemical plants in their area are entirely unprepared,[4] even though in the 1980s, more than 11,000 toxic-chemical accidents occurred in the U.S., resulting in more than 300 deaths, thousands of injuries and the evacuation of half a million people. Only a few hundred of the 32,000 U.S. fire departments have hazardous-materials teams to deal with chemical or toxic accidents.

If you are thinking of moving to a locality that has a company using hazardous chemicals or other materials, consider the related dangers and what the company and community have done to minimize risk and plan for possible emergencies.

Toxic Emissions

Disposal of toxic waste into land dumps or bodies of water has been controlled since the 1970s, but a significant portion of toxic emissions into the air is unregulated. Toxics like asbestos, fluorocarbons, methylene chloride and benzene are released from chemical, plastic and other industrial plants during manufacturing, but many toxic substances also enter the air from wood-burning, incinerators, sewage treatment plants, insecticides, household cleaning products and motor vehicles.

The EPA reported that in 1988 the manufacturing facilities it tracks released (into the air, water or land) 6.2 billion pounds of the 300 types of toxic chemicals it tracks. This was an 11 percent decrease from the 7 billion pounds released in 1987. Of the 6.2 billion pounds, 39 percent was emitted into the air.[5] The toxic emissions continued to drop in 1989; the states with the highest levels are Texas and Louisiana, followed by Ohio, Tennessee, Indiana, Illinois, Michigan, Pennsylvania, Florida and Kansas.[6]

These toxins can be inhaled or can be ingested in our water, vegetables, meat or seafood. Through a combination of all these paths into our systems, toxic substances can damage living tissue, impair the central nervous system, or cause birth defects, illness or death. Although linking a cancer to specific toxins is difficult, cancer rates in areas around petrochemical facilities releasing toxins are generally higher than the national average. In addition to being carcinogenic, many of these toxic materials are (1) mutagenic, affecting the genetic material, or (2) teratogenic, affecting the formation of fetuses.[7]

National Emissions Standards for Hazardous Air Pollutants have been established by the EPA for a few of the more common toxic releases, including asbestos, beryllium, mercury, vinyl chloride, benzene, arsenic and radionuclides, but these are only 7 of the 328 chemicals considered toxic by the EPA inventory.[8]

Table 6-2 shows the toxic emissions in each state. It reveals that Louisiana (discussed later in this chapter) releases by far the heaviest volume of toxics relative to its land area—15,000 pounds per square mile. The surprise is that Connecticut, which does not have New Jersey's image as a toxic-waste emitter, is in second place with 7,000 pounds per square mile. Although Connecticut doesn't show up among the states with the giant polluting plants, it manages to release a lot of serious toxic waste. The EPA ranks it seventh among the states in ozone depletion, despite its small size. Its chemical industry accounts for one-fourth of Connecticut's toxic-waste generation.

If we compare Table 6-2 to Table 6-5, which ranks state environmental regulation efforts, it is clear that while Louisiana and Connecticut release the greatest concentrations of toxic waste, Louisiana has been doing a lot less about it than Connecticut, at least as of 1988.

TABLE 6–2
TOXIC RELEASES BY STATE, 1988

State	Pounds '000/Sq. Mi.	State	Pounds '000/Sq. Mi.
BEST TEN		**WORST TEN**	
District of Columbia	.01	Massachusetts	3.39
North Dakota	.02	Virginia	3.54
South Dakota	.03	Florida	3.85
Nevada	.04	Tennessee	4.82
Alaska	.04	New Jersey	5.19
Colorado	.13	Rhode Island	5.21
Vermont	.17	Ohio	5.55
Idaho	.17	Indiana	5.88
New Mexico	.20	Connecticut	6.56
Oregon	.22	Louisiana	14.99

SOURCE: EPA, *Toxics in the Community 1988: National and Local Perspectives* (Washington, D.C.: EPA, September 1990), p. 138.

Solid Wastes

Managing solid wastes has been a major problem for U.S. cities and smaller communities. Most solid wastes are produced in industry, agriculture and mining; the EPA estimates that 7.6 *billion* tons of nonhazardous solid waste are produced each year by industry, compared to 160 million tons of municipal trash—i.e., household waste. Oil and gas producers, mining operations and electric utilities generate the largest amounts of non-municipal solid waste. U.S. waste production per capita is the highest in the world—three and a half pounds of municipal waste per person per day.[9]

Plastic is the fastest-growing component of municipal solid waste and the category that is probably the most controversial because of the debate over the validity of claims for biodegradability of some types of plastic.

Reform of municipal garbage collection in America is long overdue. Paper and cardboard products constitute over 40 per cent of the weight of municipal solid waste, and much of this could be readily recycled back to paper manufacturers. Yard waste, such as branches, grass clippings and leaves, is the next largest component, and is an entirely unnecessary component of municipal solid waste—grass clippings should be left on lawns or composted and leaves should be composted in gardens. Metals, glass, and plastics are the next most important components of municipal solid waste and all of these are recyclable. Municipal food waste could be composted (better still if the generators of the waste did their own composting). The remainder is a miscellaneous category of inorganic waste such as rubber, leather, wood and textiles, much of which is reusable or recyclable.

Fortunately, the closing of municipal landfills means that many local governments are requiring residents to sort their refuse. Some localities are much further along than others. Among the challenges that lie ahead are systems by which residents of large cities can handle their own waste more efficiently—for example, a composting system for urban apartment dwellers! For how can a residence be considered healthy if it contributes to a stream of refuse that is choking the community?

Waste Disposal and Reduction

Many feel that the 20,000 facilities EPA monitors are only a portion of the number of hazardous sites. When Congress in 1980 passed the Comprehensive Environmental Response, Compensation and Liability Act, nicknamed the Superfund Act, it sought to regulate the measures to be taken once hazardous waste was identified, both on the Federal and state level. But during the first five years of the Superfund plan, only 13 of the sites on the list of national priorities were closed, and for 90 percent of the sites no long-term action was initiated. Insufficient funding, a shortage of needed technology and the huge number of sites identified were the major obstacles to the effectiveness of the program.

More than half the toxic wastes from industries are being disposed of through on-site landfills, deep-well injection procedures and storage ponds, all of which are susceptible to leakage into the water supply. The rest is shipped from industrial facilities to be treated or disposed of at public sewage plants or private chemical waste sites. Each of these methods of disposal has its own hazards—the only really safe plan for the future is to cut down on the production of the hazardous chemicals and other materials.

EPA Office of Solid Waste & Emergency Response, Office of RCRA Ombudsman (Hazardous Wastes) (800) 368-5888 and (800) 557-1938 (D.C.); 7:30-4:30 ETZ, M-F. Offers limited advice, and referrals to other organizations, regarding hazardous wastes.

EPA Superfund "Hotline" (800) 424-9346; (202) 382-3000 in Washington, D.C. This line is a major contrast to the EPA's pesticide hotline, which is well staffed and helpful. The respondent to my call didn't even know the name of the EPA Administrator and lamely offered to mail information "in six to eight weeks." If this is a "hot" response, heaven forbid I should ever find out what the "cold" response is like.

Landfills and Deep-Well Injection

Landfills have been a common means of disposing of industrial and consumer wastes, both toxic and nontoxic, and about 80 percent of the garbage in the United States is landfilled. As a result, the EPA estimates that by 1995 half the landfills in the United States will be closed. Landfills are susceptible to methane gas explosions, toxic gas emissions, noxious fumes and vermin, all of which lead to reduced property values and create many problems for communities. Of the EPA's Superfund list of the worst toxic-waste sites in the country, 20 percent are municipal solid-waste landfills. Because of the problems associated with landfills, many communities and states have begun shipping their trash to other locations. The need to ship garbage elsewhere more than doubled Philadelphia's garbage disposal bill from 1984 to 1985. New Jersey ships its garbage as far away as New Mexico.[10]

Landfills are usually lined with several feet of clay or synthetic plastics to keep the waste out of the surrounding environment. A drainage system can be placed above and between the liners to collect liquids, including rainwater that enters the landfill. The liquids are pumped out and then treated. After a landfill is filled, a clay or plastic lining is placed over the disposal area.[11] Potential health and environmental hazards arise if the waste manages to seep into the soil or nearby water systems and eventually it almost always does.

Deep-well injection is a common means of disposing of dilute wastes. In 1984 the EPA banned the disposal of liquid wastes into landfills. For deep-well injection, the waste is injected into the ground at levels much deeper than where drinking water usually comes from, and impermeable layers are used to separate the wastes from the soil and ground water. But the waste can occasionally seep upward and contaminate drinking water because of poor construction and operation.

Incinerators

Americans have burned their trash since the industrial revolution, but as concern over air quality grew in the 1960s and 1970s many incinerator plants were forced to shut down. As the garbage problem continued to grow in the last decade, the incinerator industry responded with cleaner and safer incinerator facilities. Some incinerators can treat hazardous wastes, and as restrictions are being placed on landfills and deep wells, incineration is becoming more common. Several different types of incinerating processes are used: liquid injection, rotary kilns, fluidized-bed incinerators and multiple hearth incinerators. But people in the neighborhoods where incinerators are to be sited worry about residual air pollution and they often fiercely oppose the facilities.

Advocates of incinerators say that new technologies are being developed to reduce pollution and that the locality benefits from converting the waste into energy. The European "mass burn" technology is designed to burn virtually everything while filtering the exhaust of most of the remaining chemicals.[12] Supporters of the new incinerators say the high temperature of the incinerators can destroy many volatile chemicals. Subsequent steps can reduce any remaining hazardous byproducts. Advocates claim the new process greatly reduces health and environmental risks, that it is far safer than burying the waste in landfills, and that it effectively supplements reduction and recycling.

Critics respond that even minimal health risks should not be tolerated and that efforts should be focused entirely on reducing and recycling garbage. Some toxic heavy metals, acid gases and organic chemicals can be released during and after burning the waste. Metals often emitted from the facilities, such as lead, beryllium and mercury, are highly toxic and can cause cancer and nervous system disorders. Sulfur dioxide and hydrochloric acid can be released during incineration, contributing to the problem of acid rain. Many toxic chemicals found in waste can remain in the ash following incineration, and ash is often more difficult to dispose of safely than the solid waste, prolonging the problem. Incineration is also expensive.[13]

The answer may lie in careful planning of facilities to sort out the kinds of garbage that could contribute to pollution if burned. Metals could be removed before incineration both by residents and by municipal workers. As municipal waste-disposal options shrink, municipal officials are going to lose the luxury of being able to postpone a decision. You have a stake in what your officials decide.

Recycling

Recycling is gaining acceptance as one of the most environmentally sound waste-management programs. Often the initiative has come from small communities, like North Stonington, Connecticut, which established one of the first recycling programs in the state. When it came to a vote, the only opposition was from the town's trash collector. The EPA has set a goal of recycling 25 percent of the nation's solid waste by 1992, and many states have higher recycling goals.[14]

Recycling such materials as metals and paper can greatly reduce the pollutants released into the environment through the alternative methods of landfilling and incineration. It reduces the harmful effects of incineration on global warming and the greenhouse effect, and can greatly reduce energy use and the costs of extracting and processing raw materials and of manufacturing. Since burning paper results in large carbon dioxide emissions and recycling saves the trees that could absorb some of the existing carbon dioxide, paper recycling is a significant environmental step.

Recycling paper is also a less toxic procedure than making virgin paper from the pulp of trees, because it does not require many of the chemicals that are used to remove the lignin from the pulp.[15] While it is true that using and producing recycled paper does not *eliminate* the solid waste problem, it does save trees, energy, oil and water, in addition to reducing air pollution and saving landfill space. All told, *substituting recycled paper resources for virgin paper results in 74 percent less air pollution and 35 percent less water pollution for the same amount of paper while also conserving energy.* Recyclable products can include cardboard, copier paper, computer paper and other paper products. Recycling can also be used to reduce the amount of waste for such materials as glass, aluminum and some plastics.

Other Waste-Reduction Methods

The best way to reduce the amount of garbage and industrial waste is at its source. Many industries are being pressured into using more environmentally sound processes. Packaging is a large contributor to the solid-waste problem in the United States and plastics are a large part of the packaging problem. As a sign of hope, the McDonald's Corporation is revamping its policies to show more environmental consciousness, for example by replacing its bleached-white takeout bags with unbleached, brown ones.[16]

The two options for reducing the amount of plastics waste are either recycling or producing biodegradable plastics. But these two approaches may conflict. Degradable plastics can contaminate the recycled plastics when mixed together, and many fear that making degradable products hinders the more promising strategy of recycling. Recent attempts have been made to produce plastics that are either biodegradable or photo-degradable (i.e., which break down when exposed to the ultraviolet rays of the sun). Several techniques are used to produce the degradable plastics, but a danger remains that a residue, particularly toxic substances in the plastic, might be left over or released. The length of time necessary for some plastics to degrade is also creating doubts. In addition, many naturally biodegradable products such as paper or food do not always break down completely because of a lack of moisture, warmth or oxygen in landfills and degradable plastics would have similar problems.[17]

AIR POLLUTION

While *indoor* air pollution is increasingly identified as a serious health concern, outdoor air pollution affects a greater number of people and is difficult to regulate. The increasing urbanization of the United States along with the industrial expansion has led to increasing dangers to public health, directly relating to the quality of the air we breathe. The American

Lung Association estimates that air pollution from motor vehicles and industry costs the U.S. $40-$50 billion in health costs and causes some 120,000 premature deaths. Increasingly, experts worry that air pollution is becoming a global health emergency.[18] For general information on air pollution, call:

Scientists' Institute for Public Information (800) 223-1730. Available 9-7 ETZ, M-F. Provides journalists and others with referrals to U.S. experts on air pollution and other topics.

Clean Air Legislation

The Clean Air Act, originally passed in 1963 and amended in 1970 and 1977, was the first significant Federal step toward regulating air quality and reducing air pollution through Federal and state government action. Under the act the EPA established acceptable air standards, National Ambient Air Quality Standards (NAAQS), for six pollutants: carbon monoxide, ozone, nitrogen dioxide, sulfur dioxide, particulate matter and lead. Many harmful pollutants were not given NAAQS limits, and issues such as acid rain and urban smog have increased significantly, requiring new standards and considerations.[19]

Immediately following passage of the Clean Air Act, some progress was made in reducing urban air pollution. Car makers, prodded by automobile emission limits incorporating California policies, produced automobiles that were six to eight times cleaner than those made in the late 1960s and levels of vehicle-related pollutants, other than smog, declined by the mid-1980s. Also, the number of days in which air pollution standards were exceeded decreased steadily from 1970 to 1986, dropping by as much as 90 percent in the most polluted cities. The drought of the summer of 1988, however, brought high levels of air pollutants in many cities and the number of "violation days" increased from 380 days in 1986 to 1,250 days in 1988.[20]

The Bush Administration has attempted to reduce acid rain, urban smog and industrial toxic chemicals. His 1990 amendments to the Clean Air Act, although not as stringent as environmentalists wanted and phased in over many years, are the most comprehensive Federal environmental laws yet. They ban chemicals that destroy the ozone layer by the end of the 1990s and impose stricter regulations on chemicals that cause urban smog. Stricter regulations on automobile exhausts will begin in 1994, new limits on emissions from carcinogenic substances by factories and chemical plants will be in place by 2003 and new limits are put on coal-burning power plants that cause acid rain. The amendments provide a $250 million program to provide compensation and assistance to workers who may lose their jobs as a result of companies' complying with the new standards.[21]

Ozone Pollution

Ozone is the most widely accepted measure of compromised air quality and is the EPA's highest-priority air pollutant. It is visible as smog and is a major problem in many large cities, where automobiles are the major cause. Smog is generated in a chemical reaction when sunlight "cooks" volatile organic compounds and nitrogen oxides. Ozone, a highly reactive form of oxygen, becomes a pungent, bluish gas at very high concentrations. It is most commonly formed when fumes released from car exhaust, gasoline and oil, paint solvents, cleaning fluids and incompletely burned coal or wood react with sunlight. Ozone is produced year-round but is most significant during the summer, usually peaking during the afternoon.[22]

The immediate effects of high ozone levels are breathing difficulty, burning eyes, headaches and nausea. Long-term exposure to high levels of ozone can cause malfunctioning in the lungs and respiratory system and aggravate chronic heart disease. About 90 percent of the ozone we inhale remains in our lungs, causing irritation or inflammation of the lung tissue that leads to coughing, choking, shortness of breath, tightness in the chest and sore throats. The most serious adverse affects of ozone are found in children, pregnant women and the elderly. People who exercise outdoors regularly can suffer minor lung damage from inhaling ozone-polluted air, even if within the Federally accepted standards.

In 1987, the EPA estimated that 80 million Americans lived in counties where ozone levels exceeded its standards. The Clean Air Science Advisory Committee of the EPA wants stricter standards, lowering both the acceptable ozone level and the time of exposure (over which emissions are averaged). The EPA has tightened restrictions on industries producing synthetic organic chemicals, surface coatings and pesticides, but limits on such ozone sources as *paint manufacturers, dry cleaners and gas stations* have *not* been widely implemented—something to be on the lookout for in your own community.[23]

Carbon Monoxide

Another great concern for the EPA and environmentalists is carbon monoxide. Roughly 70 percent of carbon monoxide in the air comes from motor vehicle exhaust, so the levels are most severe in urban areas. Carbon monoxide is a colorless, odorless product of incomplete combustion and can occur in such natural processes as forest fires or the oxidation of methane. Other common sources of carbon monoxide emissions are wood-burning stoves and fireplaces, incineration and space heating. Carbon monoxide levels in cities are highest during rush hours and they are most dangerous during the winter months when cars run less efficiently and wood-burning stove and space heater emissions rise.[24]

When carbon monoxide is inhaled, it enters the bloodstream and replaces the oxygen in hemoglobin.[37] As the amount of oxygen in the blood is decreased, carbon monoxide can impair vision and perception, slow reflexes, impair alertness and other mental and physical capacities. It can cause drowsiness and unconsciousness, and can lead to death. Too much carbon monoxide in the blood can weaken contractions of the heart, thus reducing the amount of blood reaching other parts of the body. Persons with chronic pulmonary disease and anemic individuals are also highly vulnerable to carbon monoxide exposure. Even healthy children are more vulnerable than adults because their high metabolism means they need more oxygen. Pregnant women are also especially at risk.

Emission controls have been mandated on new cars since the late-1960s, but inspection and maintenance of automobiles is essential to maintain low carbon-monoxide levels and many states have failed to pass inspection and maintenance legislation. Ending the sale of leaded gasoline greatly reduces carbon monoxide emissions. Oil companies are developing new kinds of gasoline that burn more cleanly and efficiently.

Sulfur Dioxide

A major component of acid rain, sulfur dioxide is released in fossil-fuel combustion from such sources as coal and electric power plants and oil refineries. In addition to fuel combustion processes in power plants, other sources of sulfur dioxide are paper mills, steel plants, smelters and chemical plants. Furnaces and coal-burning stoves in the home can add to concentrations in the air. When it enters the atmosphere, sulfur dioxide can be converted into sulfuric acid aerosols and particulate sulfate compounds, which are corrosive and potentially carcinogenic. The health effects of sulfur dioxide can include extreme respiratory problems such as emphysema, bronchitis and asthma. Also, coughs and colds are often aggravated by sulfur dioxide pollution. Heart and lung disease can be exacerbated from exposure to SO_2.[25]

More than 20 million tons of sulfur are emitted into the air each year, nearly 85 percent of which come from power plants. In order to meet the NAAQS, many coal mines and factories use machines to "wash" the coal of excess sulfur. Scrubbers and desulfurization equipment are used by other industrial sources of sulfur emission. The EPA limits on sulfur dioxide most affect the Midwest and West, where many coal-fired power plants are located.[26]

Nitrogen Dioxide

A fourth pollutant regulated by the EPA's NAAQS is nitrogen dioxide. The pungent, reddish-brown gas is corrosive and a strong oxidizing agent that comes mostly from combustion in power plants and vehicular exhaust. It can also be emitted by cigarettes and gas stoves. High concentrations can be fatal, and exposure to the concentrations commonly found in the Los Angeles air have increased the rate at which tumors spread to other organs in mice, because nitrogen dioxide can impair the ability of the immune system to attack cancer cells—especially dangerous during and after surgery. Lower-level exposure to the gas can increase vulnerability to viral infections such as influenza, bronchitis and pneumonia. The effects of nitrogen dioxide are also toxic to vegetation, stunting plant growth and seed fertility in high concentrations. With sulfur dioxide, nitrogen dioxide is a precursor to acid rain and contributes to ozone pollution.[27]

Particulate Matter

Tiny particles such as smoke, dust and aerosols are produced in large quantities by industrial processes, coal- and wood-burning and automobiles. The major industrial contributors to particulate pollution are steel and cement mills, power plants and smelters. Grain-storage elevators, cotton gins, construction work, diesel engines and wood-burning stoves are other common sources of airborne particulates. Wind-blown dust can carry toxic substances such as pesticides. Many industries have installed filters and electrically charged plates to reduce the amount of emissions, and the EPA has set standards for diesel cars and trucks. The emission of particulates decreased by nearly two-thirds between 1970 and the end of the 1980s. Improved street-cleaning and paving and less agricultural and forest burning can help reduce particulate levels further.[28]

Inhalation of particulate matter can be dangerous, as many heavy metals and carcinogenic organic compounds can be carried deeply into the lungs. It can increase the severity of respiratory diseases. The smaller particulates especially can travel deep into the respiratory system and the stomach. The full effects of inhaling airborne particulates depend on what type of compounds or chemicals are being inhaled with them. They commonly cause eye and throat irritation and reduce resistance to infection. Particulate matter in the air can decrease visibility, corrode metals and other building materials, affect climate changes and damage vegetation.[29]

Lead

Lead in the air (discussed also in chapter 4) can be injurious to the environment and to people's health. It comes primarily from motor vehicle exhaust, especially in vehicles using leaded gasoline, and from lead smelting and processing plants. Lead inhaled into the system can cause serious damage to the brain, kidneys and the reproductive, circulatory and nervous systems. It affects blood formation and can accumulate in bones and tissues. At very high levels, lead poisoning can result in death, but the ambient lead levels usually account for less than 30 percent of total body exposure. The dangers are much greater for children and fetuses; high lead levels can cause brain damage and behavioral abnormalities.[30]

The EPA has restricted the amount of lead in gasoline, but many motorists still use cheaper leaded gasoline in cars made for unleaded fuel, increasing the levels of lead and other pollutants emitted.[31] Using unleaded gasoline alone will not bring the lead levels below the NAAQS, however, and other measures are needed to reduce industrial emissions.

Other Air Pollutants

Aside from the six NAAQS-regulated substances, many other gases and substances affect the quality of the urban air environment. Sulfates, nitrates and nitric oxide are some of the compounds known to degrade the quality of the air we breathe, contributing to respiratory disease and acid rain..

EPA City Air Ratings

The EPA rates cities based on a Pollution Standards Index (PSI) that is keyed to the primary NAAQS, which are 260 $\mu g/m^3$ (micrograms per cubic meter) for total suspended particulates, 365 for sulfur oxides (0.14 parts per million), 235 for ozone (0.12 ppm), 100 for nitrogen oxide (0.05 ppm) and 10,000 for carbon monoxide (9 ppm). If the PSI is below 50, it is "good." If it rises above 100, it is "unhealthful." At 200, it is so unhealthful that persons with heart or lung diseases are alerted to reduce physical activity.

EPA counts the number of days that the PSI rises above 100 at each "trend site" used for monitoring progress.

One city—Los Angeles—accounted for 206 of the 288 PSI days greater than 100 (in 1989) in the 14 metro areas shown by the EPA. Since Los Angeles has 11 trend monitoring sites, that's an average of 19 days with the PSI above 100 for each site. Using this EPA measure, Los Angeles is unquestionably the city with the worst air. At the other extreme, one of the 14 cities—San Francisco—had zero days in 1989 with the PSI above 100.

City Air Quality

To measure air quality in more of America's cities, in Table 6-3 we rank cities first by the pollutant with the most number of violations, i.e. ozone. Then the ties were broken within rankings by ranking the pollutant with the next highest frequency of noncompliance, carbon monoxide (CO). Finally, the third step was to break any remaining ties with the third most frequently noncomplying pollutant, particulates (PM10). In addition, Birmingham was out of compliance for lead (PB) and Los Angeles for nitrogen dioxide (NO2). Cities with high lead levels are usually blessed with an industrial polluter. Smaller localities that have no data with EPA's acquiescence say the reason they don't collect the information is that their historical levels (when the pollutants were tested) were too low to worry about.

Table 6-3 shows that the interdependence of pollutants may have something to do with the weather. Spokane and Anchorage report they have no ozone problem, but they do have a carbon monoxide problem. Portland, Ore., Tacoma and Seattle also don't have much of an ozone problem but do have a carbon monoxide problem. Since all these cities are clustered in the Northwest one can surmise that they are ozone-free at least partly because they don't get as much hot weather.

The cities with the worst air-quality problems are the ones with the hottest weather—Los Angeles, Riverside, Anaheim, Houston, San Diego. The East Coast cities are, however, not far behind. Some cities among the worst, like San Diego, have surprisingly poor air given that they are young cities with little heavy industry.

The nation's success at cleaning up its air over the last 50 years has been mixed. Between 1940 and 1987, the per-capita discharge for four criteria air pollutants—sulfur dioxide, volatile organic compounds (VOCs), suspended particulates and carbon monoxide—declined between 37 and 83 percent. However, during the same time, the fifth pollutant, nitrogen oxides, increased 57 percent. Suspended particulates pollution peaked in 1950; sulfur dioxide, VOCs and carbon monoxide peaked in 1970; nitrogen oxides peaked in 1978.[33]

WATER POLLUTION

A 1986 EPA survey of the quality of the nation's surface waters (rivers, streams, lakes and coastal waters) reported that 73 to 75 percent of the waterways met quality standards—but only one-fifth of the rivers and streams, one-third of the lakes and one-half of the coastal waters were tested. The tendency in the states is to focus attention on waterways most likely to be affected by pollution.[34]

Elevated levels of toxic contamination have been found in surface water

TABLE 6–3

AIR-QUALITY, THREE-STEP RANKING:
35 METRO AREAS WITH THE WORST AIR

	Ozone	CO	PM10
1. Portland, Maine	*0.13*	4	
2. Grand Rapids	*0.13*	5	
3. Wilmington	*0.13*	5	35
4. Dallas (*1.76* PB)	*0.13*	5	36
5. Fort Worth	*0.13*	6	
6. Oakland	*0.13*	6	37
7. Springfield, Mass.	*0.13*	8	31
8. Charlotte	*0.13*	8	34
9. Providence	*0.13*	8	39
10. Pittsburgh	*0.13*	8	43
11. St. Louis	*0.13*	8	*76*
12. Newark	*0.13*	9	38
13. Washington	*0.13*	9	43
14. Baltimore	*0.13*	9	44
15. San Jose	*0.13*	*12*	41
16. New York (.049 NO2)	*0.13*	*12*	*66*
17. Akron	*0.14*	7	
18. Detroit	*0.14*	8	*52*
19. Nashville	*0.14*	9	
20. Hartford	*0.14*	9	30
21. Sacramento	*0.14*	*13*	43
22. El Paso	*0.14*	*13*	*69*
23. Dayton	*0.15*	6	35
24. Milwaukee	*0.15*	6	40
25. Salt Lake City	*0.15*	8	*56*
26. Fresno	*0.15*	*12*	*76*
27. Baton Rouge	*0.16*	4	
28. Bakersfield	*0.16*	9	*79*
29. Philadelphia	*0.16*	*12*	46
30. Bridgeport	*0.18*	5	36
31. San Diego	*0.19*	*10*	
32. Houston	*0.23*	8	30
33. Anaheim	*0.24*	*11*	47
34. Riverside (.045NO2)	*0.28*	8	*93*
35. Los Angeles (*.057NO2*)	*0.33*	*18*	*64*

NOTES: The bold-and-italicized numbers are violations of the EPA's National Ambient Air Quality Standards (NAAQS).

SOURCE: EPA, *Trends Analysis* (EPA 450-4-91), 1991. Data are for 1989.[32]

in almost half the states. Metals and PCBs (polychlorinated biphenyls) are the most widely reported toxic pollutants causing harm to fish and wildlife and may be carcinogenic to humans. PCBs in New York's Hudson River have rendered several species of fish unsafe for eating and New York's harbor is one of the most polluted. Fecal coliform bacteria is a common pollutant that encourages the growth of disease-causing organisms. Other pollutants include biochemical and toxic substances that can harm aquatic life, impair drinking water and taint water used for crop irrigation.[35]

Surface water pollutants come from point sources and nonpoint sources. Point sources enter water systems at a specific "point," such as a pipe or ditch. Nonpoint sources are spread over a wide area and are difficult to trace, such as runoffs of pesticides and chemicals from agricultural areas or sewers from urban areas. Since point sources are being brought more under control, the impact of nonpoint sources is becoming more apparent. They affect 65 percent of polluted stream miles and 45 percent of polluted coastal square miles.[36]

In recent years, coastal waters have also been at risk from medical waste. According to the Natural Resources Defense Council, 19 coastal states have reported medical waste washing up on beaches. In 1988, Congress passed the Medical Waste Tracking Act that obliges all medical facilities to label and document their waste disposal so that it can be traced back to the source. However, state participation is voluntary.[37]

Ground Water

Ground water sources provide over half of the population with its supply of drinking water. Ground waters are underground water sources, such as wells, that can be tapped into by communities to serve their water needs. Nearly 68 percent of the states rely on ground water as a principal source of drinking water. Many states also depend on ground water for up to 80 percent of their agricultural irrigation.[38] Most communities in coastal regions must rely on ground water as their primary drinking water. Common contaminants of ground water are the use of fertilizers and pesticides in rural areas, industrial landfills, surface impoundments, municipal landfills and abandoned waste sites.

Two major sources of contamination are underground septic tanks and storage tanks. Sewage and nitrates are common contaminants from septic tanks. The population growth in suburban communities and other changes in housing developments and urban and suburban planning have caused septic systems to fail and their leakage into the ground water system to become worse. Many states have enacted legislation to maintain septic systems. These laws also help control contaminants—such as sewage and nitrates—that can cause health hazards when released into drinking water.

Ground water is also at risk of contamination from underground storage tanks. These tanks are commonly used to store petroleum products, most often gasoline and heating oil. Leakage from these products is the second largest source of ground water contamination. New regulations may require the removal of storage tanks that have been found to leak. They would be replaced with new ones that meet strict requirements to avoid corrosion and future leakage. Operators and owners of storage tanks must conduct periodic testing and monitoring of tanks' performance.[39]

Toxic Waste in Water

Toxic water pollutants have been linked to cancer and birth defects in humans. They can also damage aquatic life. Most of these substances come from the use of pesticides and other commercial chemical products. Metals and PCBs are the most common toxic pollutants caused by industrial waste. Texas, New Jersey and Louisiana have the most chemical companies, but Louisiana is at particular risk because in addition to its own pollutants, it also receives waste from many other states upstream along the Mississippi River. On the Mississippi between Baton Rouge and New Orleans are 93 chemical plants—this stretch of the river has been called "cancer alley" because of the high death rate from cancer believed to be caused by toxins. New Orleans, St. Louis and Memphis also show high death rates believed to be caused by toxins. Mining activities and abandoned mines also introduce metals into water systems.[40]

DDT, another pesticide, is still quite common despite its ban in the 1970s. DDT and other pesticides are infiltrated into the water supply during rainfall or irrigation when they are washed off the ground surface. DDT is especially common in the South and Southern regions of the Mississippi, where it was used on cotton. Before it was banned, DDT was also used as a household cleaning agent. Benzene and chlorine are two pollutants used in the manufacture of toilet bowl fresheners and mothballs. Benzene has been known to cause leukemia.[41]

Research and Legislation

Much has been done in recent years to clean and protect the nation's water systems. The Clean Water Act (CWA) was established in 1972 and was amended and revised in 1977, 1981 and 1987. Congress is expected to vote on further revisions in 1992. The focus is on nonpoint pollution, the largest source of U.S. water pollution.[42] CWA provides direction for EPA monitoring of industrial and municipal sewage and water-treatment systems and facilities. It also enforces Federal and state standards on the quality of ground, surface and drinking water. It provides grants, loans and information to help cities solve their waste-treatment problems and construct new treatment facilities. Almost all states have programs to monitor and protect drinking-water quality.

In May 1991 the EPA directed 79,000 utilities, virtually all U.S. water suppliers, to test tap water for lead in hundreds of thousands of homes. Some environmentalists argue that the EPA took too long to implement the CWA plan to reduce lead concentrations in drinking water.[43]

EPA Safe Drinking Water Act Hotline (800) 426-4791, (202) 382-5533 in Washington, D.C. Although the wait is sometimes ten minutes, the contractors who staff this line are courteous and competent, and offer a free booklet that they promise to get to you in three weeks. Mine arrived in a week.

Water Pollution Control Federation (800) 666-0206, 8:30-5 ETZ, M-F. Provides information on water pollution control through a technical services unit and a library. Brochures and periodicals are available.

City Water Quality

In most cities you are likely to get safer drinking water, because it is tested, than you can expect when taking your chances with wellwater. Some cities are exceptions. Parts of the New Orleans metro area have cancer rates many times the national average and the problem seems traceable to toxic wastes that are carried in part in the water.[44] New Orleans did not return our water questionnaire.

In Table 6-4 we rank drinking-water quality. The rankings are arrived at by using four measures of drinking-water quality: turbidity, chlorine, nitrates, and pH. The nitrates measure is most variable and is given the most weight, 46 percent of the overall score. Turbidity is given a weight of 24 percent. The other two factors are weighted 15 percent each.

Savannah rates No. 1, best on the water quality scale, followed by Hartford, which is on top in the important category of nitrates. Fort Wayne and Shreveport rate No. 72 and No. 71, with the most room for improvement. New York is in the middle, ranking poorly on turbidity but well on chlorine and pH. Cities like Baton Rouge and New Orleans, which are located in the "cancer alley" region, did not respond to our survey. As the EPA tightens its standards in 1992, and assuming it enforces them, differences among cities should become even smaller.

State Environmental Legislation

Table 6-5 ranks the states based on environmental conditions as opposed to policies. Hawaii rates No. 1 on environmental conditions, but a less impressive 24 on its policies. West Virginia ranks worst on environmental conditions but does slightly better on its policies.

TABLE 6—4
CITY DRINKING-WATER QUALITY

City	Score	City	Score
Savannah	0.21	Mesa	0.96
Hartford	0.33	New York	0.97
Oakland	0.40	Jersey City	1.01
Sacramento	0.45	Nashville	1.04
Newport News	0.47	Fort Lauderdale	1.05
Phoenix	0.48	Mobile	1.05
Richmond	0.57	Knoxville	1.05
Billings	0.57	Yonkers	1.07
Columbia, SC	0.61	Orlando	1.08
Raleigh	0.65	Riverside	1.08
Greensboro	0.66	Omaha	1.10
Anchorage	0.67	Minneapolis	1.12
Jacksonville	0.67	Anaheim	1.13
Worcester	0.68	Oklahoma City	1.14
Amarillo	0.71	El Paso	1.15
Stockton	0.72	Pittsburgh	1.21
Wichita	0.73	St. Louis	1.22
Salt Lake City	0.73	Toledo	1.23
Portland, ME	0.75	Denver	1.24
Milwaukee	0.75	Sioux Falls	1.25
Lincoln, NE	0.76	Wilmington, DE	1.27
Honolulu	0.78	Tulsa	1.27
Akron	0.79	Columbus, OH	1.30
Austin	0.83	Dallas	1.32
Las Vegas	0.85	Bismarck	1.36
Tucson	0.86	Los Angeles	1.36
Casper	0.88	Dayton	1.38
Springfield, MA	0.88	San Diego	1.38
Grand Rapids	0.89	Des Moines	1.39
Spokane	0.90	Kansas City	1.42
Rochester	0.91	Columbus, GA	1.43
Fort Worth	0.92	Philadelphia	1.45
Newark, NJ	0.92	Fresno	1.48
Boise	0.93	Louisville	1.49
Cleveland	0.93	Shreveport	1.63
Atlanta	0.96	Fort Wayne	1.72

SOURCE: Self-reported measurements on author's questionnaire, 1990.[45]

TABLE 6–5
ENVIRONMENTAL CONDITIONS VS. POLICIES

State	Rank, Policies	State	Rank, Policies
BEST TEN, CONDITIONS		**WORST TEN, CONDITIONS**	
Hawaii	24	Louisiana	34
Vermont	12	Indiana	27
Oregon	2	Texas	35
Maine	5	Alabama	49
Minnesota	7	Ohio	19
Massachusetts	9	Tennessee	40
Rhode Island	10	Mississippi	46
New Hampshire	20	Kansas	28
Nevada	43	Illinois	17
Colorado	26	West Virginia	45

SOURCE: Derived from Bob Hall and Mary Lee Kerr, *1991–1992 Green Index*, (Durham, NC: Institute for Southern Studies, 1991), "Final Green Index Rankings." The Conditions ranking is based on 179 environmental indicators, the Policies ranking on 77 indicators.

ACID RAIN, GREENHOUSE EFFECT, OZONE LAYER

Three currently topical environmental issues may affect the quality of life where you live or might like to live: acid rain, the greenhouse effect (global warming) and the decreasing ozone layer.

Acid Rain

Acid rain has caused debate within the Federal Government, among regions and among industries and environmentalists. In 1980 the Congress passed an Acid Deposition Act, creating a 10-year research program on acid rain under the National Acid Precipitation Assessment Program.[46]

A pH reading of 5.6 is generally considered to be the normal level of acidity in rain. "Acid rain" is any rain that has a pH of 5.0 or lower. In many parts of North America, pH readings have averaged between 4.0 and 4.5, with 4.0 being 1,000 times more acidic than distilled water. Acid precipitation is not exclusively rain; high acidic readings are found in snow and fog as well.

"Acid rain" is caused primarily by industrial releases, specifically sulfur dioxide and nitrogen dioxide. These compounds, released into the atmosphere from the burning of fossil fuels, interact with sunlight and water vapor in the upper atmosphere to form acidic compounds that often travel for many miles before returning to the earth in rain, snow, sleet or hail. When rain that contains acidic substances reaches the earth it can go through another series of chemical changes.[47]

Most hazards from acid deposition come from contamination of food and water. The EPA believes that direct contact with acid rain on the skin and internal organs carries very little health risk, but that inhalation of acid particles in acid fog could be a hazard. The Congressional Office of Technology Assessment estimates that about 50,000 deaths a year are caused in the U.S. and Canada by the same chemicals that produce acid rain. Acid rain is a common pollution problem for the New England and Mid-Atlantic regions.[48]

Research into the effects of acid rain have been primarily under the National Acid Precipitation Assessment Program (NAPAP), consisting of the various Federal agencies that relate to the environmental effects of acid deposition. Many of the pollutants that contribute to acid rain are already regulated by the NAAQS, but acid deposition can occur even if the standards are met for each of the substances.[49] Producing more fuel-efficient cars and expanding mass transit would reduce the exhaust fumes that contribute to acid deposition.

The most direct way to reduce these problems is at their sources—the utilities and industrial facilities that burn coal and oil. The cost of outfitting industries with equipment to limit chemical emissions is a strong disincentive to them. Each of the common methods of reducing sulfur dioxide—coal-switching, coal-cleaning and flue gas desulfurization[50]—is costly and of limited effectiveness. So progress in limiting the level of acid rain has been slow.

The Greenhouse Effect

The theory of the greenhouse effect has been gaining adherents in the last few years. The greenhouse effect is caused by the emission of waste gases into the Earth's atmosphere. Once these gases have accumulated they create a barrier that insulates the Earth, trapping heat. This causes the temperature of the planet to rise, known as Global Warming. A rising global temperature would drastically change weather conditions.[51]

One of the biggest problems is the atmospheric buildup of carbon dioxide, which is released during the burning of fossil fuels such as coal, oil and wood. The destruction of forests, which would otherwise have naturally absorbed carbon dioxide and emitted oxygen, contributes to this buildup. Another destructive pollutant is the family of chlorofluorocarbons (CFCs) that are emitted from aerosol sprays, air conditioners, refrigerants, the manufacturing of styrofoam and other sources. Nitrous oxides from fossil fuels and chemical fertilizers, and methane gas from organic waste, also accumulate in the atmosphere.[52]

Six things we can do to stop the effects of global warming:

- Conserve fossil fuels and develop new energy sources to substitute for them.

- Use mass transportation and natural gas rather than oil or coal.
- Protect forests and plant new ones.
- Cut down on the production of freons, chemicals used as solvents and refrigerants.
- Urge our legislators to price (or tax) energy to reflect its environmental damage.[53]
- Urge our government and the U.N. to develop international agreements whereby a country like Brazil would be rewarded by the rest of the world for being a "net oxygen exporter" because of its rainforests. This would give the country a financial incentive to end deforestation.[54]

Decreasing Ozone Layer

In 1986 a hole was discovered in the ozone layer of the Earth's atmosphere over Antarctica. While ozone at ground level is a hazardous pollutant, in the atmosphere it is a vital necessity. Stratospheric ozone forms a protective layer around the Earth, shielding it from the sun's ultraviolet rays, which are known to cause cancer. The rate of skin cancer has increased by 98 percent in the last ten years. EPA Chief William Reilly predicted in 1991 that by 2041 about 12 million Americans would develop skin cancer and that more than 200,000 of them would die. New data also show another hole developing over the North Pole. Measurements from a NASA satellite indicated that the fragile ozone layer over the U.S. has shrunk as much as 5 percent in the last 10 years.[55]

The main contributors to the rapidly decreasing ozone layer are CFCs, which linger in the atmosphere for decades and also contribute to global warming. One reason CFCs have been so widely used in industry is that they are cheap compared to other chemicals. Many steps are being taken to limit their use, such as new taxes on CFCs; Vermont has banned new cars that emit CFCs starting in 1993.[56]

CLIMATE, STRESS AND DENSITY

The two remaining, less obvious environmental issues are the local climate and degree of stress. Stress is often linked in turn to population density.

Climate

The local climate can be important in considering the healthfulness of the places we live and work.

Are people healthier in warmer or cooler climates? Warm climates are hospitable to disease and clean water is generally a scarcer commodity in warmer areas. But warm weather permits more activity, which keeps people fit and healthy. Also, cities with the least sunlight also have the most breast cancers. Vitamin D may be the link. Getting sunshine for 10 to 20 minutes a day is enough to synthesize the molecule that is catalyzed by vitamin D. Researchers worry that people may attempt to prevent breast or colon cancer by excessive sunbathing and so develop melanoma.[57]

Within the United States, people have been migrating to the South and West. Honolulu, which we rated as the healthiest city, gained over 1 percent a year in population in the 1980s. Buffalo, the least healthy, lost nearly 1 percent a year in population in the 1980s. Climate could be playing a role in both cases. In fact, even after adjusting for age, western cities as a group tend to have lower death rates than the U.S. average, while northeastern and midwestern cities have higher death rates. A statistical model suggests that annual deaths increase by .03 per thousand population for each inch of rain.[58]

Connections have been made between the temperature and the ozone pollution in cities. High temperatures are more conducive to ozone formation and the drought of 1988 saw exceptionally high levels of ozone in many cities. Wind direction (and speed) can also affect the levels of ozone pollution.

Humid areas generate lush vegetation and are also hospitable to new and old diseases. Humidity is also related to discomfort and many people move to dry areas because they have respiratory problems. The most humid cities are in Florida, Northern New York and along the lower half of the East Coast. Cities in California, Nevada, Texas and the Southwest have relatively low humidities.[59]

Urban Stress

In Table 6-6, metropolitan areas are ranked from least stressful to most stressful based on rates of alcoholism, suicide, divorce and crime.

Population Density

By population density we mean the average number of people living per square mile.[60] An overpopulated area can strain the community's ability to meet everyone's needs with limited resources. If economic and employment opportunities do not grow with a growing population, unemployment and a poor economy can be the result. The most densely populated cities are New York, Paterson, Jersey City, San Francisco, Chicago, Newark, Boston and Philadelphia. The least densely populated cities are Anchorage, Oklahoma City, Lexington, Jacksonville, Columbia, Montgomery and Nashville.

Housing shortages are also a problem for densely populated communities. Based on a study of the percentage of housing units with more than

TABLE 6–6
URBAN STRESS

Metropolitan Area	Metropolitan Area
BEST TEN	**WORST TEN**
Akron	Oklahoma City
Paterson, NJ	Phoenix
Bismarck	Fort Lauderdale
Sioux Falls	Los Angeles
Grand Rapids	San Francisco/Oakland
Syracuse	Jacksonville
Lincoln, NE	Little Rock
Buffalo	Miami
Fort Wayne	Las Vegas
Madison, WI	Reno

SOURCE: Robert Levine, "City Stress Index," *Psychology Today,* November 1988, p. 54. Akron is judged least stressful, Reno most stressful.

one person per room (excluding bathrooms, halls, kitchenettes or utility rooms), model communities have only 1 percent to 2.1 percent crowded housing units, while stressed communities have 7 percent or more crowded housing units. Among the least crowded cities are Akron, Aurora, Billings, Boise, Buffalo, Lincoln, Madison, Minneapolis, Portland (Maine), Sioux Falls, Spokane, Topeka and Virginia Beach. The most crowded cities are San Francisco, Santa Ana, Stockton, Hartford, Washington, Miami, Honolulu, Chicago, New Orleans, Jackson, Jersey City, Newark, Paterson, New York, Corpus Christi, Houston and San Antonio.

CHAPTER SEVEN

Health Services

Access to quality health care is an important factor in assuring personal well-being. This is presumably why Americans spent $2,354 per capita on health care in 1989, *three times as much* as, for example, Britain, which offers mostly *free medical care* to all of its citizens.[1]

In 1991 U.S. health spending was about $760 billion—over $2 billion a day. Not only is U.S. spending on health care the highest in the world, it has been growing rapidly. Private health services grew at a rate about *5 percent above inflation* throughout the 1980s.[2]

Americans are less satisfied than Canadians with the quality of their health care and by a large margin they are less happy with its cost. Seven out of 10 U.S. respondents told a Harris poll that too much money is spent on doctors and hospitals.

In 1970, Canada and the U.S. spent about the same percentage of their GNP on health care. But 20 years later, the U.S. was spending 50 percent more (12 percent of GNP) than Canada (8 percent) and by 2000 it may be paying twice as much if current trends continue. The Canadian national health plan uses tax money to provide medical care to everyone at no charge. The 37 million U.S. citizens with no health insurance exceed Canada's total population. Canada provides health services such as cholesterol checks and prenatal testing generally excluded from U.S. health insurance—services the poor often cannot afford. The Canadian health-care system is seen as a challenge to the U.S. system because it provides quality health care for everyone, and for less money. But its wide coverage means, among other things, long delays for elective surgery.[3]

Some states have moved to broaden health-care coverage. Eight states—Florida, Illinois, Kansas, Kentucky, Missouri, Rhode Island, Virginia and Washington—have enacted laws that waive the requirements for medical-care insurance policies to encourage private insurers to sell low-cost policies to working Americans with no health coverage. Oregon appears to be the first state to tackle the task of establishing universal health care (restricting services rather than coverage) for all citizens.[4]

New Federal legislation is on the way. The U.S. Comptroller General says that piecemeal reforms will not slow the rise in health-care spending, Rather, he says, three reforms are needed:

- insure everyone.
- develop uniform-payment rules for health-care services.
- set caps on total spending for major provider categories.[5]

Senate Democratic leaders are seeking legislation to extend health coverage to all Americans, and the Canadian model is being looked at approvingly.[6]

Meanwhile, more modest improvements in U.S. health care systems are being initiated. Federal Medicare reimbursements to hospitals for outpatient services are likely to move in 1991 to standard flat fees for certain kinds of services. The Health Care Financing Administration has proposed legislation that would change the way the government reimburses hospitals for interest and depreciation on construction and equipment purchases, to encourage hospitals with low occupancy to share equipment.[7]

As America waits for these improvements, the quality of health care varies widely among states and communities. This chapter shows how to determine where the best medical care is available. The topic is covered under three headings: medical personnel (doctors, nurses), hospitals, and health services to children (school health services and infant mortality).

MEDICAL PERSONNEL

Availability of Doctors

Overall, inhabitants of the largest U.S. metropolitan areas are served by about one doctor for every 1,000 people. But more doctors are found in cities like Boston or St. Louis, with large medical schools, where hospitals serve as training or teaching facilities. They attract young doctors completing their residency requirements. Doctors are also likely to be found in cities with "referral"—specialty—hospitals that are well-equipped to train doctors and provide needed equipment.

Boston has the highest number of doctors, more than 7 per 1,000 residents (see Table 7-1). This reflects the fact that the city has numerous medical centers and schools that serve the region and even the nation. The lack of doctors in a prosperous community like Riverside, California, which ranks at the bottom of the list with only 0.21 doctors per 1,000 residents, can be explained by the fact that Riverside is a growing community, populated by people who are looking for less expensive housing in the Greater Los Angeles area. As a bedroom community, Riverside is short on

TABLE 7–1
AVAILABILITY OF DOCTORS, METRO AREA

Metro Area	Doctors per 1,000 Pop.	Metro Area	Doctors per 1,000 Pop.
BEST TEN		**WORST TEN**	
Bridgeport	5.42	Tacoma	1.61
Boston	5.28	Montgomery	1.57
Burlington	5.25	Stockton	1.52
Raleigh–Durham	5.18	Columbus, GA	1.48
San Francisco	4.97	Charlotte, NC	1.41
Madison, WI	4.58	Las Vegas	1.40
Hartford	4.47	El Paso	1.38
Worcester	4.46	Colorado Springs	1.35
New York City	3.99	Bakersfield	1.32
Lexington, KY	3.78	Fort Worth	1.30

SOURCE: Derived from data collected and published by the American Medical Association.[8]

public facilities like hospitals and indeed its residents—many of whom work in Los Angeles—may not feel an urgent need for more hospital facilities near where they live because they have them near their work. As a community with a high percentage of young families, their medical needs (other than for pediatric care) tend to be much lower than in an older community.

So for a healthy young couple with jobs in downtown Los Angeles and basically healthy children, the number of doctors in Riverside may be more than adequate. For older people with heart ailments, it may be safer to live in communities that have more medical services.

Doctor Oversight

Doctors can make mistakes. A study of prescriptions at the Albany (New York) Medical Center showed that an average of two or more prescriptions a day were misprescribed, and nearly three out of five faulty prescriptions posed a health risk to the patient.[9]

How are consumers to know whether their doctor is mistake-prone? State and Federal agencies that run the Medicare/Medicaid programs (Department of Health and Human Services) do have a system of quality control. Participating doctors are monitored by the Medicare Peer Review Organization. These organizations function on a state level and audit doctors' records for evidence of substandard and/or unnecessary care. State Medicaid agencies have the power to sanction doctors guilty of insurance fraud. Federal agencies can also sanction doctors—they can ban doctors from participating in the Medicare/Medicaid program and may also fine doctors for specific violations.[10]

State Medical Boards control the licensing of doctors and have the power to reprimand doctors, impose fines, place doctors on probation, suspend practice and revoke licenses. However, the boards often focus on rehabilitating doctors who fall below standards, not on protecting the public. State boards rarely communicate with Federal agencies and communication among states is extremely slow, so it is easy for doctors with a string of bad mistakes on their record to cross state lines and resume practice. Many state boards do not have the resources to monitor doctors placed on probation. Oregon and Texas are the only states that actually visit doctors' offices to see that the quality of care is improving. The medical boards of Utah, Georgia and West Virginia are considered the best for their preventive strategies—they seek out substandard physicians before receiving complaints and therefore appear to have more cases of substandard physicians than other states that do not devote as much effort to monitoring doctors. The national average of disciplinary action was 4.8 actions per 1,000 physicians.[11] (See Table 7-2.)

The Drug Enforcement Administration issues licenses for doctors to prescribe controlled substances, with the authority to revoke, deny or restrict these licenses. This organization also tracks down doctors who over-prescribe or abuse scheduled drugs such as narcotics, tranquilizers and amphetamines. Malpractice insurers can cancel policies, raise rates or force physicians to restrict their practice, because without a malpractice insurance policy, it is difficult for doctors to continue their practice and in

TABLE 7–2
PHYSICIAN OVERSIGHT

State	Disciplinary Action per 1,000 MDs	State	Disciplinary Action per 1,000 MDs
BEST TEN		WORST TEN	
Georgia	8.55	New Hampshire	1.40
Iowa	8.44	Vermont	1.36
Missouri	7.90	California	1.30
Oklahoma	7.61	Texas	1.20
Nevada	7.16	Washington	1.09
Mississippi	7.03	Wisconsin	0.87
Colorado	5.98	Delaware	0.78
West Virginia	5.62	Arizona	0.55
Hawaii	5.19	Rhode Island	0.40
South Dakota	4.98	Montana	0.00

SOURCE: "State Medical Board Doctor Disciplinary Actions: 1988," *Health Letter* (Washington, D.C.: Public Citizen), September 1990.[8]

some states it is illegal. However, many states guarantee doctors insurance no matter what their former record.[12]

State medical societies and specialty societies are associations for doctors and specialists; they are not government agencies. The societies have peer-review committees to control quality and also contribute to medical discipline. They do not have the power to revoke licenses or prevent physicians from practice. The societies' main concern is protecting the interests of doctors and other members. Ultimately, the buyer of medical services in the U.S. must beware. But Table 7-2 suggests that in some states the medical consumer must be more wary than in others.[13]

Nurses

For some kinds of illnesses requiring long periods of care, and even for surgeries where pre- and post-operative care is tricky and crucial, the quality of nursing care may be as important to the patient as the quality of the M.D.s on duty. The surgeon might do a fine job, but the patient's recovery may be jeopardized if the post-operative care is inadequate.

Registered nurses cost one-fourth to one-third as much as the lowest-

---

To find and select a physician:

One approach is to contact one of the medical-referral services listed in each city's Yellow Pages under Physicians and Surgeons Information and Referral Services. Most large urban hospitals offer a referral service. Two examples follow.

Mt. Sinai Hospital Doctor Referral Service, New York City (800) MD-SINAI.

New York County Medical Society, Doctors Referral Panel (212) 399-9048.

For alternative health-care insurance and services:

Alternative Health Insurance Services, P.O. Box 9178, Calabasas, CA 91372 (818) 509-5742. Individual and Group Plans with coverage for acupuncture, naturopathy, homeopathy, chiropractic, in addition to conventional medical care.

---

paid doctors in hospitals. With economic demands and incentives to decrease the length of hospital stays, hospitals are looking for ways to substitute nursing and paramedical services for those requiring M.D.s (nurse-practitioners are paramedics who earn about half what relatively non-specialized doctors such as pediatricians get paid). More nurses are needed to supplement the amount and quality of care given in a shorter period of time. But nurses are currently in short supply, particularly in hospitals and in urban areas.[14]

The shortage may be explained by the low pay that nurses have historically received, as well as their long hours. Nurses in 1990 earned

$20,000-$25,000 a year depending on the extent of their training and specialization. Nurses, especially hospital nurses, work under extremely stressful conditions. While usually scheduled to work 40 hours a week, many nurses often work overtime because of staff shortages. Many nurses have left hospitals for work in clinics, nursing homes, schools and offices that provide better working conditions. Because of this, the average annual turnover rate of hospital nurses is 18 percent—nearly one out of five leaves every year.[15] The American Nurses Association and other nursing groups are pushing for more recognition and higher salaries for nurses' services. Many nurses today hold college degrees in nursing as opposed to simply the post-high-school training-program diploma that was more common in the past.

Nursing shortages are more prevalent in larger hospitals and in larger cities. The most populous cities (New York, Los Angeles, Chicago, San Diego, Houston) all have fewer than 6 nurses per 1,000 residents (based on registered nurses and licensed practical nurses in community hospitals). The shortage is particularly a problem in the Mid-Atlantic region, the West Coast and in states in the northern Midwest (Ohio, Illinois, Indiana, Michigan), even though these regions pay more for nurses than other regions.[16] (See Table 7-3.)

TABLE 7–3
AVAILABILITY OF NURSES
CITIES, RANKED BY NURSES PER THOUSAND RESIDENTS

City	Nurses per 1,000 Residents	City	Nurses per 1,000 Residents
BEST TEN		**WORST TEN**	
Pittsburgh	22.37	San Diego	4.20
Richmond	19.57	Yonkers, NY	3.35
St. Louis	18.88	San Jose	3.31
Dayton	16.10	Austin	3.23
Little Rock	15.81	Anchorage	2.66
Boston	15.48	Santa Ana	2.60
Miami	15.25	El Paso	2.56
Cincinnati	14.99	Aurora	1.61
Minneapolis	14.16	Virgina Beach	1.49
Knoxville	13.98	Huntington Beach	1.21

SOURCE: American Hospital Association, *Hospital Statistics, 1989–90.* The number of nurses includes only registered nurses and licensed practical nurses attached to community hospitals. Registered nurses must complete more training than licensed practical nurses. The number of nurses per 1,000 residents was calculated by the author by dividing the AHA figure for nurses as defined above by the city population. Bear in mind that urban–based nurses may serve a suburban and even regional population.

HOSPITALS

Availability of Beds

Nationwide, hospitals have a substantial surplus of beds and—the corollary—a low occupancy rate. Because of cutbacks in government funding, many hospitals are at risk of closing. The Federal Government would like to cut the cost of Medicare and Medicaid by shrinking the health-care industry without damaging the quality of care.[17] Inner-city hospitals are at particular risk because of their heavy reliance on Federal funding for Medicare/Medicaid patients. From 1986 to 1988, 150 hospitals closed—the percentage of urban hospitals that closed was only slightly smaller than the percentage of rural hospitals. The urban hospitals that closed had an average occupancy rate of 29.6 percent compared to the national average of approximately 60 percent.[18]

The number of beds per 1,000 residents is shown in Table 7-4. This is a crude measure of hospital availability. St. Louis, Pittsburgh and Richmond—all regional centers for surgery and other medical services— lead the list. At the bottom of the list are younger suburban communities near Los Angeles or Denver that rely on the central city for hospital services.

TABLE 7–4
AVAILABILITY OF HOSPITAL BEDS

City	Beds per 1,000 Residents	City	Beds per 1,000 Residents
BEST TEN		**WORST TEN**	
St. Louis	18.16	Oakland	3.77
Pittsburgh	17.50	San Diego	3.54
Richmond	15.85	El Paso	3.49
Birmingham	14.07	Yonkers	3.39
Dayton	13.93	Austin	3.06
Cincinnati	13.34	San Jose	2.85
Knoxville	13.11	Anchorage	2.50
Miami	13.08	Virgina Beach	1.53
Little Rock	13.07	Aurora	1.45
Rochester	12.89	Huntington Beach	1.36

SOURCE: American Hospital Association, *Hospital Statistics, 1989–90.* The rate of hospital beds per 1,000 residents was calculated by the author by dividing the number of hospital beds by the city population. Bear in mind that city hospitals may serve suburban and even regional populations.

Availability of beds, however, is not the only consideration. Pittsburgh, for example, is No. 2 on the beds list but is also relatively high on the occupancy-rate list (see Table 7-5). Someone seeking elective surgery in Pittsburgh may not necessarily find scheduling it such an easy task.

The fact that America generally has ample hospital beds is shown by the low occupancy rates in Table 7-5. An occupancy rate of 85 percent is considered efficient, and indeed higher occupancy rates are associated with better-quality hospital care. Only seven cities are above the 85 percent efficiency rate—five in New York State, plus Providence and Honolulu. Cities with higher occupancy rates tend to have less expensive hospital services as well as (other things being equal) better care; often, they have government programs that make medical care more affordable. A high occupancy rate is therefore a badge of honor in terms of providing medical services; the questions to raise (and which we discuss next) are whether emergency services and beds are available when needed and what the quality of the hospital is.[19]

Despite the national hospital-bed surplus, many larger cities find they have a shortage of private beds because of drug-related cases, AIDS cases and a shortage of long-term care and nursing-home facilities. This problem is particularly acute in New York, California, Florida, New Jersey and Texas, which lead the country in AIDS cases. Because hospitalized AIDS patients commonly require private or semi-private rooms for substantial periods of time, these five states are experiencing growing shortages of such hospital facilities.[20]

As we noted when looking at doctor availability in Riverside, smaller

TABLE 7–5
HOSPITAL OCCUPANCY RATE

City	Occupancy Percent	City	Occupancy Percent
BEST TEN		**WORST TEN**	
Providence	90.6	Arlington	57.7
New York	88.6	Colorado Springs	57.3
Honolulu	86.8	Lincoln, NE	57.1
Buffalo	86.2	Montgomery	56.1
Yonkers, NY	85.9	Anchorage	53.6
Syracuse	85.7	Columbus, GA	50.8
Rochester	85.5	Anaheim	49.9
Newark, NJ	82.1	Aurora	49.5
Sacramento	81.5	Santa Ana	49.5
Boston	79.9	Huntington Beach	43.2

SOURCE: American Hospital Association, *Hospital Statistics, 1989–90.*

cities within a metropolitan area often rely on the health resources of the larger city. This is why some cities appear to have insufficient resources—for example, Virginia Beach, which relies on Norfolk hospitals, and Yonkers, which relies on New York City hospitals. Some cities that appear to have a surplus of beds for their population have a high percentage of their admissions coming from outside the metropolitan area or out of state.

Emergency Services

Emergency services are changing because of advances in medical technology. Certain ambulances are now mobile intensive-care units fully equipped to initiate treatment while patients are being transported.[21] Such mobile units have helped to decrease deaths caused by heart attacks. For trauma care, accident victims are stabilized and transported to nearby trauma centers for treatment.

All hospitals with 24-hour emergency rooms must provide patients with emergency care regardless of their ability to pay. But they do not have to provide follow-up care if the patient lacks insurance. Private hospitals have the option to transfer patients to public hospitals after providing initial emergency care and/or the patient's condition has stabilized. Emergency rooms in city hospitals are typically overcrowded and understaffed. Patients not at immediate risk must often wait before receiving treatment. Poor or uninsured patients commonly have to wait six hours or more before being treated.[22]

National Emergency Medicine Association (NEMA) (800) 332-6362. Available 8-4 ETZ, M-F; answering machine after hours. Provides information and referrals for emergency medical services. Also, offers basic information on dealing with emergencies.

For all the improvement in the quality of emergency care, many cities have inadequate services. City governments must often rely on scarce Federal resources for funding. Emergency services must compete with police, schools and roads for local budget allocations. City emergency services are, however, usually better than those in rural areas where long distances to medical centers and small populations make an emergency-care system difficult to manage.

Hospital Costs

The overriding problem with U.S. health care is its costs, which are continuing to rise. Hospitals must absorb several billion dollars worth of unpaid expenses due to inadequate government funding. Hospitals and doctors must also pay about $8 billion a year in malpractice insurance, driving the cost up even more. If a hospital is on a tight budget, it can affect the quality of care. Many doctors and hospitals are reluctant to treat Medicare/Medicaid patients or patients lacking insurance.

Several states have introduced legislation to control the climbing cost of health care. Ohio and Oregon have introduced plans to cover the costs of long-term hospital care. Massachusetts has a new policy that includes tax incentives for employers to provide insurance plans for their employees. Oregon has for several years been using a ranking plan to decide what services the state will cover based on how beneficial the service is in relation to cost.[23]

Table 7-6 illustrates the hospital cost per inpatient day. These costs are as measured by the hospital and may differ from patient fees or fees covered by insurance companies or government funding. Hospitals end up absorbing a large percentage of inpatient expenses. California leads the way as the most expensive state to be hospitalized in. Anchorage's limited facilities must serve a small population spread out over a large geographic area. The lack of competition within the state keeps Anchorage's prices high. Boston is well known for its prestigious medical community, which consists of several hospitals and medical schools. Investment in state-of-the-art medical technology also drives up prices.

TABLE 7–6
COST PER HOSPITAL DAY

City	Cost per Inpatient Day ($)	City	Cost per Inpatient Day ($)
BEST TEN		**WORST TEN**	
Buffalo	450	Salt Lake City	869
Jackson, MS	467	Phoenix	871
Jersey City	479	Portland, OR	899
Yonkers, NY	485	Albuquerque	936
Greensboro	505	San Francisco	968
Grand Rapids	542	Huntington Beach	975
Omaha	546	Oakland	977
Arlington	547	Boston	1,048
Columbus, GA	550	Anchorage	1,222
El Paso	572	Santa Ana	1,234

SOURCE: American Hospital Association, *Hospital Statistics, 1989–90.*

Hospital Quality: Death Rates

Poor hospital quality is often easy to see when one arrives for treatment. But it is hard to measure. Many hospitals issue questionnaires to discharged patients asking them to evaluate their hospital experience; such surveys have proved useful for hospitals to identify their strong points and their deficiencies.

One way to assess a hospital's quality is to look at its death rates, taking into account the age of patients, their condition and other relevant factors. Data along these lines are available from a 1989 Federal survey of death rates for Medicare patients at nearly 6,000 hospitals; it found 196 hospitals with death rates that exceeded Federal projections, 3.4 percent of all hospitals. (See Table 7-7.)

TABLE 7–7
HOSPITAL DEATH RATES

Death Rates Higher than Expected

Baton Rouge, LA: Earl K. Long Memorial Hospital.
Fayetteville, AR: Fayetteville City Hospital.
Hollandale, MS: South Washington Co. Hospital.
Iola, KS: Allen County Hospital.
Lafayette, LA: University Medical Center.
Leon, IA: Decatur County Hospital.
Los Angeles: Martin Luther King Jr. General Hospital.
Memphis: Regional Medical Center.
Miami: Coral Reef General Hospital.
New York: Harlem Hospital.
Oak Forest, IL: Oak Forest Hospital.
Philadelphia: Metropolitan Hospital.
Phoenix: Maricopa Medical Center.
West Plains, MO: Ozarks Medical Center.

Plus: Other hospitals in Arkansas (1), California (2), Georgia (2), South Carolina (2), South Dakota (1), Texas (3), and West Virginia (1).

Death Rates Lower than Expected
La Jolla, CA: Green Hospital of Scripps Clinic.*
Rochester, MN: Rochester Methodist Hospital.
Buffalo: Roswell Park Memorial Institute.
Houston: M.D. Anderson Hosp./U.T. Cancer Center.*

NOTE: * = On both the better-than-average death rate list and on the "Best Hospitals" list. The death rates were higher or lower for each of the three consecutive years, 1986–88.
SOURCE: Health Care Financing Administration.[26]

A May 1991 update of this survey listed 161 hospitals with higher-than-expected death rates, including 15 hospitals that had high rates four years in a row; six were in Puerto Rico. Comparisons of hospital death rates ideally should include such relevant factors as age, gender, hospital admissions within the previous six months and reason for admission. Many hospitals have higher-than-expected death rates because of unusually sick patients, high percentages of poor patients with several ailments and the use of advanced but experimental treatments that are sought by certain patients. Hospital patients who lack medical insurance die at up to three times the rate of similar patients with insurance.[24]

Death rates are somewhat higher at public hospitals (such as city or county hospitals) and for-profit hospitals than at private hospitals affiliated with medical schools and private nonprofit hospitals. The staff of for-profit hospitals may be under cost constraints that affect how they treat patients in hospitals (the for-profit medical plans deserve praise, however, for their disease-preventing programs). The highest number of deaths occur in osteopathic hospitals, with 129 deaths per 1,000 patients; next, for-profit hospitals, with 121 deaths per 1,000 patients; next, public hospitals, 120; private nonprofit hospitals, 114; and private hospitals associated with medical schools, 108.[25]

Hospitals most likely to save and prolong lives are the ones with the largest payrolls—because they are the ones with the best trained staff (as measured by the highest percentages of board-certified specialists and registered nurses), sophisticated equipment (as measured by the presence of such facilities as a cardiac-catheterization laboratory) and *high* occupancy rates.[27] See Table 7-8. The criteria for selecting the "best" hospitals were: quality care in a wide range of medical categories (or in special areas such as cancer), well-kept facilities, up-to-date medical technology, high-powered staffs of senior physicians with national reputations in their fields, excellent nursing staffs, and a concern for working conditions.[28]

TABLE 7–8
"BEST" HOSPITALS

Ann Arbor, MI: U. Mich. Medical Center.
Atlanta: Emory Clinic, Emory U. Hospital.
Baltimore: Johns Hopkins.
Birmingham, AL: University of Alabama Hospital.
Boston: Beth Israel; Brigham; Dana-Farber; Mass. General; New England Medical Center; McLean, Belmont.
Burlington, MA: Lahey Clinic Medical Center
Chapel Hill: NC Memorial Hospital.
Charlottesville: U. of Va. Hospitals.
Chicago: Northwestern; Rush; U.C. Medical Center.
Cleveland: Cleveland Clinic; University Hospitals.

TABLE 7–8 (*continued*)
"BEST" HOSPITALS

Dallas: Baylor University Medical Center.
Denver: National Jewish Center; U. C. Hospital.
Detroit: Harper-Grace; Henry Ford Hospital.
Durham, NC: Duke University Medical Center.
Gainesville, FL: Shands Hospital, U. Fla.
Hershey, PA: M. S. Hershey Medical Center, U. Pa.
Houston: M.D. Anderson Hosp./U.T. Cancer Center.* Texas Medical Center,
    Methodist Hospital.
Indianapolis: Indiana U. Medical Center.
Iowa City: U. of Iowa Hospitals.
La Jolla, Calif.: Green Hospital of Scripps Clinic.*
Los Angeles: Cedars-Sinai; UCLA Medical Center.
Madison, WI: U. of Wisc. Hospital.
Memphis: St. Jude Children's Hospital.
Miami: Jackson Memorial, U. Miami.
Minneapolis: U. of Minn. Hospitals and Clinics.
Nashville: Vanderbilt University Hospital.
New Orleans: Ochsner Clinic.
New York: Hospital for Joint Diseases; Hospital for Special Surgery; Memorial
    Sloan–Kettering; Mount Sinai; Columbia–Presbyterian Medical Center;
    Rockefeller University Hospital; N.Y.U. Hospital.
Philadelphia: U. Pa. Hospital; Wills Eye Hospital.
Pittsburgh: Presbyterian–University Hospital.
Richmond, VA.: Medical College of Virginia Hospitals.
Rochester, MN: Mayo Clinic and Hospitals.
Rochester, NY: Strong Memorial Hospital, U. of R.
Salt Lake City: University Hospital, U. of Utah.
San Francisco: Medical Center, UCSF.
San Diego: Medical Center, UCSD.
Seattle: Fred Hutchinson Center; U. Wash. Hospital; Virginia Mason Center.
St. Louis: Barnes Hospital.
Stanford, CA: University Medical Center.
Topeka, KS: Menninger Foundation.
Tucson: University Medical Center, U. of Ariz.
Washington, DC: W. G. Magnuson Center, Bethesda.
Wilmington, DE: Alfred I. duPont Inst.

NOTE:* = On both the better-than-average death rate list and on the "Best Hospitals" list.
"Best Hospitals" from Linda Sunshine and John W. Wright, *The Best Hospitals in America*
(New York: Avon Books, 1989, first printed 1987).

RECREATIONAL SERVICES

One of the important health-related services a city can offer its residents is access to recreational facilities. The range of services varies widely among cities, as may be seen in the city-by-city summaries in Chapter 9.

A good measure of public recreational opportunities is the number of sports fields and courts maintained by the city. Table 7-9 counts football fields, soccer fields, baseball fields, basketball courts and tennis courts, divided by city population.

Amarillo (pop. 166,000) is in first place with 488 of these sports facilities, i.e., 294 of them per 100,000 population. At the other extreme, New York City (pop. 7,353,000) provides 1,388 of these facilities, or 19 per 100,000 population. Another way of putting this is to observe that New York City has 2.8 times the number of these sports facilities to serve a population that is 44 times larger. This lack of facilities is more serious in a congested city like New York than in the younger cities on the West Coast that have failed to provide enough public facilities but have no shortage of open space, e.g., on the waterfront.

HEALTH SERVICES TO CHILDREN

School Health

Public-school systems play a key role in promoting the welfare and healthiness of school-age children. By requiring immunizations, vaccinations and physical examinations for children prior to admission, schools create a

TABLE 7–9
PUBLIC RECREATIONAL-SPORTS FACILITIES

BEST TEN		WORST TEN	
Amarillo	294	San Francisco	41
Winston-Salem	235	Nashville	37
Virginia Beach	211	Fresno	37
Sioux Falls	209	Patterson	35
Billings	199	Los Angeles	31
Flint	167	Birmingham	28
Louisville	165	Boston	27
Bismarck	164	Anaheim	26
Burlington	148	San Jose	23
Dayton	147	New York	19

SOURCE: Derived from cities' responses to author's questionnaire.

healthy environment for learning and growth. However, not all children have equal access to good health-care services, any more than they all do to a good education. While many school systems require students to be inoculated against diseases before enrollment, only some provide the immunization services. Because of limited budgets for city schools, many students are inadequately immunized. Immunization rates for U.S. children rank behind 14 other nations and the immunization rates for nonwhite children are behind those of 48 nations.[29]

Public schools must also offer a variety of preventive health services to their students. Most schools test hearing, vision and speech, and for scoliosis and learning disabilities. Less common are mental health examinations and "well-child" physical examinations. Early detection, screening, follow-up procedures and prevention are of great importance in child health care.

Health-education programs are responsible for promoting preventive health and health information to children. The subjects most often taught in health-education classes are nutrition, hygiene, illnesses, smoking, and drugs and alcohol. Many states require an alcohol-awareness test before issuing a driver's license. Many schools teach sex education as part of their health curriculum, but not all offer information about birth control. Very few schools offer in-school clinics where students can receive birth-control counseling and contraceptives. A 1989 study found that of seven industrialized countries, the United States had the highest rate of teen-age pregnancy.[30]

Larger cities, reacting to the frequency of pregnant teen-agers, have begun to offer in-school services and referral systems to help them from dropping out and to insure that they receive prenatal care. Many states require that Family Life be taught in health classes. Schools also offer specific subjects relevant to health problems in their particular area. In Miami, skin cancer is common and students are taught awareness and prevention as part of their health-education curriculum.

AIDS education is taught in roughly a third of the cities that responded to our survey of school health programs. Many more are in the process of designing and installing an AIDS curriculum. Those that do offer AIDS education are constantly updating their courses to make them more comprehensive and available for all grade levels. AIDS education in these cities is usually mandated by state legislation. With the growing number of AIDS cases, education beginning at an early age assumes greater importance.

A program first developed in 1979 called Teenage Health Teaching Modules (THTM) for use at the secondary level was intended to educate students, families and communities about health issues and thus improve their attitudes and behavior. It was found to reduce the risk of disease and injury among young people.[31]

School-health programs are heavily reliant on city budgets and financing. Some cities allocate more funds for health education than others, reflecting the number of grades in which health courses are offered and the variety of health services the schools are able to provide students.

Table 7-10 ranks the health services offered in the public school systems of different cities. Similar to their rankings for other health services, St. Louis and Boston are ranked at the top of the list for having the most comprehensive school-health programs; Cleveland and Grand Rapids have the least comprehensive programs of the cities for which we have information.

How successful are school-health programs? Because young mothers are especially at risk of losing their children, one measure of success might be infant-mortality figures. In-school programs are an important mechanism for steering pregnant teen-agers to the sources of prenatal information and help. Since school-health services are often governed by state guidelines and requirements, it is appropriate to look at this subject from a state perspective.

Infant Mortality

The U.S. infant-mortality rate was 9.1 deaths per thousand births in 1990, the lowest ever, but higher than the rate in 22 other nations. Japan's infant-mortality rate is half that of the U.S.

TABLE 7-10
SCHOOL-HEALTH SERVICES, CITIES*

City	Rank Personnel	Programs	City	Rank Personnel	Programs
BEST TEN			**WORST TEN**		
1. St. Louis	4	1	78. Anaheim	67	60
2. Hartford	1	4	79. Birmingham	69	60
3. Paterson	3	4	80. Fort Wayne	70	60
4. Boston	10	2	81. Cleveland	51	82
5. Newark	2	16	82. Bismarck	59	79
6. Jersey City	5	21	83. Fresno	66	74
7. Des Moines	8	21	84. Mobile	70	74
8. Norfolk	22	7	84. Oklahoma	65	79
9. Savannah	9	21	86. Amarillo	74	74
10. Charlotte	26	7	87. Grand Rapids	68	82

* Cities ranked from most personnel/programs to fewest.

NOTE: The first column is a combined ranking of the cities; 1 means the city offers the most school-health *personnel and programs*. The *personnel* column ranks resources for school health; a 1 indicates the city with the highest personnel input. The *programs* column ranks school-health service programs; a 1 indicates the city with the most school-health programs.

SOURCE: Author's questionnaires, self-administered by officials in the responding cities.[32]

Infant-mortality rates vary widely, depending on where you live and who you are. The highest rates are in larger inner cities where underprivileged mothers obtain inadequate prenatal health care. The 1990 infant-mortality rate for blacks is projected at 16.6, almost twice the white rate. The pattern of high infant-mortality rates for blacks is repeated in each of the states. In Alabama, the infant-mortality rate is 12.2—8.8 for whites and 19.0 for blacks. Infant-mortality rates are *lower for both whites and blacks in urban areas in Alabama than for rural areas*, yet average infant mortality rates are lower in rural areas. The reason is that blacks are more concentrated in urban than rural areas (see Table 7-11).[33]

Although infant deaths are decreasing, little progress is being made in reaching the 24 percent of U.S. women who are not getting adequate prenatal care. Medical improvements have helped reduce infant deaths, but the incidence of premature and low-birth-weight babies remains high.[34]

New Hampshire shows up as No. 1 for "other" (nonblack, nonwhite) birth rates, with a rate of only 5.9 deaths per 1,000 live births. But since this category is a small one, Massachusetts is more deservedly the leader on the

TABLE 7–11
INFANT MORTALITY, BY STATE, 1987
DEATHS UNDER 1 YEAR, PER THOUSAND LIVE BIRTHS

State, Area/Race	Deaths per Thousand	State, Area/Race	Deaths per Thousand
BEST ELEVEN		**WORST TEN**	
New Hampshire, Other	3.3	New Mexico, Blacks	19.8
Massachusetts, Rural	6.2	Delaware, Blacks	20.0
Massachusetts, Whites	6.6	Michigan, Other	20.1
Connecticut, Urban Places	7.0	Pennsylvania, Other	20.5
Hawaii, Rural	7.0	Illinois, Blacks	20.6
Nebraska, Rural	7.2	District of Col., Other	21.0
Iowa, Rural	7.2	Michigan, Blacks	21.4
Massachusetts, All Areas	7.2	Pennsylvanis, Blacks	22.3
Connecticut, Whites	7.3	District of Col., Blacks	22.8
New Jersey, Rural	7.3	Vermont, Blacks	33.3
New Jersey, Whites	7.3		

NOTE: Each state is rated for whites, blacks and other, plus rural, urban and all areas. With 50 states and D.C., the total would be 306 (51 × 6) instead of 301, except for the following two facts: (1) No figures are shown for D.C. urban and rural because it is all urban; and (2) No figures are shown for blacks in North Dakota, Idaho or Montana, because the number of live births in this category was too small to be significant.

SOURCE: Derived by the author from data in U.S. Department of Health and Human Services, *Vital Statistics*, 1987 (1990).

infant mortality list. Its rural and white rates are No. 2 and No. 3 at 6.2 and 6.6 deaths per 1,000 live births, and the "all areas" (i.e., all races, too) rate is No. 8 with 7.2 deaths per 1,000. Although Massachusetts deserves credit for being the No. 1-ranked state in the U.S., its rate is higher than the Japanese national infant-mortality rate of only 5.

The other state listings among the top 10 are Connecticut urban, No. 4 with 7.0 deaths per thousand; Hawaii rural, also No. 4 with 7.0; Iowa and Nebraska rural with a 7.2 rate, and Connecticut whites and New Jersey rural and whites with a 7.3 rate. Maine and Rhode Island also show up well statistically. On the bottom end of the scale, Vermont blacks have the highest infant-mortality rate in the nation, 33.3 deaths per thousand life births. In other words, the odds of a black baby born in Vermont dying before its first birthday are one in 30. This is in the same category as China and is higher than Malaysia, North and South Korea, Romania, the Soviet Union, Sri Lanka and Yugoslavia. However, this could be an aberration for the year 1987 because the number of blacks in Vermont is small.

The District of Columbia is next to the bottom with 22.8 deaths per thousand black baby births; it also has a rate of 21.0 deaths per 1,000 "other" baby births. All of the 14 worst mortality rates are in the "black" or "other" category. Michigan and Pennsylvania appear twice. To put an infant-mortality rate of 20 or more in perspective, it is higher than such less-privileged countries as Bulgaria, Chile, Taiwan, Cuba, Czechoslovakia, Portugal, Puerto Rico and Spain.[35]

Several factors contribute to the infant-mortality rate in the largest cities. Women living in poverty often cannot afford doctors' visits. Smoking, drinking and drug abuse during pregnancy contribute to low birth weight, which puts a newborn child at risk. Babies with birth weights of less than 5.5 pounds account for almost 60 percent of infant deaths. Children born with low birth weights are more likely to suffer brain hemorrhages, infection, pneumonia and other complications. Some low-weight infants must be rehospitalized and may require surgery or suffer from handicaps.[36] The number of pregnant women with AIDS or with the AIDS virus is rising, and they pass the virus on to their children.

One out of every three pregnant women receives insufficient prenatal care. Because of the high number of Medicaid recipients and uninsured persons living in inner city areas, access to early prenatal care is limited. Doctors are reluctant to treat women on Medicare or without insurance. Many cities offer some form of assistance for prenatal care, but not nearly enough to fill the need. Chicago and Washington offer free care for poor women and free transportation to and from public health clinics. Los Angeles offers prenatal care at little or no charge but is so overloaded with patients that women can wait up to four months for an appointment. In New York, women may have to wait up to six weeks, in Washington, from six to ten weeks. A recent study by the White House Task Force on Infant

Mortality concluded that one-fourth of the 40,000 infant deaths that occur each year are preventable. Improved prenatal care could also help prevent vision and hearing loss, mental retardation and other handicaps that occur in newborns; besides the socioeconomic status of the mother, prenatal care is the most important determinant of the health of a child.[37]

Four Key Indicators of Good Community Health Services

To sum up, look for the following four signs of good health services in your community, or one you are thinking of moving to:

1. *Prompt emergency medical services.* U.S. cities on the whole do well on this score. Rural areas are worse off, depending on volunteer services that vary in quality, on the distance to the nearest emergency room and on the quality and experience of the emergency room staff. In the cities, professionally staffed ambulances are usually on their way quickly and well-equipped trauma centers that get a lot of experience do a good job on the serious cases. Doctors are more plentiful relative to population in the big cities with large hospitals and because of the concentration of people they can get the necessary experience to treat complex ailments. The best-qualified nurses are more plentiful in middle-sized cities because nurses can manage better there on their modest incomes.

2. *Access to care.* Government health coverage is restricted to the indigent and elderly. True, while the quality of inner-city public hospitals often leaves much to be desired, someone who is poor and seriously sick or injured is probably better off at the nearby emergency room of a city hospital than attempting to get care in a rural environment. But for intermediate and chronic cases, which are more common, the U.S. medical environment is harsh for the more than 30 million people who are uninsured and for the millions more who are underinsured. The time has come for the Federal Government to institute the previously mentioned May 1991 recommendation of U.S. Comptroller General Bowsher for *universal health insurance.* It would reduce the enormous indirect burdens on the society that result from lack of universal access to medical care. To make it affordable, Bowsher recommends uniform-payment rules for health-care services and caps on total spending for major provider categories, such as hospitals, physicians and technology.[38]

3. *Health screening.* If you are younger and bringing up a family, you may care more about the availability of preventive-health services. Especially for children, one important service is a systematic screening program (as well as immunizations) to focus needed medical attention on treatable health problems. Almost all schools

have at least some crude screening tests. The better screening programs go beyond vision and hearing tests and look for learning disabilities, treatable speech problems, scoliosis and mental-health problems.
4. *Health education.* Health education—for adults as well, but especially for school children—is a crucial component of public health. The quality of health education varies widely among schools.

CHAPTER EIGHT

Accidents

The United States is becoming safer from accidents—during the 1980s the death rate from accidents dropped 21 percent. Ironically, in a decade noted for a deregulatory climate in Washington, it was largely through the accumulation of Federal laws requiring improved auto safety features like seat belts, and other product and workplace safety laws (as well as supplementary state laws enforcing speed limits and use of seat belts), that the 1980s saw more progress in reducing accidental deaths than in any other decade of the century.[1]

An "accident" is an event that produces unintended injury, death or property damage. It may be contrasted with diseases or physiological malfunction such as heart attacks or diabetes and with suicide (which is an intended event). Each year, accidents cause nearly 100,000 preventable deaths and nearly 10 million disabling injuries (see Table 8-1).

As we saw in Chapter 5, fatal accidents rank as the fourth-leading cause of death in the United States after heart disease, cancer and strokes. But fatal accidents are the *No. 1* cause of death for children and youths aged 1 to 24 years.

DISTRIBUTION OF FATAL ACCIDENTS

Motor-vehicle accidents account for half of accidental deaths and also for most of the costs due to accidents. Home-related accidents are next. They take about half as many lives as motor-vehicle accidents and result in twice as many disabling injuries. Fatal accidents in public places follow closely behind, while accidental death at work is the fourth major class of fatal injuries (Table 8-1). It's not necessarily true that work is safer than the home—the accident-prone elderly and children tend to be home-bound.

Consumer Product Safety Commission (800) 638-CPSC, (800) 638-8270 (Alaska, Hawaii), (800) 492-8104 (Maryland), 24 hours. Provides recorded information on recalls, corrective actions and product safety. Also directs callers to operators who can accept complaints about unsafe products.

TABLE 8–1
DEATHS AND DISABLING INJURIES FROM ACCIDENTS, 1989

Type of Accident	Deaths	Change From 1988	Disabling Injuries
1 Motor Vehicle	46,900	−4%	1,700,000
Work	3,900		200,000
Public	42,900		1,500,000
2 Home	22,500	0%	3,400,000
3 Public*	19,000	+3%	2,400,000
4 Work*	6,500	−4%	1,500,000
Total	94,000	−2%	9,000,000

NOTES: * = Non-motor-vehicle. Type of accident: The figures for deaths in the four categories do not add up exactly to the total because of double-classification and rounding errors. Disabling injuries: A disabling injury is defined as one that incapacitates the victim beyond the first date of injury. Injuries are not reported on a national basis, so the totals shown are estimated based on studies that have developed ratios of disabling injuries to deaths in each category of accident. Public accidents: A public accident is one that occurs neither at home nor at work, and excludes all motor-vehicle accidents. Public motor-vehicle accidents: Motor-vehicle fatalities and injuries that occur neither at home (a relatively insignificant 200 fatalities a year and fewer than 10,000 disabling injuries) nor at work (and do not involve workers driving or riding on the job).

SOURCE: Derived from National Safety Council, *Accident Facts*, 1990, p. 1.

The accidental-death rates in 1989 for work (per 100,000 population) and motor-vehicle use (per 100 million miles) were the lowest on record. Motor-vehicle deaths declined 20 percent. The biggest drop was among young drivers 15 to 24 years old, a sign that new laws such as raising the minimum age for drinking to 21—and public-education programs warning teen-agers and adults not to drink and drive—are working. The death rate from work-related accidents, such as falls and motor-vehicle crashes, dropped 29 percent. While deaths from public accidents were up 3 percent, the number of such accidents, which include falls, drownings and plane crashes, was down 22 percent relative to population. Home-related death rates declined 16 percent, and that figure would have fallen further were it not for an increase in the number of fatal drug overdoses.(See Table 8-2.)

TABLE 8–2
TYPES OF FATAL ACCIDENTS, 1989

Year	Motor Vehicle	Falls	Drown- ing	Fires/ Burns	Food/ Objects	Fire- arms	Poison*	Poison (Gas)
1989	46,900	12,400	4,600	4,400	3,900	1,600	5,600	900

* Liquid and solid.

SOURCE: National Safety Council, *op. cit.*, p. 32.

COST OF ACCIDENTS

Accidents that lead to death or disabling injuries not only drain victims and their relatives emotionally, but also deplete them financially. People not involved in the accident suffer and the nation as a whole suffers from a loss in productivity. The cost for all accidents, including vehicle accidents and fires, came to $148.5 billion in 1989.[2] (See Table 8-3.)

Wage losses due to accidents lead to losses in productivity, since a worker's wages contribute to the wealth of the nation. This figure was computed from actual wages lost for nonfatal injuries and projected earnings lost for fatalities and permanent disabilities. Medical expenses of $23.7 billion include doctor fees, hospital charges, medicine costs, emergency medical service and future medical expenses.

Insurance administration costs, $28.4 billion, is the insurance company's cost of doing business, which does not include premiums paid and claims paid out. The latter is rather identified as compensation for losses such as wages, medical expenses and property damage. Not included are administrative costs of health maintenance organizations and property damage claims in home and public accidents.

Property damage from motor-vehicle accidents added up to $26.8 billion, while monetary losses from building, home and public fires amounted to $9.4 billion. Indirect losses as a result of work accidents, i.e., the money value of time lost by workers giving first aid to injured workers, time spent filling out accident reports and time lost due to production slowdowns, are estimated at $22.5 billion.

Work-related Accidents

Between 1912 and 1989, the rate of accidental work-related deaths was down 81 percent, from 21 per 100,000 population to 4 per 100,000. The most dangerous industries historically are mining, agriculture and construction. But not only has the death rate in these industries been falling,

TABLE 8–3
COST TO NATION OF ACCIDENTS

Category of Cost	Cost ($billions)
Wage Loss	$ 37.7
Medical Expenses	$ 23.7
Insurance Administration Cost	$ 28.4
Property Damage in Motor-Vehicle Accidents	$ 26.8
Fire Loss	$ 9.4
Indirect Loss, Work Accidents	$ 22.5
Total, all accidents	$148.5

SOURCE: National Safety Council, *op. cit.*, pp. 2–3.

but also the number of deaths, even though the number of workers in some areas has increased dramatically.

In a ranking of cities that had the highest accidental death rates at construction sites, compiled by the Occupational Safety and Health Administration, New York topped the list (deaths per billion dollars' worth of construction). The construction industry has been encountering growing safety problems. Reasons that have been advanced for New York's extremely high death rate at construction sites are (1) a lack of qualified state and Federal inspectors, (2) a shortage of other safety checks and (3) corruption in the New York industry.[3]

Motor-vehicle accidents are the leading cause of death among people who are working. In 1989, 3,900 deaths, or 38 percent of deaths at work, were attributed to motor-vehicle accidents (someone driving a company car on official business would be considered on the job; a commuter driving to work would not be).[4] In addition, motor-vehicle accidents at work caused 1.7 million injuries in 1989, of which 60,000 resulted in some permanent impairment. The most frequent injuries occurred to the back, followed by the thumb or finger, and the leg.

Even more deaths and injuries occur off the job (car accidents while driving to and from work; vacation travel and so forth) in a ratio of 3.5 to 1 for deaths and 1.6 to 1 for injuries. Production time and money lost due to off-the-job accidents totaled 60 million days and $45.8 billion in 1989. For on-the-job accidents, the total time lost in 1989 was 75 million days, but the future time loss due to 1989 accidents was estimated to be 90 million days!

While we can be pleased with the reduction in accidents at work, they are still too costly not to continue to make accident-prevention a top workplace priority.

Home Accidents

Your home is the most likely place to cut your hand, break your leg, hit your head or suffer some other disabling injury.[5] In 1989 total injuries in the home came to 3.4 million, meaning one of 73 people in the U.S. was disabled for at least one day.

Falls. Falls are the No. 1 cause of accidents at home. Persons over 75 years of age are most vulnerable to injuries and deaths from falls—most commonly on stairs or from ladders and roofs. Over half of all accidental deaths in the home—6,600 out of 12,400—were the result of falls. Stairs and steps are considered by the Consumer Product Safety Commission to contribute to the largest number of injuries (572,000) and to be the second most hazardous group of products made after allowing for severity of injuries.[6]

Drowning. In 1989, 4,600 deaths occurred as a result of drowning (2,800 in public waters and 600 in swimming pools and bathtubs). Home drowning deaths account for 13 percent of all types of drowning deaths and 2.7 percent of home deaths. Babies are the most vulnerable, followed by the elderly.

Other common home-related deaths include electrocution, fires and poisoning. They affect mostly children and the elderly.

Childhood Accidents

Daylight saving time is the prime season for children's accidents because they are outside playing for more hours of the day. Each year more than 1,200 children under the age of 14 drown. Swimming pools are the main culprit. Fences should be installed around pools so that small children cannot climb in. No child should swim alone and swimming lessons by qualified instructors are highly recommended.[7]

Bicycles are also a main cause of childhood accidents. Every day at least one child dies and 1,000 are injured in bike accidents. Many suffer head injuries that affect them for the rest of their lives. Most of these accidents can be prevented by simply following safety rules. Above all, children should always wear helmets; so should adults.[8]

Playgrounds should be well padded with rubber mats, fine gravel, artificial turf or wood chips.

Public Accidents

Public-accident numbers do not include motor-vehicle related deaths, but the number of deaths still add up to 19,000. Most of them occur to persons 75 years old and over, and most are caused by falls, drowning, air transport and fires.

Many injuries occur as a result of sports activities. Among the five most frequent causes of product-related injuries (the No. 1 cause is steps, as mentioned elsewhere), four are sports—bicycles (430,000), football (403,000), baseball (401,000) and basketball (349,000). Of these, basketball injuries are the least severe. Some of the injuries are fatal—swimming accounts for a high proportion of the fatalities.

Deaths from storms in the U.S. totaled 289 between September 1988 and August 1989. Of the total, 67 deaths occurred from lightning, 43 from flash floods, 31 from tornadoes, 27 from thunderstorm winds and 27 from non-flash floods.

Deaths from water transport include falls and burns as well as drownings. More than nine out of ten drownings involved occupants of small boats. Drinking and driving is a major problem, but so is drinking and boating. Half of all boating deaths involve alcohol.

Despite regular reports of airplane crashes, the common knowledge that flying is safer than driving is still true: per passenger mile, it is still far more dangerous to ride in a car than a scheduled commercial airplane. Passenger deaths in scheduled air services totaled 273 in 1988, according to the National Transportation Safety Board. Although the number of deaths increased from 1987 to 1988, the rate of fatalities per 100 million passenger miles actually decreased. (See Table 8-4.)

Safety varies with types of flying. For all general aviation, including nonscheduled flights, recreational, instructional and private business flights and crop dusters, the number of accidents per 100,000 hours of flight declined from about 14 in 1980 to 9 in 1989. Within that general category, accidents by on-demand air taxi (small planes hired by individuals) has peaked at 5.5 in the years 1981, 1983 and 1985, but to a low of 3 in 1990. On commuter planes, including regional commercial flights and usually seating fewer than 30 people, accidents dropped from 3 in 1980 to 0.6 in 1990. Accidents on private planes flown for business purposes reached a high of 4.7 in 1983 and leveled down to 3.5 in 1989. For corporate-owned planes flown by professional pilots, accidents dropped from 2 in

TABLE 8–4

PASSENGER DEATHS AND DEATH RATES, 1978, 1983, 1988
RATES PER 100 MILLION PASSENGER–MILES

Year	Passenger Cars/Taxis		Buses		Railroad Trains		Scheduled Airlines	
	Deaths	Rate	Deaths	Rate	Deaths	Rate	Deaths	Rate
1978	28,035	1.26	28	0.03	13	0.12	175	0.09
1983	22,739	0.98	49	0.05	4	0.04	17	0.01
1988	25,614	1.19	44	0.03	2	0.02	273	0.01

SOURCE: National Safety Council, op. cit., p. 90.[10]

1980 to less than 1 in 1989. Major airlines, not including charters, have the fewest number of accidents and have been at the near-zero mark over the 10-year period.[9]

Auto Accidents

Automobiles and other motor vehicles are the principal means of transportation in America. Today more Americans drive more cars more miles than ever before.[11] A dramatic boom in the American work force in the last few decades has consequently led to a dramatic increase in the number of auto commuters.

Other than the usual headaches of traffic jams, what are the real hazards of traffic to our safety and health? One might expect that just the sheer volume of traffic in metropolitan areas would contribute to greater numbers of fatal accidents, but surprisingly the greatest dangers for automobile users exist outside the city.

Motor-vehicle deaths are well ahead of fatal work-related, home and public accidents. A motor-vehicle death occurs on average once every 11 minutes and an injury every 18 seconds,[12] for a total in 1988 of 34.2 million motor-vehicle accidents. The total cost of these accidents comes to approximately $89 billion annually. In 1988, the average bodily injury insurance claim amounted to $8,736, a 146 percent increase from 1979.

The nature of auto accidents differs between highly populated urban areas and sparse rural areas. Most fatal accidents occur in rural areas, whereas nonfatal-injury accidents and property damage occur mostly in urban areas. Table 8-5 shows where and on which type of roadways the accidents occur.

TABLE 8–5
MOTOR–VEHICLE ACCIDENTS BY CLASS OF TRAFFICWAY, 1989

Classification of Trafficway	Fatal Accidents	Classification of Trafficway	Fatal Accidents
URBAN		**RURAL**	
Local streets (%)	43.0	County roads (%)	35.4
State roads (%)	20.6	State roads (%)	32.9
Interstate (%)	17.7	U.S. routes (%)	14.8
U.S. routes (%)	12.7	Interstate (%)	11.5
County roads (%)	4.8	Local streets (%)	4.6
Major arterial (%)	0.5	Major arterial (%)	0.3
Other (%)	0.7		
Total, Urban	14,500	Total, Rural	26,800

SOURCE: National Safety Council, *op. cit.*, pp. 59.

Although the number of alcohol-related traffic fatalities (ARTFs) has decreased since 1982, alcohol-impaired driving remains a serious public-health problem, with over 22,000 ARTFs in 1989. The rate of decline has indeed slowed due to factors such as changes in (and stricter enforcement of) state laws, increases in the minimum legal drinking age in 35 states from 1982 through 1987, increased media attention resulting in increased public awareness and an increased number of programs directed against drinking and driving.[13]

Table 8-6 shows the distribution of accidental motor-vehicle deaths by states, with a rate based on 100 million passenger miles traveled. The highest rate of fatalities in 1989 was 3.5 deaths per 100 million miles in New Mexico, followed by four states with 3.3 deaths per 100 million: Arkansas, Mississippi, Nevada and West Virginia.

The lowest fatality rates per 100 million miles in 1989 were 1.4 in North Dakota and 1.5 in New Jersey.

STATES AND INTERSTATE HIGHWAYS

Long interstate highways pose a special risk to drivers. Even though city highways may seem more dangerous because of the proximity of cars, long stretches of interstate highways outside of city limits are more risky, because drivers travel faster and are more likely to doze at the wheel.

TABLE 8–6

**ACCIDENTAL MOTOR–VEHICLE DEATH RATES BY STATE, 1989
RATES PER 100 MILLION PASSENGER-MILES**

State	Accidental Death Rate	State	Accidental Death Rate
BEST TEN		WORST TEN	
North Dakota	1.4	Oregon	2.5
New Jersey	1.5	North Carolina	2.5
Minnesota	1.6	Georgia	2.5
Connecticut	1.6	Arizona	2.6
Virginia	1.7	Idaho	2.8
Rhode Island	1.7	South Carolina	3.2
Massachusetts	1.7	West Virginia	3.3
Maine	1.7	Nevada	3.3
Washington	1.8	Mississippi	3.3
Delaware	1.8	Arkansas	3.5
		New Mexico	3.5

SOURCE: National Safety Council, *op. cit.*, p. 69.

In regional terms, the more sparsely populated parts of the country are more dangerous on interstate highways: Western states had the most fatal accidents for every mile traveled, followed by the South, Midwest and Northeast, which was the safest part of the nation's interstate system to drive on. Table 8-7 shows states ranked by fatal accidents on interstate highways.

The most dangerous state, based on rates per miles traveled, is New Mexico, although more highly populated states such as California and Texas have much higher numbers of deaths. Of the 1,345 counties with interstates, San Miguel county, east of Santa Fe, saw the most fatal accidents per mile traveled.

One of the major reasons New Mexico highways are so deadly is the state's acute shortage of state police officers; yet no state has more roads than New Mexico—11,000 miles of them. Compounding that is the state's high speed limit of 65 mph and the pervasiveness of drunk driving. In 1989, 57 percent of highway deaths in New Mexico were alcohol-related, compared to a nationwide average of 50 percent.[14]

To a large extent, road safety depends on how strongly drinking and speeding laws are enforced by the state. Even though all states currently have a minimum drinking age of 21, certain states enforce the law much more vigorously. Massachusetts has no shortage of police on the highways, and that helps make it the safest state in the country to drive in. The state police there pride themselves on their stringent speed-limit enforcement, diligent crackdown on drunk driving and computer tracking of drivers with unsafe records.

TABLE 8—7

FATAL–ACCIDENT RATES ON INTERSTATES, BY STATE RANKED BY RATE PER 100 MILLION PASSENGER MILES, 1988–89

Rank	Death Rate	Rank	Death Rate
BEST TEN		WORST TEN	
D.C.	0.36	Utah	1.59
Massachusetts	0.50	Delaware	1.61
Wisconsin	0.56	Idaho	1.79
Connecticut	0.59	Mississippi	1.82
Minnesota	0.59	Montana	1.83
Maryland	0.64	Arizona	1.85
Ohio	0.67	Nevada	2.08
Michigan	0.68	Wyoming	2.13
Oregon	0.73	Alaska	2.16
Indiana	0.74	New Mexico	2.47

SOURCE: Pesce, *loc. cit.*

THE DEADLIEST INTERSTATES

Surprisingly, the *lower* volume of traffic on interstate highways contributes to the high mortality rates. Like the snakes that hypnotize birds before swallowing them, the long snakes of open roads appear to put drivers to sleep or at least dull the edge of their alertness. (See Table 8-8.)

Idaho's Cassia County, a sparsely populated area where I-84 goes south into northern Utah, is the deadliest stretch of highway in the country and I-15, going from Pocatello, Idaho through a steep pass into Salt Lake City, is the fourth most deadly. Both of these highways have dangerous crosswinds blowing at up to 80 mph, whipping up snow in winter and dust in summer and causing blinded motorists to pile into one another. I-15 also has a very steep stretch through a mountain pass.

TABLE 8–8

INTERSTATE HIGHWAY SAFETY RANKED BY FATALITIES PER 100 MILLION PASSENGER MILES, 1988–89

State	Interstate No.	County	Fatalities
BEST TEN			
Oklahoma	44	Mayes	2.64
Texas	45	Madison	2.64
Utah	80	Tooele	2.64
Texas	37	Live Oak	2.65
Georgia	75	Turner	2.66
Montana	15	Beaverhead	2.67
Texas	10	Fayette	2.69
Texas	35	Frio	2.69
California	15	San Bernardino	2.70
Vermont	91	Windsor	2.70
WORST TEN			
Mississippi	59	Lamar	5.55
Louisiana	59	St. Tammany	5.65
Texas	10	Reeves	5.96
Utah	70	Emery	5.99
New Mexico	10	Grant	6.67
Texas	10	Pecos	6.68
Idaho	15	Clark	6.73
Nevada	80	Lyon	7.19
New Mexico	25	San Miguel	7.51
Idaho	84	Cassia	8.86

SOURCE: Pesce, *loc. cit.*

Falling asleep is a central factor in 200,000 to 400,000 accidents each year. Sleep experts say that one-third of truck drivers on the road at any time may be too tired to stay awake or respond quickly enough to avert an accident. While Federal regulations require interstate truck drivers to break their trips periodically, the regulations are difficult to enforce; meanwhile, state regulation of in-state drivers is spotty.

Non-Interstate Highways

Interstate highways can be dangerous, but the other highways accounted for 89 percent of the 45,555 traffic deaths in 1989.[15] The counties with the lowest population density had the highest fatality rates: 65 percent of all deaths caused by auto accidents occurred in rural areas.[16] South Carolina had the worst record in terms of fatalities on non-interstate roads (city and state highways and local roads)—in 1988 and 1989, 1,900 people died on these roads. Of all the counties in the United States, the riskiest one to drive through was Esmeralda, Nevada.

In recent years, drugs have become a contributing factor in automobile accidents. Nearly one in four New York City drivers aged 16 to 45 who die in motor vehicle accidents have used cocaine within 48 hours of the accident.[17]

Experts advise those who intend to drive long distances to get enough sleep, not just the night before, but also for several days before the date of departure. Do not drink alcohol within three hours of driving. Some experts urge drivers not to drink at all the day before, because alcohol can have long-lasting effects on alertness and judgment. Many advise long-distance drivers to stop often, even once an hour, just to stretch and walk around.

Cities

The most populous cities, such as New York, Los Angeles and Chicago, do not even rank among the 500 counties with the highest fatal accident rates. Compared with other urban areas, the six most populous cities rank extremely well (see Table 8-9).

Another major reason for the sharp difference between rural and urban motor-vehicle death rates is the response time for medical aid. Since rural regions have fewer hospitals, response time for vehicle accidents is at least twice that in more populated urban regions.[18] For instance, in Nevada the average response time was nearly 28 minutes, which doesn't help much given the fact that, according to the American Automobile Association, the first 15 minutes are the most critical. Getting the victim to a hospital within an hour of the accident, called "the golden hour," is vital for that person's survival. Unfortunately, with Federal spending on state transportation down and state revenues falling below expectations, many states don't have enough "med-evac" vehicles.

TABLE 8–9

DEATHS FROM ACCIDENTS, BY METRO AREA

Metro Area (% from Car Accidents)	Accident Deaths per 100,000	Metro Area (% from Car Accidents)	Accident Deaths per 100,000
BEST TEN		**WORST TEN**	
Albuquerque (32.2%)	11.9	Mobile (48.1%)	43.0
Hartford (64.7%)	15.5	Greensboro–	
Springfield, MO (63.8%)	15.9	Winston-Salem (47.7%)	43.6
Honolulu (40.5%)	22.5	Memphis (47.7%)	44.9
Madison, WI (52.5%)	22.7	Tucson (52.4%)	44.3
Columbus, OH (45.1%)	23.9	Shreveport (43.5%)	46.3
Lincoln, NE (35.3%)	24.2	Birmingham (51.1%)	46.6
Charlotte (50.0%)	25.3	Columbia, SC (48.2%)	47.2
Washington (47.1%)	26.0	Montgomery (44.8%)	47.4
Anaheim–		Riverside–	
Santa Ana (62.3%)	26.5	San Bernardino (66.2%)	47.8
		Toledo (59.8%)	48.1

SOURCE: U.S. Department of Health and Human Services, *Vital Statistics of the U.S., 1987,* Volume II, Part B, Mortality, Table 8–8.

Auto Safety Legislation and Features

The combination of Federal and state car safety laws is having a beneficial effect. Most states have mandatory seat-belt laws. Seat belts by themselves are not adequate for addressing the problem of highway deaths and injuries.[19] Lap/shoulder belts are effective in low- to moderate-speed crashes (up to 25 mph head-on), but at higher speeds belted occupants may hit steering columns, windshields and dashboards, especially with their faces and heads.

All 1990 cars were required to be equipped with air bags on the driver's side or automatic safety belts.[20] The combination of an air bag plus a seat belt is a much more effective restraint system than either device alone. The National Highway Traffic Safety Administration says that if 50 percent of people involved in crashes were using seat belts about 4,400 deaths and 73,000 moderate-to-critical injuries could be prevented each year.

Different car models have different safety records, but according to the Insurance Institute for Highway Safety (IIHS), large cars are still the safest in a crash.[21] In a series of crash tests at 5 mph, 16 small four-door 1990 cars sustained extensive damage. The Honda Civic DX performed the best among the 16 cars.

The good news overall is that yearly death rates from motor-vehicle accidents have gone down steadily almost every year.[22] The total number of accidents has risen, but so has the number of registered vehicles and vehicle miles traveled. Thus the total deaths per 100 million miles has decreased dramatically. Many factors, such as the availability of modern hospitals and emergency medical service, have contributed to the decline.

Eight Ways to Avoid the Most Common Accidents

1. *Don't climb on unsteady platforms*, whether ladders, chairs or tables; especially, don't overreach on a platform; pass this safety habit on to your children.
2. *Teach your children driver safety;* encourage them to take more than the bare minimum of driving lessons before they venture out alone.
3. *Don't drive when road conditions are poor.*
4. *Keep your car well maintained.*
5. *Support law enforcement on the highway;* it saves lives. Radar-detectors are a bad investment at any price.
6. *Insist your children wear bicycle helmets* and wear one yourself.
7. *Be aware of the risks of team sports, swimming and skiing* and warn your children to take normal precautions.
8. *Wear protective clothing when using a chain saw* (sturdy shoes, long pants and long-sleeved jacket, goggles and silencers for the ears). Then, proceed with care.

CHAPTER NINE

The Health of Cities

In this chapter, we review basic health-related data for metropolitan areas and cities. The figures are based primarily on two sources:

- Federal Government data, such as rates of mortality, homicides, robberies and accidents, and a labor-market measure of economic health,
- Information obtained directly from state, county and city officials on the environment, health services, recreational facilities and school health services.

The names of all local contacts cited in the text of the city summaries that follow are derived from questionnaires the author sent to each city. While I sometimes disagree with them on matters of detail, the public servants who took the trouble to answer my questions carefully are worthy of the greatest respect. Listing their names is in part an effort to recognize them for the work they do on a daily basis to improve your health.

The data and rankings based on them are derived from the following sources:

Death Rates: The number of metro-area deaths relative to population is useful as an overall measure of how healthy a city is, when adjusted for the median age of residents. The heart-attack and cancer rates are also age-adjusted. Infant-mortality rates are for the entire state—appropriately enough, since public-health services are generally a state-and-county function—and represent deaths in the first year of life per 1,000 live births in 1987. The mortality rates were all derived from data for 1987 published in *U.S. Vital Statistics 1987*, Volume II—Mortality, Part B, published in 1989 (a later edition was delayed by Federal budget cuts and wasn't available in 1990 when we did our research). Contact: Department of Health and Human Services, Public Health Service (202) 436-8500. For background on these figures, please refer to Chapter 1 for general mortality data; Chapter 5 for heart-attack and cancer data, and Chapter 7 for infant-mortality rates.

Public Safety: Safety hazards include violence or accidents. Four measures of public safety are provided. Homicides are a good indicator of the seriousness of violence, although most homicides are among friends and relatives and are hard for the police to prevent except by controlling the proliferation of weapons. Homicide data are for 1989, as reported in FBI, *Crime in the United States, 1989* (published 1990), pp. 330–358. Robbery rates are a better measure of the likelihood of stranger-to-stranger street crime, which is easier for the police to prevent. The data are also for 1989 and the source is the same as for homicides. Suicide and accident rates are from *Vital Statistics of the U.S.*, already cited. Some accident data are also from the National Safety Council. Further discussion of homicide, robbery and suicide data is in Chapter 5. Further discussion of accident data is in Chapter 8.

Economic Health: The area's economy affects health in many ways, including access to health services and levels of stress. The metropolitan statistical area population—the primary metro area if there is a choice between primary and consolidated, which is the case in large cities—is for 1988, from a report on estimates by the Census Bureau in 1989, using June 1989 definitions of metro areas established by the Office of Management and Budget. Of the three measures of economic health calculated by the author, two are based on data in a special Bureau of Labor Statistics printout for November 1988 and November 1990 (provided in February 1991) and the third on small-business growth data in *Inc.* Magazine, March 1990. Further background on this subject is provided at the end of Chapter 1.

Environment: Data on air and water quality and hazardous waste are important because they warn residents of conditions that can cause illness and even death. The data were reported by the cities or counties themselves in 1990, on a questionnaire sent by the author. We show the frequency of "exceedances" (violation of maximum legal concentrations) of ozone. Hazardous-waste data include location of EPA Superfund sites, commercial disposal sites and other hazardous-waste sites and information on city recycling laws and programs. Under weather we provide a general synopsis of the city's weather factors—average temperature, relative humidity, precipitation and snowfall (the source is the National Oceanic and Atmospheric Administration, *Comparative Climatic Data Through 1987*). Further background on environmental measures is provided in Chapters 2-4 and especially 6.

℞ **Health Services:** Data on basic health facilities—the number of doctors, nurses and hospital beds in each city—were derived from two sources: (1) doctors (M.D.s only, excludes those employed by the Federal Government, metro data) per thousand population is from the American Medical Association, *Physician Characteristics and Distribution in the U.S.* (Chicago: AMA, 1987); and (2) nurses and hospital beds per thousand population (community hospitals only, city data) is from the American Hospital Association, *Hospital Statistics 1989–1990* (Chicago: AHA, 1990). Rates per thousand inhabitants were calculated by the author by dividing the number of doctors, nurses or beds by the metro or city population as reported by the Census Bureau. Most of the remaining information about health services is provided by the cities or counties themselves in response to the author's questionnaires: emergency hotlines and health-education programs, neighborhood clinics and centers; number of neighborhood health clinics; community mental health centers and emergency medical facilities and their accessibility to the handicapped from public transit; preventive health programs and services sponsored by the city, including prenatal and infant medical care, food provision, vaccinations for children, blood pressure testing, cholesterol testing, AIDS testing and family planning; treatment programs including city-sponsored programs for drug rehabilitation, alcoholism, mental health therapy and sexually transmitted diseases. For further background on these programs, see Chapter 7.

🏃 **Recreation:** In their responses, many city officials focused on their plans for a new stadium or spectator-sports team. Our interest is in participatory, not spectator, sports. The local baseball, football and soccer fields plus basketball and tennis courts are the "criteria facilities" referred to in each city summary that has the necessary data. To rank them, the author divided the total number of facilities by the population. The percentage of parkland compared to total city area is also provided by city officials; we requested that they exclude state and Federal parkland to obtain a measure of local recreational commitment. Water-sport facilities, where available, are also described, along with other recreational activities indicated on the author's questionnaires. For further background, see Chapter 7.

👪 **School-Health Education and Services:** Cities have a unique opportunity to intervene on behalf of the health of their pupils through screening and health-education programs. A measure of the extent of health services in this area is provided by a count of how many desirable school-health education and health-care programs the school system offers, such as screens and tests, vaccinations, mental-health examinations, well-child examinations, hearing tests, vision tests, speech therapy, scoliosis and learning disabilities. Treatments offered in the city's public schools (medical, dental and psychiatric) are also indicated. We also calcu-late the number of health-care personnel assigned to the schools, weight-ing a physician-pediatrician ($85,000 hospital salary) as 4, a psychologist as 3, a nurse practitioner as 2, a registered nurse as 1.5 and other health aides and licensed practical nurses as 1; these ratios roughly correspond to salary differentials for hospital personnel as provided to the author from *The American Journal of Nursing* and hospital references by the American Hospital Association (Library Reference Desk, 312-280-6000). Note that nurses' salaries vary by region, with the south-central region tending to be lowest and the Northeast and west coast the highest. For further back-ground on this subject, see the end of Chapter 7.

Disclosure: We wrote to every city for information in 1989 and followed up for a full year. In 1991 we sent the city summary to every city and to every official who had previously responded. Even so, information is missing. We are surprised that some cities will spend mil-lions of dollars on economic development but won't take a few minutes to respond to a free opportunity to put their best foot forward. Possibly in some cases the nonrespondents believe that no information would be better for them than even a varnished version of the truth. The reader may wish to take note of the disclosure factor as a general indicator of city responsiveness—bearing in mind that an unresponsive city hall can be very bad for your health. The last box in the panel at the top of each entry indicates the degree of cooperation we obtained from each city.

Based on the information we have collected for each of the above catego-ries, we developed the following rating system to permit ready acces-sibility of the reader to our assessments:

✔ The "best" rating ("excellent"), this generally means that the metro area or city (depending on the category and context) is in the top third of those we looked at, although we have not always made an effort to ensure that the ratings were evenly distributed three ways. These communities are doing something right and are worthy of emulation.

✓ The "middle" ("good") rating, this generally means the city or metro area is in the middle third of the cities we looked at. These cities are average and may be on their way to being the cities to emulate in the future.

✗ The "worst" ("poor") rating, this generally means the city or metro area is in the bottom third of the cities we looked at. They have problems, which should be of concern *both* to people who are thinking of moving to these places and the people who already live there.

? The "inadequate information" rating, this generally means the city or metro area did not provide information or the source we used for data did not have the city in it. A question mark for the first rating reflects the fact that we calculated the age-adjusted death rate only for 100 cities; it does not reflect on the city or metro area. Question marks in other categories generally reflect poorly on the city's responsiveness as summarized in the last rating on disclosure.

Akron, OH

⚰	☠	$	⬆	℞	🏃	🏕	?
✓	✓	✓	✓	✓	✓	**?**	✓

Akron (Summit County) is at the bottom of the second third of 100 major cities in its age-adjusted death rate. Cities in Ohio have an infant-mortality rate of 10.3 and are therefore a less favorable environment for pregnant mothers than rural areas, which have an infant-mortality rate of 7.8. The state's infant-mortality rate in rural areas is very low (16/301, 2.5 deaths per thousand births lower than in urban areas). The rate for minority groups is high (238/301 for blacks, nearly double the rate for whites), because a high proportion of the state's minorities live in cities; this pushes the city infant-mortality rate above the state average. Contact: Neil M. Casey, Biostatistician, Akron City Health Department, #117, 177 South Broadway, Akron, OH 44308 (216) 375-2976.

	Number	Rank
Age-Adjusted Death Rate	0.43	66/100
Heart Attacks	0.15	67/100
Cancer	0.08	64/100

Akron's homicide rate is slightly higher than average, ranking 65th out of 111 metro areas. Its robbery and accident rates are significantly above average, among the 20 highest metro areas. But the suicide rate is among the 20 lowest.

Incidence per 1,000 Pop.	Number	Rank
Homicides (1989)	0.09	65/111
Robberies (1989)	3.35	91/111
Suicides	0.10	18/100
Accidents	0.38	84/100

$\boxed{\$}$ Akron's 1988 metro population was 654,000, 62nd out of 113 metro areas. Its unemployment rate of 4.8 percent (November 1990) ranks 44th out of 113 metro areas. This rate is down from 5.1 percent two years earlier—a significant achievement during a period when many cities were suffering from higher unemployment rates, especially since Akron's labor force grew over 4 percent during the period. For the long term, the relative lack of entrepreneurship in the area (83rd of 113 metro areas) is a negative factor. Contact: Mayor Donald L. Plusquellic, City of Akron, 166 S. High St., Akron, OH 44308.

$\boxed{\spadesuit}$ **Air Quality:** Akron has come a long way from its days as a town known for its rubber factories. It has seen a 5–10 percent decrease over the 1985–90 period in most air pollutants, such as airborne particles, sulfur dioxide, carbon dioxide and lead, none of which exceeded the EPA's national ambient air quality standards in 1988. Ozone, which exceeded the Federal standard of 0.12 ppm for one hour or more on no fewer than 21 days (a particularly high number for a middle-sized city) in 1988, seems to have been brought under control. Exceedances dropped to 4 in 1989 and to 0 in 1990. Someone seems to care about the air. Contact: Jerry J. Garro, Air Monitoring Officer (Room 340), Akron City Health Department, 117 South Broadway, Akron, OH 44308 (216) 375-2480.

Water Quality: New programs to reduce water turbidity and for better circulation for higher chlorine concentrations have been instituted, and as of April 1991 no significant problems with the water supply have been detected. Contact: Frank Slaton, Director of Environmental Health (Room 438), Akron City Health Department, 177 South Broadway, Akron, OH 44308 (216) 375-2405.

Weather: Akron is a relatively cool city with an average annual temperature of 49.5, with 125 days per year when the temperature falls below 32. Annual precipitation is about average at 35.9 inches.

Average Daily Temperature (degrees F)	49.5
High	59.0
Low	39.9
Average Humidity	
Morning (percent)	80
Afternoon (percent)	60
Annual Precipitation (inches)	35.9
Average Total Snowfall (inches)	48.3
Ozone days over 0.12 ppm (1 hour, 1988)	21

$\boxed{\text{R}\!\!\!/}$ Akron sponsors 50 health-education campaigns in all the common areas—on such issues as AIDS, sexually transmitted diseases, prenatal care, mosquito control and open burning. It has emergency hotlines for all of the common subjects except suicide. Smoking is prohibited on public transportation and partially restricted in private and public offices and in restaurants. The Akron area seems well supplied with medical resources and provides a full range of preventive-health services. On the face of it, the relatively high infant-mortality rates in Ohio cities do not appear to stem from problems with overall services in Akron, and the availability of neighborhood clinics is a positive sign for the distribution of health services throughout the community. Contact: C. William Keck, M.D., M.P.H., Akron City Health Department, #215, 177 South Broadway, Akron, OH 44308 (216) 375-2960.

Health Resources per 1,000 Pop.	Number	Rank
Hospitals	7.75	35/91
Nurses	9.47	25/90
Doctors	2.04	79/113

Akron has 95 sports fields/courts per 100,000 residents, ranking 30th out of 79 cities. It has an impressive array of recreational facilities and a large park area (a high 10 percent of land area) within which to pursue them. Its facilities include 100 baseball fields, 30 football and soccer fields, 67 basketball courts, 54 tennis courts, 1 golf course and 2 swimming pools. Contact: Pattie A. Urdzik, Recreation Bureau Manager, City of Akron, 1420 Triplett Boulevard, Akron, OH 44306 (216) 375-2804.

Parkland/Total City Area (percent)	10
Aerobics classes	yes
Arts and craft classes	yes
Hiking or exploration groups	yes

Akron school children in Kindergarten through the 11th grade are offered all common health-education programs. But students are not provided with any medical, dental or psychiatric treatment. We did not receive enough information to assign a rating. Contact: Fred Schuett, Health and Physical Education Curriculum Specialist, Akron City Schools, 65 Steiner Ave., Akron, OH 44301 (216) 434-1661, ext. 3268.

Albuquerque, NM

RIP	⤵	$	♠	℞	🏃	👥	?
✔	X	✓	X	✓	✓	?	✓

Albuquerque (Bernalillo County) residents are in the top third of longevity—i.e., in the bottom third of age-adjusted death rates. It also has a low rate of cardiovascular disease. The state has a low infant-mortality rate among whites and in the cities, but a very high rate among blacks (the other racial groups are in between).

	Number	Rank
Age-Adjusted Death Rate	0.63	33/100
Heart Attacks	−0.84	5/100
Cancer	−0.13	33/100

Albuquerque has the lowest accident rate of 100 metro areas, but the fourth-highest suicide rate. The robbery rate is average, but the homicide rate is high.

Incidence per 1,000 Pop.	Number	Rank
Homicides (1989)	0.10	77/111
Robberies (1989)	2.12	58/111
Suicides	0.20	97/100
Accidents	0.11	1/100

Albuquerque's 1988 metro population was 493,000, 79th out of 113 metro areas. Its economic health at the end of 1990 was good, ranking 46th of 113 metro areas. Its unemployment rate ranks 44th, change in unemployment 40th (the labor force declined slightly faster than employment) and its enterprise 66th. Contact: Mayor Louis Saavedra, City of Albuquerque, City Hall, Albuquerque, NM 87103.

Air Quality: The ozone level in Albuquerque is stable, but very close to exceeding federal standards. Carbon monoxide is trending down slightly. The level of total suspended particulates is dependent on the annual rainfall. Contact: Steve Walker, Manager, Air Pollution Control Division, Environmental Health Department, PO Box 1293, One Civic Plaza, Room 3023, Albuquerque, NM 87103.

Weather: Albuquerque's average annual temperature is slightly above average at 56.2, but the nights are cool (it's located at the foot of the Sandia mountains) and the city still experiences an average of 120 days per year when the minimum daily temperature falls below 32. The city is extremely dry with a normal annual precipitation of only 8.2 inches.

Average Daily Temperature (degrees F)	56.2
High	70.3
Low	42.1
Average Humidity	
Morning (percent)	60
Afternoon (percent)	29
Annual Precipitation (inches)	8.12
Average Total Snowfall (inches)	10.9
Ozone days over 0.12 ppm (1 hour, 1988)	0

℞ Albuquerque did not respond to the health services survey. Information on basic health resources suggests a scarcity of the emergency hospital services that low-income groups rely on.

Health Resources per 1,000 Pop.	Number	Rank
Hospital beds	4.46	76/91
Nurses	5.76	63/90
Doctors	2.99	25/119

The city has a relatively small parkland area. Compared to other cities it is long on golf courses, basketball courts and tennis courts, and short on baseball fields. The city's Therapeutic and Special Services Program works with Handicapped children and adults to help improve motor functions. Contact: Mike Walker, Director, City of Albuquerque, Parks and Recreation Department, PO Box 1293, Albuquerque, NM 87103.

Parkland/Total City Area (percent)	1.8
Aerobics classes	yes
Arts and craft classes	yes
Hiking or exploration groups	yes

The city did not respond to the school-health survey, which is too bad given the wide range in the previously mentioned infant-mortality rates in the state.

Amarillo, TX

🪦	🏃	$	↟	℞	🏃	🏖️	?
?	✓	✓	✓	X	✔	X	✔

🪦 Amarillo (Potter County) was not rated using the age-adjusted death rate. Texas has low infant-mortality rates in rural areas and among whites; the rates are high in cities and among minority populations.

	Number	Rank
Infant Mortality (Texas)		
All Areas	9.1	90/301
Blacks	15.1	235/301
Other	13.5	220/301
Rural	7.9	24/301
Urban Places	9.7	125/30
Whites	8.3	46/301

🏃 Amarillo's robbery rate is below average, but homicides are above average. The fact that Amarillo is not a big tourist spot suggests that the homicides tend to be among friends and relatives.

Incidence per 1,000 Pop.	Number	Rank
Homicides (1989)	0.09	65/111
Robberies (1989)	1.38	30/111

$ Amarillo's 1988 metro population was 196,000, 107th out of 113 metro areas. Its economic health at the end of 1990 was below average, ranking 67th of 113 metro areas. Its unemployment rate ranks 55th, change in unemployment 15th (the labor force contracted by 3.4 percent, nearly 1 percentage point more than the decline in employment) and its enterprise 111th. Contact: Mayor Keith Adams, City of Amarillo, PO Box 1971, Amarillo, TX 79186.

↟ **Air Quality:** The area has no significant air-quality problems. Airborne particles are influenced by dust storms. Contact: Eli Bell, Director, Texas Air Control Board, 6330 Hwy 290 East, Austin, TX 78756.

Hazardous Waste: Potter County has no hazardous-waste disposal sites. Contact: Mike Kennedy, Director of Public Works, City of Amarillo, PO Box 1971, Amarillo, TX 79186.

Water Quality: Amarillo's drinking water supply comes from surface and ground water sources. The pH of the drinking water is 8.1. The city has added amendments to its Safe Drinking Water Act. Contact: Mike Kennedy, Director of Public Works, City of Amarillo, TX 79186.

Weather: Amarillo's average daily temperature is above average at 57.2. Precipitation is slightly below average at 19.1 inches annually.

Average Daily Temperature (degrees F)	57.2
High	70.7
Low	43.8
Average Humidity	
Morning (percent)	73
Afternoon (percent)	45
Annual Precipitation (inches)	19.1
Average Total Snowfall (inches)	15.3

℞ Amarillo provides all basic public health-education programs and emergency hotlines. The city initiated a wellness council to increase public awareness of disease prevention. Smoking is prohibited on public transportation and in medical facilities through anti-smoking laws. Smoking is partially restricted in restaurants, public offices and private offices with public contact. Contact: Robert J. Carson, Public Health Administrator, Amarillo Bi-City-County Health Department, PO Box 1971, Amarillo, TX 79186.

The city offers a variety of classes and group activities such as sports skills, storytelling, arts and crafts, bicycle safety, firearms safety and swimming lessons. Amarillo has an abundance of sports facilities which include 200 baseball fields, 138 basketball courts, 125 volleyball courts, 98 football/soccer fields, 52 tennis courts, 5 running tracks, 4 swimming pools and 3 golf courses. Volleyball is one of the most popular sports, having a total of 92 leagues throughout the year. Softball is also very popular. Contact: Strick Watkins, Director of Parks and Recreation, City of Amarillo, PO Box 1971, Amarillo, TX 74106-1971.

Parkland/Total City Area (percent)	4.3

To serve 27,000 students in the public school system are 15 nurses and one consulting physician; a part-time nurse is only available in 30 percent of the schools. Health-education programs are offered to students in grades 9-12. These programs include nutrition, hygiene, illnesses, smoking, drugs and AIDS education. No medical, dental or psychiatric treatment is provided for students. Contact: Dr. John Williams, Superintendent, Amarillo Independent School District, 1616 South Kentucky, Amarillo, TX 79106.

Anaheim, CA

🪦	🚷	$	🌲	℞	🎭	👪	?
✓	✓	✔	✓	✓	✓	✗	✔

Anaheim (Orange County) has an average age-adjusted mortality rate. Infant-mortality rates for California are high among minorities and in urban areas.

	Number	Rank
Age-Adjusted Death Rate	−0.22	45/100
Heart Attacks	0.27	73/100
Cancer	0.06	61/100

Anaheim has the 10th lowest accident rate. Rates for homicide and robbery are also below average.

Incidence per 1,000 Pop.	Number	Rank
Homicides (1989)	0.06	39/111
Robberies (1989)	1.76	42/111
Suicides	0.12	45/100
Accidents	0.26	10/100

 Anaheim's 1988 metro population was 2,257,000, ranking 17th out of 113 metro areas. Its economic health at the end of 1990 was good, despite recent layoffs, ranking 29th of 113 metro areas. Its unemployment rate ranks 29th, change in unemployment 84th (employment declined faster than the labor force) and its enterprise 8th. Contact: Mayor Ben Bay, City of Anaheim, PO Box 3222, Anaheim, CA 92805.

Hazardous Waste: Anaheim has no active or inactive waste sites. It generated about 40,000 tons of hazardous waste in 1986. Of this, half came from a single location and consisted of a pile of shredded-automobile waste that in 1990 was still on-site pending a final decision on disposal. Half-a-dozen permanent household hazardous-waste-collection sites are a current priority for the county. Unfortunately, illegal dumping of hazardous waste on public and private properties has increased alarmingly. Contact: Steven Wong, Hazardous Waste Management Program, Div. of Environmental Health, Orange County Health Department, 1719 West 17th Street, Santa Ana, CA 92702; and Tom Graham, Fire Inspector, Anaheim Fire Department, Fire Prevention Bureau.

Weather: The Anaheim primary metro area, part of the Los Angeles consolidated metro area, generally enjoys a two-season (summer-winter) climate. Summer is characterized by morning lows of 61 degrees and afternoon highs of 81 degrees; the average winter morning low is 47 degrees, but the temperature usually rises to about 67 by afternoon. Dry weather is the rule, with relative humidity averaging slightly more than 50 percent yearly. The area average yearly rainfall of 14 inches occurs during the cooler season (November-April). Snow is a rarity, except in the outlying mountains and elevated desert regions.

Smoking is prohibited on all Anaheim public transportation and partially restricted in restaurants, private offices and public offices. The County Health Care Agency deploys mobile vans to administer immunizations (especially measles) and provide HIV testing. Public awareness campaigns are in effect against AIDS, sexually transmitted diseases, drugs, alcohol and hypertension. The city offers basic health-education programs to the public, including child safety, hypertension and drunk driving. Emergency hotlines are available for child abuse, suicide, AIDS information and sexual assault. The county is involved in a major program to discourage tobacco use among residents, particularly young people and ethnic populations. Health-care services are provided by bilingual staff speaking Chinese, Korean, Vietnamese, Cambodian, Laotian, Hmong, Spanish and other languages. Orange County has no hospital, but a unique partnership between the county and private hospitals provides a medical-care program for indigents. A new shelter for abused, abandoned and neglected children was built using funds from the county and the private sector. The Orange County Health Care Agency provides numerous health services in the City of Anaheim including: counseling, nurse health visits to residents, AIDS outreach, an International Refugee Assistance Project, a multi-service center for the homeless, drug and alcohol treatment, substandard-housing inspections and correction, monitoring of radiation, disposal of infectious wastes and a child-guidance center. Contact: Dr.

Thomas Prendergast, Orange County Health Care Agency, 515 N. Sycamore Street, Santa Ana, CA 92701.

Health Resources per 1,000 Pop.	Number	Rank
Hospital beds	4.71	71/92
Doctors	2.66	44/113

Anaheim operates three swimming pools, a multipurpose stadium, a nature center, four community recreation buildings, two senior centers and a human-service center. The city has traditionally used its school facilities to offer recreational programs, but as many schools convert to year-round classes, the city is now being left with a deficiency in indoor recreational space. Contact: Christopher Jarvi, Director, Anaheim Parks, Recreation, & Community Services, 200 South Anaheim Blvd., Anaheim, CA 92805.

Parkland/Total City Area (percent)	2.5

The Anaheim public-school system employs seven nurses for 13,500 students in kindergarten through sixth grade. These nurses work part-time in 100 percent of the schools. All common health-education programs are offered to students in grades K-6. No medical, dental or psychiatric treatment is provided for students. Contact: Dr. Mary Ellen Blanton, Deputy Superintendent, Anaheim City School District, 890 South Olive Street, Anaheim, CA 92805.

Anchorage, AK

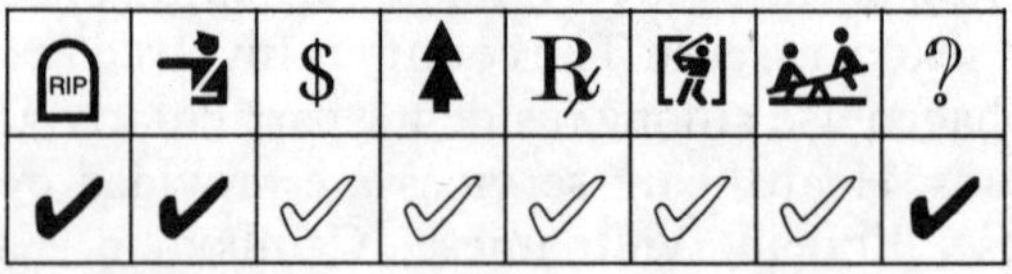

Anchorage (Borough County) has the second best age-adjusted death rate, after Honolulu. Infant-mortality rates for Alaska are low among blacks and whites, but relatively high among other minorities. Infant-mortality rates are almost the same in urban and rural areas.

	Number	Rank
Age-Adjusted Death Rate	−3.24	2/100
Heart Attacks	−0.81	7/100
Cancer	0.64	6/100

 Accident rates are high in Anchorage. Homicide, robbery and suicide rates are below average.

Incidence per 1,000 Pop.	Number	Rank
Homicides (1989)	0.05	27/111
Robberies	1.22	25/111
Suicides	0.11	38/100
Accidents	0.35	72/100

$ Anchorage's 1988 metro population was 218,000—103rd out of 113 metro areas. Its economic health at the end of 1990 was average, ranking 56th of 113 metro areas. Its unemployment rate ranks 51st, change in unemployment 5th (employment rose 4.9 percent while the labor force rose only 2.9 percent) and its enterprise 106th. Contact: Mayor Tom Fink, PO Box 196650, Anchorage, AK 99519-6650.

Air Quality: Anchorage violated air quality standards for only two pollutants, particulate matter and carbon monoxide. During extended dry periods, particulates become a problem. Carbon monoxide reaches elevated levels during the period from October through March, when temperature inversions and light winds trap pollutants close to the ground. Average daily carbon monoxide concentrations have dropped 50 percent since 1983 and the number of days in violation of National Ambient Air Quality Standards decreased to five in 1989 from 49 in 1983. Contact: Steve Morris, Program Manager, Air Quality, Municipality of Anchorage, Department of Health and Human Services, PO Box 196650, Anchorage, AK 99519-6650.

Water Quality: Water in Anchorage is supplied 80 percent by surface water (reservoirs) and 20 percent by ground water. Surface water sources are processed through the Ship Creek Water Treatment Facility and the Eklutna Water Treatment Facility. Samples from wells, water treatment plants and individual households are collected and tested in a state-certified lab. AWWU conducts more than 12,000 quality control tests each year. All public water supplies in Alaska meet the stringent quality standards of the ADEC (state) and EPA (federal). Contact: Mark Preyo, General Manager, Anchorage Water and Wastewater Utility, PO Box 196650, Anchorage, AK 99519-6650.

Weather: Anchorage is a frigid city, with an average daily temperature of only 35.3. It is also a dry city, with a normal precipitation of 15.2 inches annually.

Average Daily Temperature (degrees F)	35.3
High	42.4
Low	28.2
Average Humidity	
Morning (percent)	72
Afternoon (percent)	63
Annual Precipitation (inches)	15.2
Average Total Snowfall (inches)	68.6
Air Pollution Index (percent of mean)	99

℞ Anchorage sponsors health-awareness campaigns on AIDS and sexually transmitted diseases and the five major issues affecting teens, which are teen pregnancy, illiteracy, school drop-outs, juvenile crime and substance abuse. The city offers all basic health-education programs except anti-drug and prenatal and infant care. The city provides emergency hotlines for suicide and AIDS information. Anti-smoking laws in Anchorage prohibit smoking on public transportation and in public offices and partially restricts smoking in restaurants and private offices. Contact: Jeanne Wolf, Manager, Community Health, Department of Health and Human Services, PO Box 196650, Anchorage, AK 99519-6650.

Health Resources per 1,000 Pop.	Number	Rank
Hospitals	2.50	87/92
Nurses	2.66	85/90
Doctors	2.32	64/113

Anchorage's natural environment offers a wide variety of recreational facilities ranging from dog-sled trails to lighted ski trails for night skiing. Skiing facilities are particularly extensive. The city also has a winter sports facility, 121 miles of bike trails, and 50 tennis courts. Indoor and outdoor ice rinks accommodate hockey players and skaters. Water facilities include 4 beaches, 6 indoor swimming pools, small nonmotorized boating areas and fishing lakes. Contact: Bill Lindsey, Manager, Municipality of Anchorage, Parks and Recreation Division, PO Box 196650, Anchorage, AK 99519-6650.

Parkland/Total City Area (percent)	1.1

For the approximately 40,000 enrolled in the public school system, there are 60 nurses and 27 psychologists. 18 full-time nurses staff 24 percent of the schools and 56 part-time nurses staff the other 76 percent of the schools. Health-education programs are available to students in grades K-6 and 8. The city also has an AIDS education program. Contact: Robert A. Hall, Director, Municipality of Anchorage, Health and Human Services, PO Box 196650, Anchorage, AK 99519-6650.

Atlanta, GA

⌂RIP	⤴	$	↟	℞	🏃	👥	?
✔	✗	✔	✓	✓	✓	✗	✔

Atlanta (Fulton County) has a relatively low age-adjusted mortality rate. Infant-mortality rates for Georgia are high among minorities and in urban areas. Infant-mortality rates for whites are also high.

	Number	Rank
Age-Adjusted Death Rate	−1.69	12/100
Heart Attacks	−0.71	10/100
Cancer	−0.45	10/100

 Atlanta has high homicide, robbery and accident rates. Suicide rates are average.

Incidence per 1,000 Pop.	Number	Rank
Homicides (1989)	0.15	98/111
Robberies (1989)	4.29	101/111
Suicides	0.12	53/100
Accidents	0.35	70/100

Atlanta's 1988 metro population was 2,737,000—9th out of 113 metro areas. Its economic health at the end of 1990 was good, ranking 35th of 113 metro areas. Its unemployment rate ranks 64th, change in unemployment 58th (the labor force grew faster than employment) and its enterprise 5th. Contact: Mayor Maynard Jackson, City of

Atlanta, 55 Trinity Ave., S.W., Atlanta, GA 30335. Or: Tom Harris, same address (404) 330-6100.

Air Quality: In the 1985–90 period pollution levels changed little, despite major reductions in the volatile organic compounds that, along with nitrogen oxides, contribute to the formation of ozone. The Federal Pollutant Standards Index was 51.9 in 1986, rose to 54.5 in 1987, then dropped slightly below 50 into the "good" air quality zone in 1988 and 1989, but went up again to 51.3 (in the "moderate" zone) in 1990. Contact: Bob Collom, Chief, Air Protection Branch, Georgia Dept. of Natural Resources, 205 Butler St., #1162, Atlanta, GA 30334 (404) 656-6900.

Hazardous Waste: There are no hazardous-waste sites in Fulton County. All disposal of hazardous waste in the state of Georgia ceased prior to October 1, 1988. Contact: John Taylor, Branch Chief, Land Protection Branch, Georgia Dept. of Natural Resources, Floyd Towers East, #1154, Atlanta, GA 30335 (404) 656-7800.

Water Quality: 100 percent of Atlanta's water supply comes from surface water (reservoirs). Contact: Rob Rivers, Director, Bureau of Water, City Hall, Atlanta, GA 30315 (404) 330-6080.

Weather: Its elevation of 1,050 feet above sea level makes Atlanta the nation's second highest large city. Nonetheless, though the local climate does experience four distinct seasons, Atlanta is generally a warm, humid area.

Average Daily Temperature (degrees F)	61.2
High	71.3
Low	51.1
Average Humidity	
Morning (percent)	82
Afternoon (percent)	56
Annual Precipitation (inches)	48.6
Average Total Snowfall (inches)	1.9
Ozone days over 0.12 ppm (1 hour, 1988)	23

Fulton County sponsors 16 health-awareness campaigns which address AIDS and other sexually transmitted diseases, teen pregnancy, infant mortality, child health and child safety, maternal health, family planning, substance abuse, routine and emergency mental health, mental retardation, hypertension, the environment, TB, nutrition and supportive living. Other programs include an extensive outreach program, a street team for substance abuse and WIC (Women, Infants and Children) food packages for the homeless. Basic health-education programs and emergency hotlines are provided by the city. Smoking is prohibited on public transportation and partially restricted in public offices. Contact: Dr. William R. Elsea, Commissioner, Fulton County Health Dept., 99 Butler St., S.W., Atlanta, GA 30303 (404) 730-1200.

Health Resources per 1,000 Pop.	Number	Rank
Hospital beds	11.80	13/92
Nurses	13.64	11/90
Doctors	1.99	84/113

Atlanta provides 40 baseball fields, 35 football/soccer fields, 80 basketball courts, 100 tennis courts, 5 golf courses, 5 running tracks and 22 swimming pools. It sponsors a summer camping program for youth between 6 and 15 called Camp Best Friends. Contact: Jim Washington, Director, City of Atlanta Dept. of Parks, Recreation and Cultural Affairs, Garnett Station Place, #501, 236 Forsyth St., S.W., Atlanta, GA 30303 (404) 653-7091.

Parkland/Total City Area (percent)	3.6

For the 62,386 students in its schools, the school system employs 34 nurses, 4 physicians on a contractual basis, 20 psychologists and 28 social workers. Of the nurses, 32 are full time in all the middle schools, all the high schools and the vocational school. The remaining two nurses are itinerant for the exceptional-children program. The elementary schools are serviced by public-health nurses. All common health-education programs are offered to students in grades K-12. No medical, dental or psychiatric treatment is provided for students. Contact: Samuel A. Wallace, Coordinator, Health Services/Atlanta City Schools, 2960 Forest Hill Drive, S.W., Atlanta, GA 30315 (404) 827-8613.

Austin, TX

RIP	✈	$	🌲	℞	🏌	👪	?
✔	✓	✓	✓	✗	✓	?	✓

Austin (Travis County) has a relatively low age-adjusted mortality rate. Texas has low infant-mortality rates in rural areas and among whites; rates are high in cities and among minority populations.

	Number	Rank
Age-Adjusted Death Rate	−1.47	16/100
Heart Attacks	−0.49	17/100
Cancer	−0.32	18/100

 Austin has slightly higher-than-average suicide and accident rates and below-average homicide and robbery rates.

Incidence per 1,000 Pop.	Number	Rank
Homicides (1989)	0.07	46/111
Robberies (1989)	1.52	33/111
Suicides	1.02	62/100
Accidents	0.35	69/100

$ Austin's 1988 metro population was 747,000—58th out of 113 metro areas. Its economic health at the end of 1990 was below average, ranking 63rd of 113 metro areas. Its unemployment rate ranks 44th, change in unemployment 27th (employment grew slightly while the labor force shrunk slightly) and its enterprise 100th. Contact: Mayor Lee Cooke, City of Austin, PO Box 1088, Austin, TX 78767.

Air Quality: Despite significant growth over the past five years, the ozone level has remained within acceptable EPA standards. Contact: Doyle Pendleton, Deputy Director for Monitoring, Texas Air Control Board, 12124 Park 35 Circle, Austin TX 78753.

Hazardous Waste: On Home Chemical Waste Collection Day, 380 drums of hazardous waste were collected from homes. Information on hazardous-waste sites is unavailable. Contact; Marvin Erickson, Acting Director, Fire Department, PO Box 1088, Austin, TX 78767.

Water Quality: Austin's water supply comes entirely from surface water such as reservoirs. Recent increases in total hardness, chloride and sulfate are due to changes in source water. Contact: Randy Gross, Water and Wastewater Department, PO Box 1088, Austin, TX 78767.

Weather: Austin has a pleasant climate, with an average of 300 sunny days per year. In winter the temperature does not often dip below freezing. The normal daily temperature range during winter is from 42 to 62 degrees Fahrenheit. In summer the range is between 73 and 94 degrees.

Average Daily Temperature (degrees F)	68.1
High	78.6
Low	57.5

Average Humidity	
Morning (percent)	83
Afternoon (percent)	56
Annual Precipitation (inches)	31.5
Average Total Snowfall (inches)	1.1
Ozone-days over 0.12 ppm (1 hour, 1988)	0

℞ The city has some interesting new health programs. For example, in 1990 nursing assistants were hired to do some of the duties of regular nurses, thereby providing more nurse hours. Additional staff were also added to increase child health programs and a new Health Education Coordinator position was created to oversee and coordinate all health-education programs in the community. The city created a pilot chronic-disease screening program targeting those of the young and middle-aged black population who do not typically receive routine health care. It also sponsors a mass immunization program, a teen pregnancy-prevention program and a Woman and Infant Children awareness program. The city offers all common public health-education programs. Emergency hotlines are provided for child abuse, suicide and AIDS information. Also provided is a community mental health center crisis line. Austin has an anti-smoking law. Smoking is prohibited on all public transportation and partially restricted in restaurants and public and private offices where smoking is allowed only in designated areas. Contact: Dr. Solbritt Murphy, Health and Human Services Department, PO Box 1088, Austin, TX 78767.

Health Resources per 1,000 Pop.	Number	Rank
Hospital beds	3.06	87/92
Nurses	3.23	84/90
Doctors	1.87	91/113

Many varied programs are available through the school systems (including universities and colleges) and through the private sector. Public sports facilities include 106 tennis courts, 64 swimming pools, 62 baseball fields, 46 basketball courts, 22 football/soccer fields and 4 golf courses. Participation in sports leagues is high with 250 volleyball, 200 softball, 50 tennis and 50 basketball leagues. The city boasts 39 miles of hike-and-bike/jogging trails. A 3.3 mile Veloway, a 20-foot-wide asphalt surface with curbing, is scheduled for completion in 1991. Recreation facilities include a living history farm, 1 nature center and 3 senior citizen activity centers. The city offers several classes in aerobics, visual and performing arts, gymnastics, personal development and hiking. Contact: Charles Jordan, Director, Parks and Recreation Department, PO Box 1088, Austin, TX 78767.

Parkland/Total City Area (percent)   7.5

 Austin did not return a school-health questionnaire.

Bakersfield, CA

RIP	⌧	$	♠	℞	🚑	👥	?
?	✓	x	✓	x	?	?	x

 Bakersfield's (Kern County) age-adjusted death rate was not computed. The state has a low infant-mortality rate for whites, while that of blacks is high at 246/301. The rate for urban areas is also considerably higher than that of rural ones because most of the state's blacks live in the cities.

Bakersfield has average homicide and robbery rates.

Incidence per 1,000 Pop.	Number	Rank
Homicides (1989)	0.09	63/111
Robberies (1989)	2.02	56/111

$ Bakersfield's 1988 metro population was 520,000—77th out of 113 metro areas. Its economic health at the end of 1990 was very poor, ranking 110th of 113 metro areas. Its unemployment rate ranks 111th, change in unemployment 107th (employment declined faster than the labor force) and its enterprise 82nd. Contact: Clarence E. Medders, City of Bakersfield, 1501 Truxton Avenue, Bakersfield, CA 93301.

Air Quality: Industrial and oil field combustion equipment have switched to cleaner-burning fuels, such as natural gas. Contact: William Roddy, Air Pollution Control Officer, 2700 M Street, Suite 275, Bakersfield, CA 93301.

Weather: The average daily temperature is a warm 65.6. Precipitation is extremely low, averaging 5.7 inches annually.

Average Daily Temperature (degrees F)	65.6
High	77.7
Low	53.3
Average Humidity	
Morning (percent)	65
Afternoon (percent)	38
Annual Precipitation (inches)	5.7
Average Total Snowfall (inches)	Trace
Ozone-days over 0.12 ppm (1 hour, 1988)	5

℞ Discouragement of smoking has become an increasing priority in Bakersfield. Programs to help the public quit smoking have been started. The city has all the common emergency hotlines and health-education programs.

 The city did not return a recreation questionnaire.

 The city did not return a school-health questionnaire.

Baltimore, MD

⚰ RIP	🏃	$	🌲	℞	🏃	👥	?
X	X	✓	X	✔	✓	✓	✔

⚰ RIP Baltimore (Baltimore County) ranks among the least healthy metro areas—in the bottom quartile on the age-adjusted mortality rate. However, its heart-attack rate is low; it's the cancer rate that is high. Maryland has a very high infant-mortality rate for blacks, while that of whites is relatively low. The rate for urban areas is also considerably higher than that of rural ones, since most of the state's minorities live in the cities.

	Number	Rank
Age-Adjusted Death Rate	0.66	73/100
Heart Attacks	−0.47	19/100
Cancer	0.24	81/100

Baltimore has a high robbery rate, 10th highest of 111 metro areas. The accident rate is average and the suicide rate is in the lowest third, perhaps reflecting the Roman Catholic origins of this city (Lord Baltimore's family, the Calverts, sought a refuge for Catholics), although Catholics now constitute fewer than 20 percent of the population.

Incidence per 1,000 Pop.	Number	Rank
Homicides (1989)	0.14	96/111
Robberies (1989)	4.45	102/111
Suicides	0.11	27/100
Accidents	0.33	58/100

Baltimore's 1988 metro population was 2,342,000—15th out of 113 metro areas. Its economic health at the end of 1990 was below average, ranking 67th of 113 metro areas. Its unemployment rate ranks 75th, change in unemployment 91st (employment declined while the labor force increased slightly) and its enterprise 15th. Contact: Mayor Kurt L. Schmoke, City of Baltimore, Office of the Mayor, City Hall, Baltimore, MD 21202.

Weather: Even though Baltimore is not very far south, the proximity of the ocean helps keep the winters relatively mild. The summers are hot and humid, with a month's worth of days in the 90s.

Average Daily Temperature (degrees F)	55.1
High	65.0
Low	45.1
Average Humidity	
Morning (percent)	77
Afternoon (percent)	54
Annual Precipitation (inches)	41.8
Average Total Snowfall (inches)	21.9

Smoking is restricted to designated areas in restaurants and other public buildings. The city has all the common health-education programs and all the common emergency hotlines. Baltimore is well supplied with health resources—in the top 25 cities for hospital beds and nurses and in the top 15 for doctors. The presence of Johns Hopkins University is a major asset. Contact: Elias Dorsey, Commissioner of Health, Baltimore City Health Department, 303 East Fayette Street, Baltimore, MD 21202 (301) 396-4392.

Health Resources per 1,000 Pop.

Health Resources per 1,000 Pop.	Number	Rank
Hospital beds, community hospitals, city	8.98	23/92
Nurses, community hospitals, city	10.90	19/90
Doctors, metro	3.51	14/113

Baltimore has extensive sports fields and facilities, including 223 baseball fields, 172 basketball courts and 115 tennis courts. For sports leagues the city has 69 softball, 66 soccer, 78 baseball, 32 basketball and 5 volleyball leagues. Baltimore's harbor provides a rowing center, 2 boat launches and 1 fishing pier. There are special programs available for the mentally and physically handicapped and for senior citizens. These programs include swimming, nature walks, indoor and outdoor track and field training, craft design and pre-school care. The city has been reevaluating its recreational programs. Contact: Marilyn J. Perritt, Director of Recreation and Parks, 222 East Saratoga Street, Baltimore, MD 21202.

Parkland/Total City Area (percent)	11
Aerobics classes	yes
Arts and craft classes	yes
Hiking or exploration groups	yes
Other Activities: rowing, fishing, crabbing, canoeing, roller skating, bowling, dance (tap, ballet), soccer clinics, theatre.	

To serve 110,000 students (grades K-12) in the public school system, are 61 nurses, 2 physicians, 30 health aides and 10 nurse practitioners. A full-time nurse available in ten percent of the schools and a part-time nurse in 90 percent. Contact: John Santelli, M.D., M.P.H., Director of School and Adolescent Health, Baltimore City Health Department, 303 East Fayette Street, 2nd Floor, Baltimore, MD 21202.

Baton Rouge, LA

⚰️	🏃	$	🌲	℞	🚶	👫	?
✓	X	✓	?	X	?	?	XX

Baton Rouge (East Baton County) ranks in the middle on overall health, the average age-adjusted mortality rate. Louisiana has a very low infant-mortality rate for whites (30/301), while the rate for blacks ranks very high at 265/301. The rate for rural areas is also lower than that of urban ones, but even the rate for rural areas is substantially higher than the rate for whites alone.

	Number	Rank
Age-Adjusted Death Rate	−0.21	46/100
Heart Attacks	0.09	62/100
Cancer	0.05	59/100

The city has high rates for homicide and accidents, but a relatively low number of robberies.

Incidence per 1,000 Pop.	Number	Rank
Homicides (1989)	0.12	89/111
Robberies (1989)	1.72	39/111
Suicides	0.13	61/100
Accidents	0.37	82/100

$ Baton Rouge's 1988 metro population was 536,000—75th out of 113 metro areas. Its economic health at the end of 1990 was below average, ranking 58th of 113 metro areas. Its unemployment rate ranks 106th, change in unemployment 1st (employment grew 2.7 percent while the labor force declined, yielding a decline in unemployment, as in New Orleans, from 8.4 percent to 5.4 percent) and its enterprise 60th. Contact: Mayor Tom McHugh, City of Baton Rouge, City Hall, Baton Rouge, LA.

Weather: Baton Rouge is warm and wet, with an average daily high of 78, and an average annual precipitation of 55.8.

Average Daily Temperature (degrees F)	67.5
High	78.0
Low	57.0

Average Humidity
    Morning (percent)   88
    Afternoon (percent)   59
    Annual Precipitation (inches)   55.8
    Average Total Snowfall (inches)   0.1

The city did not respond to the health services survey.

Health Resources per 1,000 Pop.	Number	Rank
Hospital beds	6.49	49/91
Nurses	6.57	56/90
Doctors	1.64	102/113

The city did not respond to the recreational facilities survey.

The city did not respond to the school-health survey.

Billings, MT

🪦	🏊	$	🌲	℞	🥾	🛝	?
?	✓	✗	✔	✓	✔	✔	✔

Billings (Yellowstone County) was not rated using the age-adjusted death rate. Montana has a high infant-mortality rate for minorities (224/301), while the rate for whites is below average. The urban rate is much higher than the rural one since most of the state's minorities live in the cities. The infant-mortality rate is not shown for blacks because Montana has too few black children for the death rate to be significant, in the view of the Federal Government.

	Number	Rank
Infant Mortality (Montana)		
All Areas	10.0	143/301
Other	13.9	224/301
Rural	8.9	77/301
Urban Places	12.0	198/301
Whites	9.3	100/301

Billings is ranked extremely well for robberies and a little lower than average for homicides.

Incidence per 1,000 Pop.	Number	Rank
Homicides (1989)	0.07	48/111
Robberies (1989)	0.49	5/111

$ Billings' 1988 metro population was 116,000—111th out of 113 metro areas. Its economic health at the end of 1990 was below average, ranking 81st of 113 metro areas. Its unemployment rate ranks 62nd, change in unemployment 52nd (the labor force grew by a whopping 8.1 percent, outpacing employment's 7.8 percent growth) and its enterprise 89th. Contact: Mayor James Van Arsdale, City of Billings, PO Box 1178, Billings, MT 59103.

Air Quality: Major industries have taken voluntary steps to reduce emissions. As a result, concentrations of carbon dioxide have steadily fallen. Contact: Steve Duganz, Director, City-County Air Pollution Control, 3306 2nd Ave. North, Billings, MT 59101.

Water Quality: All of Billings' water supply comes from surface-water reservoirs. The pH of the drinking water is 7.72. Contact: Gerald Underwood, Director, Public Utilities Department, PO Box 30958, Billings, MT 59111.

Weather: Billings is a cool city (average daily temperature of 46.7) and a dry one (precipitation of only 15.1 inches annually).

Average Daily Temperature (degrees F)	46.7
High	57.9
Low	35.4
Average Humidity	
Morning (percent)	66
Afternoon (percent)	44
Annual Precipitation (inches)	15.1
Average Total Snowfall (inches)	56.7
Ozone days over 0.12 ppm (one hour)	0

℞ Smoking is partially restricted in restaurants and public offices and prohibited on public transportation. The city has all the common health-education programs and all the common emergency hotlines as well as those for victims of domestic violence, community help, rape crisis and runaways. Contact: Dr. George Sheckleton, City-County Health Department, Yellowstone County Courthouse, Billings, MT 59101.

Billings' sports facilities include 65 baseball fields, 36 tennis courts, 17 football/soccer fields, 15 basketball courts, 6 golf courses and a cross country running track. Every year in April there is a three-part Peaks to Prairie race. It includes a race of 8.4 miles from 8,000 feet to 5,800 feet, a 42-mile bike race and 22-mile canoe race down the Yellowstone River. Contact: Mike Hinks, Director, Parks, Recreation & Public Lands, 510 North Broadway, Billings, MT 59101.

Parkland/Total City Area (percent)   9

To serve 15,137 students in the public-school system (grades K-12) are 10 RNs and 2 LPNs, 13 psychologists and 2 health clerks. A part-time nurse is available in all of the schools. The city has all the common health-education programs as well as those on AIDS education, human growth & development and family life. Dental treatment and vision-assistance programs are provided for students. Contact: Department of Pupil Services, Billings Public Schools, 915 North 30th Street, Billings, MT 59102.

Birmingham, AL

⚰️	⚡	$	↑	℞	🏃	👥	?
X	X	✓	✓	✓	X	X	✔

Birmingham (Jefferson County) residents have a high age-adjusted death rate, ranking 82nd out of 100 cities. They have a high cancer rate and a relatively low heart disease rate. Infant-mortality rates in Alabama are high; only whites taken alone are below 10 deaths per thousand live births.

	Number	Rank
Age-Adjusted Death Rate	9.26	82/100
Heart Attacks	−0.03	32/100
Cancer	0.17	75/100

Birmingham residents have a relatively low suicide rate but the metro area has quite a high robbery rate and one of the highest homicide rates. Birmingham has the 5th highest accidental-death rate of 100 metro areas.

Incidence per 1,000 Pop.	Number	Rank
Homicides	0.15	99/111
Robberies	2.74	76/111
Suicides	0.12	42/100
Accidents	0.47	96/100

$ Birmingham's 1988 metro population was 923,000—53rd out of 113 metro areas. Its economic health at the end of 1990 was good, ranking 38th of 113 metro areas. Its unemployment rate ranks 56th, change in unemployment 27th (its employment growth slightly outpaced the labor force growth) and its enterprise 50th. Contact: Mayor Richard Arrington, City of Birmingham, 710 North 20th Street, Birmingham, AL 35703.

Air Quality: Birmingham had 6 days of ozone exceedances in 1988. Contact: Robert Ferguson, Director of Environmental Services, Jefferson County Board of Health, 1400 6th Avenue South, PO Box 2648, Birmingham, AL 35202.

Weather: Birmingham is warm and wet, with an average daily temperature of 62, an average humidity of 84 percent in the morning, and an annual precipitation of 52.2 inches.

Average Daily Temperature (degrees F)	62.0
High	72.7
Low	51.3
Average Humidity	
Morning (percent)	84
Afternoon (percent)	57
Annual Precipitation (inches)	52.2
Average Total Snowfall (inches)	2.4
Ozone-days over 0.12 ppm (one hour)	6

℞ The Jefferson County Department of Health provides all common emergency hotlines and health-education programs. In recent years, the County has placed greater emphasis on access to care through neighborhood clinics. One such clinic is based in a school. Birmingham has anti-smoking laws that partially restrict smoking in restaurants, public and private offices and on public transportation. Contact: Dr. Mary Ann Pass, Deputy Health Officer, Jefferson County Board of Health, PO Box 2646, Birmingham, AL 35202.

Health Resources per 1,000 Pop.	Number	Rank
Hospital beds	15.85	4/92
Doctors	2.71	41/113

The park board helps sponsor a rugby team that plays against teams from all over the Southeast. Birmingham has 50 baseball fields, 22 football/soccer fields, 3 golf courses, 10 running tracks and 16 swimming pools. The city operates 52 softball leagues, 7 basketball leagues, 7 volleyball leagues and 9 tennis leagues. The city also provides a special day camp for the mentally retarded. Contact: Melvin Miller, Director, Parks and Recreation Board, 400 Graymont Avenue, Birmingham, AL 35204.

Parkland/Total City Area (percent)	2.4
Aerobics classes	yes
Arts and craft classes	yes
Hiking or exploration groups	yes

The city employs six full-time nurses and an audiologist for the 41,135 students in its school system. Each nurse is responsible for an average of 13 schools. All common health education topics are taught between Kindergarten and ninth grade. The school system requires but not administer immunizations. Contact: Dr. Cleveland Hammonds, Superintendent, Birmingham Board of Education, PO Box 10007, Birmingham, AL 35202.

Bismarck, ND

🪦	🚴	$	🌲	℞	🏃	👥	?
?	✔	✔	x	✓	✔	x	✔

Bismarck (Burleigh County) was not rated using the age-adjusted death rate. North Dakota has a very low infant-mortality rate (ranking 67th out of 301), which is higher in urban areas but is still better than most other states. But the ranking for nonwhites is much higher, 222nd out of 301 (no infant-mortality rate is shown for blacks because too few black babies were born in the state to permit meaningful statistical analysis, in the view of the Federal Government). Contact: Dr. William Buckingham, Health Officer, City of Bismarck, Family Practice Center, 515 East Broadway, Bismarck, ND 58502.

Bismarck is one of the safest cities in the country, with the lowest robbery rate and the 2nd lowest homicide rate.

Incidence per 1000 Pop.	Number	Rank
Homicides (1989)	0.01	2/111
Robberies (1989)	0.09	1/111

| $ | Bismarck's 1988 metro population was 86,000—112th out of 113 metro areas. Its economic health at the end of 1990 was excellent, ranking 21st of 113 metro areas. Its unemployment rate ranks 6th, change in unemployment 7th (employment increased 3 percent, nearly twice the rate of growth of the labor force) and its enterprise 90th. Contact: Mayor Bill Sorensen, City of Bismarck, City Hall, Bismarck, ND 58502.

Hazardous Waste: There are no hazardous wastes sites in the county. All hazardous waste is disposed of by private firms. Contact: Jack Hegedus, Director of Fire & Inspections, City of Bismarck Fire & Inspection Department, 1020 East Central Avenue, Bismarck, ND 58502.

Water Quality: Bismarck's drinking water supply comes from surface water (Missouri River). Contact: Jack Hegedus, Director, Fire & Inspections Department, 1020 East Central Avenue, Bismarck, ND 58502.

Weather: Bismarck is a cool city, with a high humidity, low precipitation (15.4 inches annually), but a high average snowfall at 41 inches.

Average Daily Temperature (degrees F)	41.3
High	53.5
Low	29.1
Average Humidity	
Morning (percent)	80
Afternoon (percent)	57
Annual Precipitation (inches)	15.4
Average Total Snowfall (inches)	41.0
Ozone-days over 0.12 ppm (1 hour, 1988)	NA

℞ The public-transit system is not accessible to the handicapped, but buses are available to the elderly and handicapped through various private organizations. The city recently started a program of cholesterol screening and free blood-pressure screening (many clinics are at work sites in the community). Smoking is partially prohibited in restaurants, on public transportation and in public and private offices. The city provides all common emergency hotlines and health-education programs. Contact:

Doris Fischer, Director of Bismarck-Burleigh Nursing Service, 221 North 5th, PO Box 5503, Bismarck, ND 58501.

The City of Bismarck offers 24 baseball fields, 7 football/soccer fields, 34 basketball courts, 23 tennis courts, 2 golf courses, 5 running tracks, 3 swimming pools, a beach and 2 public boat ramps. It also has a gymnastics center, a 3-hole junior golf course, 11 miles of walking-jogging-bicycle trails (used by up to 1,000 people per day in nice weather), a civic center, a city auditorium, a full service camp ground, two indoor-ice arenas, one recreation center, 12 outdoor skating rinks, 24 horseshoe courts, an amusement park, one indoor and one outdoor archery range, one indoor rifle/pistol range, a horse arena, weight facilities and 8 racquetball courts. In 1986 the District started a new Matching Grants Program, whereby clubs and organizations operating within Park District facilities can apply for matching grants up to $5,000 for program operation and facility development. Of interest is the historical interpretative site of a Native American Indian Village. The Bismarck Parks and Recreation District offers over 450 classes, leagues, and special event opportunities for a variety of age groups, abilities, and skills. In addition, the city has many unique recreation facilities such as the Tom O'Leary Complex, which contains a golf course, a driving range, two putting greens, tennis courts and other facilities and the VFW All Seasons Arena, with an indoor ice arena, curling rink and activity rooms. Contact: Steve Neu, Director, Bismarck Parks and Recreation District, 215 North 6th Street, Bismarck, ND 58502.

Parkland/Total City Area (percent)	19
Aerobics classes	yes
Arts and craft classes	yes
Hiking or exploration groups	yes

For a total of 10,500 students (grades K-12) in the public school system, there are three psychologists available. No nurses are available in the schools. A new AIDS curriculum was recently added for grades four and five. All common health-education courses are offered in grades K-8 and are electives in high school. Contact: Dr. Sharon Johnson, Assistant Superintendent, Curriculum and Secondary Schools, Bismarck Public Schools, 400 Avenue E, Bismarck, ND 58502.

Boise, ID

RIP	⫧	$	♠	℞	🏃	👫	?
✔	✔	✔	✓	X	✓	X	✔

Boise (Ada County) has a low age-adjusted death rate, mostly attributable to its low cancer rate, 13th of 100 metropolitan areas. Infant-mortality rates for Idaho are slightly higher than the median rate for all states. Too few black babies were born in Idaho to permit a meaningful statistic for this category, but the "other" nonwhite category was identical to the rate for whites.

	Number	Rank
Age-Adjusted Death Rate	−1.27	18/100
Heart Attacks	0.01	56/100
Cancer	−0.36	13/100

Boise has the lowest homicide rate and second lowest robbery rate of 111 large metropolitan areas. But, at the same time, it has the third highest suicide rate. Boise has a relatively high accident rate, reflecting the very high traffic-accident rate on its highways.

Incidence per 1,000 Pop.	Number	Rank
Homicides (1989)	0.01	1/111
Robberies (1989)	0.24	2/111
Suicides	0.21	98/100
Accidents	0.32	39/100

Boise's 1988 metro population was 201,000—106th out of 113 metro areas. Its economic health at the end of 1990 was good, ranking 30th of 113 metro areas. Its unemployment rate ranks 9th, change in unemployment 52nd (the labor force grew slightly more than employment, but neither changed much) and its enterprise 59th. Contact: Mayor Dirk Kempthorne, City of Boise, Office of the Mayor, PO Box 500, Boise, ID 83701-0500.

Air Quality: Carbon monoxide levels downtown have been decreasing over the past five years. The wood stove curtailment program administered by the City of Boise with advice from the IAAB appears to be effective. Contact: Dave Pisarski, State of Idaho Air Quality Bureau, 450 West State Street, Boise, ID 83720.

Hazardous Waste: There are no active or inactive waste sites in Ada County on the EPA's National Priorities List for "Superfund" in 1990. The first annual home hazardous-waste collection day was held on June 10, 1989. Waste oil pick-up at the curbside began in the summer of 1989 for all city customers. Contact: Robert Finch, Director, Public Works Department, PO Box 500, Boise, ID 83701.

Water Quality: 100 percent of Boise's water supply is ground water. Contact: Division of Environmental Quality, Boise Field Office, 801 Reserve Street, Boise, ID 83712.

Weather: Boise's average daily temperature is about average at 51.1. Precipitation is low at 11.7 inches annually.

Average Daily Temperature (degrees F)	51.1
High	62.8
Low	39.3
Average Humidity	
Morning	69
Afternoon	43
Annual Precipitation (inches)	11.7
Average Total Snowfall (inches)	21.4

℞ Boise provides all common emergency hotlines except for sexually transmitted diseases. It provides all common health-education programs. Anti-smoking laws in Boise partially restrict smoking in restaurants and public offices and on public transportation. Smoking is not restricted in private offices. Contact: Hewey Reed, Director, Central District Health, 145 Orchard, Boise, ID 83704.

Boise offers 18 softball fields, 18 football/soccer fields, 36 basketball courts, 19 tennis courts, 5 swimming pools and 12 outdoor horseshoe pitches. It sponsors 8 basketball leagues, 5 volleyball leagues, 9 softball leagues and 2 flag football leagues. One of the city's parks, Boise River Greenbelt, covers approximately 86 acres along the river through Boise. It links a golf course and six major parks which when fully developed will offer close to 800 acres of public open space. Wildlife can be spotted along the entire length of the Greenbelt. Contact: Director, Boise Park System, PO Box 500, Boise, ID 83701-0500.

Parkland/Total City Area (percent)	2.7
Aerobics classes	yes
Arts and craft classes	yes
Hiking or exploration groups	yes

Boise offers all common health-education programs in grade 9, except for sex education. The public school system employs 17 nurses and 12 psychologists for 22,601 students. It has a consulting contract with two physicians. There are part-time nurses available in 98 percent of the schools and full-time nurses in 1.3 percent of the schools. Dental treatment is provided for students. Contact: Barney Parker, Superintendent, City Independent School District, 1207 Fort Street, Boise, ID 83702.

Boston, MA

RIP	🏃	$	⬆	℞	🏃	🪑	?
X	✔	X	?	✔	X	✔	✓

The primary Boston metro area includes close-in suburban areas such as Cambridge and Somerville. The age-adjusted death rate for the primary metro area is higher than average, ranking in the worst third of 100 metro areas. The explanation is not hard to find—both age-adjusted heart attacks and cancer rank in the worst fifth of metro areas. Boston appears to be a leading example of how lifestyle contributes to the early deaths of Americans generally. A strong public-health effort by the state of Massachusetts has produced a very low infant-mortality rate in rural areas and among whites (2nd and 3rd lowest). Even the urban areas are 13th lowest. But among blacks the rate is high, ranking 226th of 301 rated states and groups.

	Number	Rank
Age-Adjusted Death Rate	0.55	69/100
Heart Attacks	0.39	80/100
Cancer	0.25	82/100

Boston has relatively low rates of homicide, suicide and accidents. It does, however, have a high number of robberies.

Incidence per 1,000 Pop.	Number	Rank
Homicides (1989)	0.04	21/111
Robberies (1989)	2.91	82/111
Suicides	0.08	12/100
Accidents	0.27	13/100

$ Boston's 1988 metro population was 2,845,000—8th out of 113 metro areas. The City of Boston (in Boston-Suffolk County) is part of the consolidated metro Boston area consisting of Boston; Brockton, MA (population 185,000); Lawrence-Haverhill, MA-NH (population 375,000); Lowell, MA-NH (260,000); Nashua, NH (172,000), and Salem-Gloucester, MA 258,000). The primary metro area's economic health at the end of 1990 was poor, ranking 100th of 113 metro areas. Its unemployment rate ranks 74th, change in unemployment 104th (employment fell by over 4 percent while the labor force dropped only 1.8 percent) and its enterprise 68th. Contact: Mayor Raymond L. Flynn, City of Boston, Boston City Hall, Boston, MA 02201.

Manchester's 1988 metro population was 150,000—108th out of 113 metro areas. Its economic health at the end of 1990 was poor, ranking 104th of 113 metro areas, a change in fortune from a few years ago when it was a burgeoning outpost of Boston's prosperity. Its unemployment rate ranks 95th, change in unemployment 113th (the worst situation among all the cities—employment dropped by 2.9 percent while the labor force increased 1.9 percent) and its enterprise 63rd.

↟ **Hazardous Waste:** No legal disposal site for hazardous waste dumping remains in Massachusetts in 1990. A proposal for a hazardous waste incinerator was under review in late 1990. It would be located about 20 miles southeast of Boston. Contact: Superintendent, Hazardous Waste, c/o Office of the Mayor, Boston City Hall, 1 City Hall Plaza, Boston, MA 02201.

Water Quality: In 1988, drinking water was declared unsafe in 40 Boston grade schools and water in 19 schools contained lead levels just below the Environmental Protection Agency limits. As a result the city was forced to ship in bottled water to half the elementary schools.

Weather: The weather is varied and unpredictable. Situated on Massachusetts Bay at the mouths of the Mystic and Charles rivers, Boston is surrounded on three sides by water. The city's wet and changeable weather is largely determined by the Atlantic's sea breezes. The city receives a great deal of rain and snow, with an average of 128 days a years having some precipitation. Boston is also the second windiest city in America (after Corpus Christi), with winds averaging over 12 miles per hour.

Average Daily Temperature (degrees F)	51.5
High	59.0
Low	43.9
Average Humidity	
Morning (percent)	72

Afternoon (percent)   58
Annual Precipitation (inches)   43.8
Average Total Snowfall (inches)   41.5

℞ | The city did not return a public-health questionnaire. It has the highest ratio of doctors to population of 69 cities for which we have this information, the 6th highest number of nurses and the 20th highest number of hospital beds, reflecting its strong teaching hospitals.

Health Resources per 1,000 Pop.	Number	Rank
Hospital beds	10.42	20/92
Nurses	15.48	6/90
Doctors	5.28	2/113

The City of Boston has 50 baseball fields, 5 football/soccer fields, 75 basketball courts, 24 tennis courts, 2 golf courses, 6 running tracks and 20 swimming pools. The city recently added four Tot Lot playgrounds and a recreational facility for children to Boston Parks. The central city is quite small relative to the metropolitan area, which has many more public facilities. The area is also blessed with a large number of first-rate university facilities that are frequently available to outsiders for a fee. Contact: Donald Gillis, Director, Neighborhood Services, Boston City Hall, 1 City Hall Plaza, Boston, MA 02201.

The school system offers all common health-education topics in grades K through 12, plus special programs on AIDS, tuberculosis, self-esteem, depression and suicide. It employs 80 nurses, 1 physician and 50 psychologists. A full-time nurse is available in 25 percent of the schools and a part-time nurse in the rest of the schools. Medical, dental and psychiatric treatment is provided for students. Contact: Michael Grady, M.D., Program Director, Boston Public Schools, 26 Court Street, Boston, MA 02108.

Bridgeport, CT

⚰️RIP	🏃	$	🌲	℞	🏚️	🏕️	?
✔	✓	X	✔	✔	?	✔	✓

Bridgeport (Fairfield County) is a healthy metro area. It has the fifth lowest age-adjusted death rate of 100 metropolitan areas. Both its age-adjusted cancer rate and heart disease rate are among the 15 lowest. The state's infant-mortality rate varies widely between whites, with a low 7.3 deaths per thousand live births, and blacks, with 19.5 per thousand.

	Number	Rank
Age-Adjusted Death Rate	−2.63	5/100
Heart Attacks (Bridgeport-Stamford)	−0.61	14/100
Cancer (Bridgeport-Stamford)	−0.45	09/100

The city's suicide and accident rates are also low but its robbery rate is high, among the highest 20 metro areas, and the homicide rate is higher than the median.

Incidence per 1,000 Pop.	Number	Rank
Homicides	0.10	73/111
Robberies	3.88	97/111
Suicides (Bridgeport-Stamford)	0.07	6/100
Accidents	0.28	17/100

$ Bridgeport's 1988 metro population was 444,000—84th out of 113 metro areas. Its economic health at the end of 1990 was poor, ranking 102nd of 113 metro areas. In mid-1991 Bridgeport sought protection from its creditors under a bankruptcy filing. Its unemployment rate ranks 76th, change in unemployment 103rd (employment declined while the labor force grew) and its enterprise 81st. Contact: Mayor Mary Moran, City of Bridgeport, 45 Lyon Terrace-B, Bridgeport, CT 06604.

Air Quality: The air has improved in recent years as measured by carbon monoxide, sulfur dioxide, acidity and particulate matter. Contact: Leslie Carouthers, Commissioner, State Department of Environmental Protection, 165 Capitol Avenue, Hartford, CT 06106.

Weather: Bridgeport's average daily temperature is close to average at 51.9 degrees. The city has a high annual precipitation at 41.6 inches.

Average Daily Temperature (degrees F)	51.9
High	59.7
Low	43.9
Average Humidity	
Morning	76
Afternoon	60
Annual Precipitation (inches)	41.6
Average Total Snowfall (inches)	25.4
Ozone-days over 0.12 ppm (1 hour, 1988)	18

℞ Bridgeport offers all common health-education programs, and all common emergency hotlines except for sexually transmitted diseases. The city has public-awareness campaigns concerning blood pressure, AIDS and infant mortality. Smoking is prohibited on public transportation and partially prohibited in public and private offices. Contact: Tim Callahan, City of Bridgeport Health Department, 752 East Main Street, Bridgeport, CT 06608.

The city did not respond to the survey of recreational facilities.

 Bridgeport offers all common health-education topics. For 19,781 students (grades K-12), it provides 27 nurses, one physician and one nurse practitioner. A full-time nurse is available in 11 percent of the schools and a part-time nurse is available in the rest of the schools. Dental treatment is provided for students. Bridgeport is undergoing a severe financial crisis resulting in a reduction of school-health personnel. Contact: Maureen Kunkel, M.D., Bridgeport Health Department, 752 East Main Street, Bridgeport, CT 06608.

Buffalo, NY

🪦	🛌	$	↟	℞	🏃	👥	?
X	✔	✓	?	✓	?	?	XX

🪦 Buffalo (Erie County) has the highest age-adjusted death rate of the 100 metropolitan areas we compared—as might be expected from the fact that it has the highest age-adjusted heart-disease *and* cancer rates of these 100 areas. We used the primary Buffalo metropolitan area. Buffalo has the highest *unadjusted* rates as well—the only metropolitan area with over 3 deaths per thousand population from cancer and the only one with over 4 deaths per thousand from heart attacks. The consolidated Buffalo area adds in Niagara Falls, NY (population 216,000). Statewide, infant-mortality rates are higher in cities than in rural areas (12.3 vs. 7.8) and are higher for blacks than whites (17.2 vs. 12.3). Contact: Dr. Ralph Citron, Commissioner of Health, Erie County Health Department, 95 Franklin Street, Buffalo, NY 14202 (716) 858-6327.

	Number	Rank
Age-Adjusted Death Rate	4.23	100/100
Heart Attacks	0.98	100/100
Cancer	2.14	100/100

 Buffalo's homicide rate is relatively low, but its accident rate is in the highest quartile.

Incidence per 1,000 Pop.	Number	Rank
Homicides	0.04	25/111
Robberies	2.17	61/111
Suicides	0.13	56/100
Accidents	0.36	76/100

$ Buffalo's 1988 metro population was 959,000—50th out of 113 metro areas. Its economic health at the end of 1990 was good, ranking 41st of 113 metro areas. Its unemployment rate ranks 34th, change in unemployment 19th (the labor force declined 1.4 percent while employment grew slightly) and its enterprise 88th. The really good economic news for Buffalo is that it has been discovered by prospering Torontonians as a city with relatively low labor and real estate costs. Contact: Mayor James D. Griffin, City of Buffalo, 65 Niagara Square, Buffalo, NY 14202.

Hazardous Waste: The Western New York area, which includes Buffalo, developed the first hazardous-waste situation catastophic enough to attract national attention to the health risks of inactive hazardous-waste sites. In the Love Canal area of the City of Niagara Falls, just north of Buffalo, chemical burns appeared on children playing near the waste-disposal site. Several companies in the chemical-industry areas near Love Canal and the Forest Glen Trailer Park were identified as disposing of such chemicals as aniline and phenothiazine, which are byproducts of processing rubber and photographs. Erie County has a hazardous-waste site at Wide Beach in Brant. The soil is contaminated from PCB oils. Contact: Richard M. Tobe, Commissioner of Environment & Planning,

Erie County Department of Environment & Planning, 95 Franklin Street, Buffalo, NY 14202 (716) 858-6716.

Weather: The city's average daily high temperature is close to average at 55.8. Annual precipitation is high at 37.5 inches, with much of that coming in the form of snow (92.3 inches of snow annually).

Average Daily Temperature (degrees F)	
High	55.8
Low	39.3
Average Humidity	
Morning (percent)	80
Afternoon (percent)	63
Annual Precipitation (inches)	37.5
Average Total Snowfall (inches)	92.3

 Buffalo is well supplied with health facilities, ranking 8th of 69 areas in doctors and 18th in nurses. The county provides all common health-education programs and emergency hotlines. Its hotlines include Tel-Med and cancer information. Other specific health issues the county addresses are AIDS, sexually transmitted diseases generally, smoking cessation, infant and maternal care, nutrition and medically indigent. The Erie County Health Department converted one of its health centers into an exclusively maternal and infant care center. Contact: Dr. Ralph Citron, Commissioner of Health, Erie County Health Department, 95 Franklin Street, Buffalo, NY 14202.

Health Resources per 1,000 Pop.	Number	Rank
Hospital beds	NA	
Nurses	12.19	18/90
Doctors	2.92	29/113

 The city did not respond to the recreational-facilities survey.

The city did not respond to the school-health survey.

Burlington, VT

⚰️	⛏️	$	🌲	℞	🖼️	🛏️	?
X	✔	✓	?	✔	✔	?	X

 Burlington (Chittenden County) is in the bottom quartile in age-adjusted death rates, despite being in a less-congested part of the country with clean air and water. All of the death rates we focus on are below average except age-adjusted ischemic heart disease, which is higher than average. We might speculate that the local dairy industry encourages high-fat diets that contribute to high blood cholesterol and cardiovascular diseases. Though Vermont has few blacks, those that had children in 1987 suffered from the highest infant-mortality rate in the nation, 33.3 per thousand live births.

	Number	Rank
Age-Adjusted Death Rate	0.74	76/100
Heart Attacks	0.05	57/100
Cancer	−0.21	26/100

Burlington has the 7th lowest rate for robberies. Rates for homicide and suicide are also extremely low.

Incidence per 1,000 Pop.	Number	Rank
Homicides (1989)	0.05	21/111
Robberies (1989)	0.51	7/111
Suicides	0.10	17/100
Accidents	0.32	35/100

$ Burlington's 1988 metro population was 129,000—109th out of 113 metro areas. Its economic health at the end of 1990 was below average, ranking 72nd of 113 metro areas. Its unemployment rate ranks 21st, change in unemployment 97th (the labor force grew by 3.4 percent, faster than employment, which grew by only 1.6 percent) and its enterprise 65th. Contact: Mayor Peter Clavelle, City of Burlington, City Hall, Burlington, VT 05401.

Weather: Burlington is a cool city with an average daily temperature of 44.1. Precipitation is high at 33.7 inches, as is annual snowfall at 77.9 inches.

Average Daily Temperature (degrees F)	44.1
High	53.6
Low	34.6
Average Humidity	
Morning	77
Afternoon	59
Annual Precipitation (inches)	33.7
Average Total Snowfall (inches)	77.9

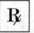 A public-health questionnaire was not returned.

Burlington provides 9 baseball fields, 11 football/soccer fields, 14 basketball courts, 22 tennis courts, 1 golf course, 1 running track, 3 swimming pools, 1 marina, 99 campground sites, 14 miles of bike paths and 6 community gardens. It operates 8 softball leagues, 6 basketball leagues, 3 volleyball leagues, 2 tennis leagues and 3 soccer leagues. It offers a special Senior Fitness Program, composed of cardiovascular and stretching exercises. The community recreation Task Force is currently working with architects on a design for a recreation center. Contact: Donald Bessler, Director, Burlington Parks and Recreation Department, 216 Leddy Park Road, Burlington, VT 05401 (802) 864-0123.

Parkland/Total City Area (percent)	8.5
Aerobics classes	yes
Arts and craft classes	yes
Hiking or exploration groups	yes
Other Activities: Athletic activities	
for youths and senior-citizen	
recreation events.	

The city did not respond to the school-health survey.

Casper, WY

⚰️RIP	🏃	$	⬆	℞	🏃	👫	?
?	✔	x	✓	✓	✓	✓	✔

 Casper (Natrona County) was not ranked on the age-adjusted death rate. Wyoming has a high infant-mortality rate among minorities. The lowest infant-mortality rate is in rural areas of the state.

Casper's homicide rate is 25th lowest of 111 metro areas, and its robbery rate is third lowest of 111 metro areas.

Incidence per 1,000 Pop.	Number	Rank
Homicides (1989)	0.05	25/111
Robberies (1989)	0.27	3/111

$ Casper's 1988 metro population was 65,000—113th out of 113 metro areas. Its economic health at the end of 1990 was poor, ranking 92nd of 113 metro areas. Its unemployment rate ranks 87th, change in unemployment 50th (the labor force grew faster than employment) and its enterprise 90th. Contact: City Manager, Thomas O. Forsland, City of Casper, City Hall, Casper, WY.

Air Quality: Casper is in compliance with all Federal and state standards. The total amount of suspended particulates has declined in the last 10 years, but went up in 1988 in part because of the forest fires in Yellowstone Park in September 1988. Contact: Charles A. Collins, State Department of Environmental Quality, Air Quality Control Division, Herschler Building, Cheyenne, WY 82002.

Hazardous Waste: All hazardous waste in Casper is shipped out of town. An annual hazardous-household-waste collection is sponsored. Contact: Michael D. Haigler, City of Casper Public Works Department, 200 North David Street, Casper, WY 82601.

Water Quality: 25 percent of the drinking water in Casper comes from surface water such as reservoirs and 75 percent comes from ground water such as wells. Contact: David W. Hill, Board of Public Utilities, 200 North David Street, Casper, WY 82601.

Weather: Casper is a cool city with an average daily temperature of 45.2. Precipitation is low at 11.4 inches annually, but snowfall is very high at 81.4 inches.

Average Daily Temperature (degrees F)	45.2
High	58.3
Low	32.1
Average Humidity	
Morning (percent)	71
Afternoon (percent)	44
Normal Precipitation (inches)	11.4
Average Total Snowfall (inches)	81.4

R̟ The Health Department has a full-time health educator. The city provides health-education programs for CPR training, AIDS education, anti-smoking, prenatal and infant care and sexually transmitted diseases. Emergency hotlines are provided for child abuse, suicide AIDS information and family violence. The city has an anti-smoking law that prohibits smoking in public offices and partially restricts it in restaurants and private offices. Contact: Jill Anderson, Director, City-County Health Department, 1200 East 3rd Street, Casper, WY 82601.

Casper ranks 38th out of 82 cities on recreational facilities per 1,000 residents. It has 8 softball fields, 9 baseball fields, 4 soccer fields and 15 tennis courts. The Casper Recreation Center offers crafts, dances, sports and fitness classes and weight training.

The public-school system employs 14 nurses, four psychologists, a physical therapist, an occupational therapist, speech therapists and social workers for its 12,386 students. There is a nurse full-time in the two high schools. The nurse is present 75 percent of the time in the four junior high schools and 25 to 50 percent present in the elementary schools, depending on their size. All students are provided with basic health-education programs. No medical, dental, or psychiatric treatment is provided for students. Contact: Claranne Cannon, Natrona County School District, 970 North Glenn Road, Casper, WY 82601.

Charleston, WV

🪦	🏊	$	⬆	R̟	🏃	👥	?
X	✓	X	✓	✓	?	✔	✓

Charleston (Kanawha County) ranks a high 86th in the age-adjusted mortality rate and an unhealthy 96th in deaths resulting from cancer. West Virginia has a high infant-mortality rate among minorities and in urban communities. Lower infant-mortality rates are found among whites and in rural areas of the state.

	Number	Rank
Age-Adjusted Death Rate	1.34	86/100
Heart Attacks	0.06	58/100
Cancer	0.72	96/100

Charleston has below-average rates of robberies (23rd lowest of 111 metro areas) and suicide (35th lowest). Rates for homicide (74th out of 111 metros) and accidents are slightly above average for the metro areas.

Incidence per 1,000 Pop.	Number	Rank
Homicides (1989)	0.10	74/111
Robberies (1989)	1.20	23/111
Suicides	0.13	35/100
Accidents	0.35	66/100

Charleston's 1988 metro population was 261,000—98th out of 113 metro areas. Its economic health at the end of 1990 was poor, ranking 84th of 113 metro areas. Its unemployment rate ranks 96th, change in unemployment 15th (employment grew by 3.8 percent, compared to labor force, which grew by 2.7 percent) and its enterprise 96th. Contact: Mayor Kent Strange Hall, City of Charleston, 501 Virginia Street, Charleston, WV 25301.

Air Quality: The city exceeded national standards for ozone 7 days in 1988. Contact: Joyce Nessif, Air Quality Data Administration, West Virginia Air Pollution Commission, 1558 Washington Street, Charleston, WV 25311.

Weather: The average temperature is slightly above the U.S. average at 54.8 degrees. Precipitation is very high at 42.4 inches annually.

Average Daily Temperature (degrees F)	54.8
High	65.5
Low	44.0
Average Humidity	
Morning (percent)	82
Afternoon (percent)	56
Normal Precipitation (inches)	42.4
Average Total Snowfall (inches)	32.7
Ozone, Days over 0.12 ppm (1 hour, 1988)	7

The city provides all basic health-education programs and emergency hotlines. Drinking and driving is a major concern of the city. It provides Holiday Care Cab program and a Night Lock-up and a breakfast program. It has no laws restricting smoking as of the time the city responded to our questionnaire, but it does have an anti-smoking educational program. Contact: Dr. Donald M. Rosenberg, Director, Kanawha County/Charleston Health Department, 108 Lee Street, Charleston, WV 25301; 304-348-8069.

The city did not respond to the recreational services survey. The city operates 10 recreation centers and two parks, one of which has a golf course and a swimming pool.

The 35,788 students in the public school system are served by 23 nurses, 10 psychologists, 1 physician, 4 dental hygienists, 1 occupational therapist and 1 physical therapist. Health education is offered to students in grades K-12. The school system also has an AIDS education program. Dental treatment is provided for students. Contact: Roberta Stuck, Director, Health Services, Kanawha County School District, 200 Elizabeth Street, Charleston, WV 25311.

Charlotte, NC

Charlotte (Mecklenberg County) metro area includes Gastonia, North Carolina and Rock Hill, South Carolina. North Carolina has high infant-mortality rates among minorities and in cities. The Charlotte metro area ranks 4th on the age-adjusted mortality rate, suggesting good longevity prospects for its residents. Contact: Stephen R. Keener, M.D., Assistant Health Director, Mecklenberg County Health Department, Disease Control/Epidemiology, 2856 Beatties Ford Road, Charlotte, NC 28202.

	Number	Rank
Age-Adjusted Death Rate	−2.84	4/100
Heart Attacks	−0.47	18/100
Cancer	−0.65	5/100

Charlotte has the 3rd lowest suicide rate and the 8th lowest accident rate. Rates for homicide (25th highest) and robbery (37th highest), however, are both in the highest third.

Incidence per 1,000 Pop.	Number	Rank
Homicides (1989)	0.12	87/111
Robberies (1989)	2.72	75/111
Suicides	0.07	3/100
Accidents	0.25	8/100

$ Charlotte's 1988 metro population was 1,112,000—42nd out of 113 metro areas. Its economic health at the end of 1990 was good, ranking 31st of 113 metro areas. Its unemployment rate ranks 34th, change in unemployment 78th (the labor force grew faster than employment) and its enterprise 9th. Contact: Mayor Sue Myrick, Office of the Mayor, 600 East 4th Street, Charlotte, NC 28202-2839.

Weather: The climate is moderate, with long spring and fall seasons. Very hot summer conditions (90 degrees and above) occur about one-third less often than in southern Florida. About twice a year the temperature approaches 100 degrees. Temperatures fall below the freezing point on an average of one half of the winter days. Snow accumulation rarely exceeds six inches annually.

Average Daily Temperature (degrees F)	60.0
High	70.5
Low	49.4
Average Humidity	
Morning (percent)	83.0
Afternoon (percent)	54.0
Normal Precipitation (inches)	43.2
Average Total Snowfall (inches)	5.80

℞ The city did not return a public-health questionnaire.

Health Resources per 1,000 Pop.	Number	Rank
Nurses, community hospitals, city	8.15	38/90
Doctors, metro area	1.41	108/113

Charlotte has extensive sports facilities that include 130 tennis courts, 128 basketball courts, 87 baseball fields, 49 football/soccer fields and 5 swimming pools. Basketball is a favorite sport, with 183 sports leagues. Softball, volleyball and tennis are also popular. An especially popular program features two-week summer day camps, which have served 4,520 young people and offer field trips, swimming, sports, games, art, dance, nature, crafts and music. There is also a six-week Youth Fun and Fitness & Sports camp (ages 6-12) sponsored by the NRPA and the President's Council on Physical Fitness & Sports. Other activities include the Festival in the Park, the Ultra Swim Meet and the Park Watch Program. Improvements have been made on the playgrounds in Reedy Creek Park and on the York Road Renaissance Park Complex and a Right of Ways/Tree program was initiated. Contact: Marvin F. Billups, Jr., Director, Parks and Recreation Department, 600 East 4th Street, Charlotte, NC 28202.

Parkland/Total City Area (percent)   2.9
Aerobics classes   yes
Arts and craft classes   yes
Hiking or exploration groups   yes

For a total of 75,201 students (grades K-12) in the public school system, there are 27 nurses, two physicians, 90 psychologists, three social workers, one nutritionist and three dental hygienists. There is a full-time nurse present in all schools. Health education is taught in grades K-10. Topics include family living, mental health, environmental health, consumer health, safety/first aid and growth & development. Substance abuse prevention is taught in grades 11 and 12. In 1990, new policies were adopted for AIDS and the use/possession of drugs and illegal substances. Also, a team was formed to promote fitness/wellness among the staff. No medical, dental or psychiatric treatment is provided for students. Contact: Margaret P. Griehsbach, Assistant Superintendent, Charlotte-Mecklenburg School System, PO Box 30035, Charlotte, NC 28230.

Chattanooga, TN

⚰ RIP	🏊	$	🌲	℞	🚴	👫	?
X	✔	✔	✓	X	?	?	X

Population statistics for Chattanooga (Hamilton County) include the surrounding area in Georgia. Tennessee has some of the highest infant-mortality rates in the nation for minorities. Infant-mortality rates among whites are fair. Contact: Wayne Wormsley, Health Statistician, Chattanooga-Hamilton County Health Department, 921 East 3rd Street, Chattanooga, TN 37403.

	Number	Rank
Age-Adjusted Death Rate	0.40	63/100
Heart Attacks	−0.16	40/100
Cancer	0.09	65/100

Chattanooga has the 15th lowest suicide rate of 100 metro areas. Homicide (33rd lowest) and robbery rates are also below average, but accident rates are relatively high.

Incidence per 1,000 Pop.	Number	Rank
Homicides (1989)	0.05	33/111
Robberies (1989)	1.83	45/111
Suicides	0.09	15/100
Accidents	0.41	87/100

$ Chattanooga's 1988 metro population was 438,000—85th out of 113 metro areas. Its economic health at the end of 1990 was excellent, ranking 18th of 113 metro areas. Its unemployment rate ranks 51st, change in unemployment 34th (the labor force shrunk faster than employment) and its enterprise 12th. Contact: Mayor Gene Roberts, City of Chattanooga, Municipal Building, Chattanooga, TN 37402.

Air Quality: Chattanooga has a diversified economy with a historically strong manufacturing base. It has cleaned up its air without closing down its economy. In the early 1960s, the city's air quality was ranked among the worst in the country. In 1989 and 1990 Chattanooga had no ozone exceedances and as of 1991 complies with all Federal air-quality standards. Contact: Robert H. Colby, Director, Chattanooga-Hamilton County Air Pollution Control Bureau, 3511 Rossville Blvd., Chattanooga, TN 37407.

Water Quality: Of the city's water supply, 60 percent comes from surface reservoirs, 5 percent from ground water wells and 35 percent from natural springs. A Water Quality Committee was created by the County Commission. Statistics are not available concerning the chemical contents of the drinking water. Contact; Bob Jerardi, Environmental Health Director, Chattanooga-Hamilton County Health Department, 921 East 3rd Street, Chattanooga, TN 37403.

Weather: Chattanooga has warm summers, with the temperature and humidity broken by short-lived thunderstorms, and cool winters due to the Cumberland mountains that protect the area from cold air from the northwest.

Average Daily Temperature (degrees F)	59.4
High	70.5
Low	48.3
Average Humidity	
Morning (percent)	85
Afternoon (percent)	56
Normal Precipitation (inches)	52.6
Average Total Snowfall (inches)	4.2
Ozone, Days over 0.12 ppm (1 hour, 1988)	2

℞ A comprehensive primary-care need assessment was initiated to help identify gaps in health-care service delivery. Also, a new community-based Homeless Clinic was established in 1988. The media and business have become actively involved in public health awareness activities and education. All basic health-education programs and emergency hotlines are provided by the city. Smoking is a serious concern of the city and is prohibited on public transportation and partially prohibited in restaurants and in both public and private offices. Several interesting new programs have been developed for minority AIDS education, indigent health, black infant mortality, "Just Say No" programs in schools and drunk-driving-prevention programs. Contact: William Ulmer, Director, Community Health Services Department, Chattanooga-Hamilton County Health Department, 921 East 3rd Street, Chattanooga, TN 37403.

Health Resources per 1,000 Pop.	Number	Rank
Hospital beds, community hospitals, city	9.78	22/92
Nurses, community hospitals, city	10.43	22/90
Doctors, metro area	1.88	90/113

 The city did not respond to the recreational-facilities survey.

 The city did not respond to the school-health survey.

Chicago, IL

RIP	🚫	$	🌲	℞	🏃	👥	?
X	X	✔	✔	✔	✔	X	✔

RIP The Chicago (Cook County) consolidated metro area consists of the primary metro area of Chicago, plus the primary metro areas of Aurora-Elgin, IL (population 352,000), Gary-Hammond, IN (604,000), Joliet, IL (377,000), Kenosha, WI (120,000) and Lake County, IL (494,000). Illinois has one of the highest infant-mortality rates among blacks. Infant-mortality rates for other minorities and urban communities are also high. Chicago's age-adjusted mortality rate ranks an unhealthy 90th.

	Number	Rank
Age-Adjusted Death Rate	1.67	90/100
Heart Attacks	0.59	85/100
Cancer	0.39	88/100

Chicago has a very high homicide rate, 92nd of 111 metro areas, and has the fourth-highest robbery rate, 108th of 111 metro areas, exceeded only by Miami, New York City and Los Angeles. Suicide rates are below average for the metro areas, accident rates above average.

Incidence per 1,000 Pop.	Number	Rank
Homicides (1989)	0.13	92/111
Robberies (1989)	5.62	108/111
Suicides	0.12	32/100
Accidents	0.35	64/100

Chicago's 1988 primary metro population was 6.216 million—3rd out of 113 metro areas. Its economic health at the end of 1990 was excellent, ranking 28th of 113 metro areas. Its unemployment rate ranks 76th, change in unemployment 34th (employment grew faster than the labor force) and its enterprise 70th. Contact: Mayor Richard M. Daley, City of Chicago, 121 North LaSalle Street, Room 507, Chicago, IL 60602.

Air Quality: Chicago came into attainment for carbon monoxide in 1991. For particulates, the city is in attainment for every neighborhood except near a group of steel and coking plants. It remains in nonattainment for ozone, in part because of three exceedance-days in 1988 (which continue to bulk in importance in EPA attainment formulas). Chicago has had no ozone exceedances in 1990 or through mid-June 1991. Contact: Environmental Control Division, Consumer Services, City of Chicago; and Henry L. Henderson, Law Department, City of Chicago, 180 North LaSalle Street, Chicago, IL 60601, 312-744-7340.

Hazardous Waste: The City of Chicago has few Superfund sites because the city's drinking water does not come from groundwater, so that groundwater contamination is not taken into account by Federal/state authorities in scoring Chicago waste sites for the National Priority List. The Chicago facilities that have received Superfund attention are those that threaten hazardous releases into the air; the responding actions by the city are to remove surface and above-ground sources of pollution. The available data on hazardous waste generation include the entire county. The total amount of hazardous waste generated within or shipped into Cook County during 1989 (the latest year available in mid-1991 when we went to press) was 3.3 million tons. Of this, 20,000 tons were shipped out of the county for disposal and 32,000 tons were treated or disposed of on-site. The remaining tonnage was treated within Cook County at a hazardous-waste incinerator, a hazardous-waste landfill and a variety of other treatment facilities that neutralize or otherwise manage the waste. Contact: Illinois

Environmental Protection Agency; Environmental Control Division, Consumer Services, City of Chicago; and Henry L. Henderson, Law Department, City of Chicago, previously identified.

Water Quality: Chicago draws its water from intakes under Lake Michigan, one mile offshore. The water is then processed through one of the city's two water-purification facilities. On March 15, 1991, pH was somewhat excessive at 8.1 (fewer than one-third of the cities are higher); nitrates were below the median, at 0.19 to 0.21 ppm, and turbidity was average at 0.20 to 0.25.

Weather: Chicago's climate has been classified as continental, meaning hot summers and cold winters. During the summer, periods of high heat and humidity may last for several days. The moderating effects of Lake Michigan at times keep the city as much as 10 degrees cooler than outlying areas.

Average Daily Temperature (degrees F)	49.2
High	58.7
Low	39.7
Average Humidity	
Morning (percent)	80
Afternoon (percent)	60
Normal Precipitation (inches)	33.3
Average Total Snowfall (inches)	39.8

℞ A proposal entitled "Chicago and Cook County Health Care Action Plan" was submitted to the Governor, Mayor and County Board President, which would make health care more accessible to the citizens of the city. Basic health-education programs and emergency hotlines are provided by the city. Smoking is prohibited on public transportation and partially restricted in restaurants, private and public offices and the airport. Contact: Richard M. Krieg, Ph.D., Acting Director, City of Chicago Department of Health, Richard J. Daley Center, Room 219, Chicago, IL 60602.

Health Resources per 1,000 Pop.	Number	Rank
Hospital beds, community hospitals, city	4.90	69/92
Nurses, community hospitals, city	4.81	75/90
Doctors, metro area	1.41	27/69

Chicago rates 45th out of 82 cities on the provision of sports facilities, much better than New York City or Los Angeles. It offers 222 football/soccer fields, 99 soccer fields (30 of them indoors), 522 baseball diamonds, 1,164 basketball backboards (translating to 582 courts) and 716 tennis courts. In addition, it offers 6 golf courses, 89 swimming pools, 29 track fields, 355 volleyball fields, 4 bridle paths, 121 ice-skating rinks, 32 bathing beaches, 19 bicycle paths, 8 harbors, 4,772 boat moorings (252 of them dry), 2,233 dinghy spaces and 2 zoos. The 561 Chicago parks, occupying over 7,000 acres, are owned and operated by the Chicago Park District, a special state-chartered governmental entity with its own taxing and bonding authority. Its property lies wholly within the City of Chicago and includes 26 miles of frontage on Lake Michigan, the largest concentration of accessible public land in the Great Lakes Basin. In addition to the city's parkland, Cook County owns 67,000 acres of forest and open land. Contact: Chicago Park District and Cook County Forest Preserve.

To serve 407,422 students in the public school system (grades K-12) are 202 nurses and 8 full-time physicians plus 27 contractual physicians and one part-time pediatric neurologist. A part-time nurse is available in 99 percent of the schools, but a full-time nurse is available in fewer than .05 percent of them. An interesting new program provides medical review and consultations and extends related services to all medically fragile students who are home-bound or in physically handicapped schools. Health education is taught to students in grades 5-12. No medical treatment is provided. The school system has adopted a policy of requiring a physical and immunization on entry. The school system also offers (1) wellness programs for employees, (2) Health Fairs for blood pressure and cholesterol screening, and blood-sugar testing, and (3) operates a smoking-cessation clinic in cooperation with the Chicago Lung Association. Contact: Ted D. Kimbrough, General Superintendent, Chicago Public Schools, 1819 West Pershing Road, Chicago, IL 60609.

Cincinnati, OH

RIP	⤵	$	▲	℞	🖼	👥	?
X	✔	✔	?	✓	?	?	XX

The consolidated Cincinnati (Hamilton County) metro area includes Hamilton-Middletown, OH (population 276,000); the primary Cincinnati metro area consists only of Cincinnati and nearby suburbs plus suburban areas (including Covington) in northern Kentucky and in southeastern Indiana, but stops to the north at the edge of the Hamilton-

Middletown primary metro area. Cincinnati's age-adjusted mortality rate is a high 74th. Ohio has high infant-mortality rates among minorities and low rates among whites and in rural communities.

	Number	Rank
Age-Adjusted Death Rate	0.69	74/100
Heart Attacks	0.28	74/100
Cancer	0.37	87/100

 Homicide, robbery, suicide and accident rates in Cincinnati are all below average.

Incidence per 1,000 Pop.	Number	Rank
Homicides (1989)	0.06	36/111
Robberies (1989)	1.46	32/111
Suicides	0.12	35/100
Accidents	0.32	29/100

$ Cincinnati's 1988 metro population was 1.45 million—29th out of 113 metro areas. Its economic health at the end of 1990 was excellent, ranking 19th of 113 metro areas. Its unemployment rate ranks 14th, change in unemployment 12th (employment grew by 4.1 percent, a full 1 percent faster than the labor force) and its enterprise 74th.

Weather: The climate is quite livable, with about 100 days a year at or below freezing. There is about a month's worth of 90-degree days each year. Rainfall is concentrated in storms in the winter and spring. Weather statistics are for the Greater Cincinnati Airport, which is nearby in Kentucky.

Average Daily Temperature (degrees F)	53.4
High	63.5
Low	43.2
Average Humidity	
Morning (percent)	81
Afternoon (percent)	60
Normal Precipitation (inches)	40.1
Average Total Snowfall (inches)	23.6

 The city did not respond to the health-services survey.

Health Resources per 1,000 Pop.

	Number	Rank
Hospital beds, community hospitals, city	13.34	6/92
Nurses, community hospitals, city	14.99	8/90
Doctors, metro area	2.62	46/113

 The city of Cincinnati offers 4,751 acres of parkland, along with 2,395 additional acres set aside in 195 recreation areas. The city did not respond to the recreational-facilities survey.

The city did not respond to the school-health survey.

Cleveland, OH

⚰️RIP	🏃	$	🌲	℞	🏌️	👫	?
X	✓	✓	✓	✓	✓	X	✓

Consolidated Cleveland (Cuyahoga County) includes Akron, OH (population 647,000) and Lorain-Elyria (population 268,000). Ohio has high infant-mortality rates among minorities and low rates among whites and in rural communities. Cleveland's age-adjusted death rate ranks a high 87.

	Number	Rank
Age-Adjusted Death Rate	1.43	87/100
Heart Attacks	0.97	95/100
Cancer	0.47	89/100

Homicide and robbery rates in Cleveland are somewhat above average for the 111 metro areas while suicide and accident rates are slightly below average.

Incidence per 1,000 Pop.

	Number	Rank
Homicides (1989)	0.10	71/111
Robberies (1989)	2.69	73/111
Suicides	0.12	41/100
Accidents	0.32	37/100

$ Cleveland's 1988 metro population was 1,845,000—24th out of 113 metro areas. Its economic health at the end of 1990 was good, ranking 45th of 113 metro areas. Its unemployment rate ranks 36th, change in unemployment 30th (employment grew by 1.7 percent, versus 1.3 percent for the labor force) and its enterprise 83rd. Contact: Mayor Michael Wright, City of Cleveland, 601 Lakeside Avenue, Cleveland, OH 44114.

Water Quality: Cleveland's total drinking water supply comes from surface water (Lake Erie), which is currently blessed with an absence of organic contaminants. The pH of the drinking water is 7.5. The problems of discoloration in a few parts of the water-supply system are often handled through a cleaning and lining program. Contact: Don J. Heuer, P.E., Consulting Engineer, Department of Public Works, 1201 Lakeside Avenue, Cleveland, OH 44114.

Weather: As cold air from Canada moves south, it is warmed by Lake Erie. The result is that Cleveland is warmer than its Canadian neighbors in winter but is cloudy and is hit with a lot of snow (54 inches compared to only 24 inches in Cincinnati, which has a higher rainfall). The lake also keeps down summer temperatures.

Average Daily Temperature (degrees F)	49.6
High	58.5
Low	40.7
Average Humidity	
Morning (percent)	79
Afternoon (percent)	62
Normal Precipitation (inches)	35.4
Average Total Snowfall (inches)	54.1

R Prevention programs—including AIDS testing and provision of food to the poor and elderly—are supported by outside funding. Health-education programs are offered in the areas of CPR training, AIDS education, Anti-smoking, anti-drug, prenatal and infant care and family planning. The city provides all basic emergency hotlines. The city has particularly stringent anti-smoking laws. Smoking is completely prohibited in restaurants, private and public offices and on public transportation. Contact: Daisy Alford, Director, Health and Human Services, 1925 St. Clair Avenue, Cleveland, OH 44114.

Health Resources per 1,000 Pop.	Number	Rank
Hospital beds, community hospitals, city	11.32	16/92
Nurses, community hospitals, city	13.25	12/90
Doctors, metro area	3.26	18/113

[icon] The city's sports facilities include 162 tennis courts, 150 baseball fields, 75 basketball courts, 43 swimming pools and 25 football/soccer fields. Sixteen recreation centers service other activities. The city offers a special senior aquatics program, to which many seniors are referred to by their doctors. The city also holds senior Olympics, with over 5,000 participating. Contact: W. Laurence Bicking, Director, City of Cleveland, Department of Parks, Recreation & Properties, 1220 East 6th Street, Cleveland, OH 44114.

Parkland/Total City Area (percent)   5.1

[icon] For the 72,000 students in Cleveland's public school system there are 44 full-time nurses, 6 physicians and 2 social workers. Chemical dependency assessment counselors are present in 3 high schools. Health education is taught in the 9th grade. No medical, dental or psychiatric treatment is provided for students. Hearing tests are conducted by a speech therapist. Contact: Betty L. Mantzell, Supervisor, Health Services, Cleveland Public Schools, 10600 Quincy Avenue, Room 200, Cleveland, OH 44106.

Colorado Springs, CO

RIP	[icon]	$	[icon]	R	[icon]	[icon]	?
✔	✔	✓	X	X	?	X	✓

[icon] Colorado Springs (El Paso County) ranks a good 11th with its age-adjusted mortality rate. Colorado Springs also has the 7th lowest cancer rate among 100 metro areas. Colorado infant-mortality rates are high among minorities and relatively low among whites and in rural communities.

	Number	Rank
Age-Adjusted Death Rate	−1.94	11/100
Heart Attacks	−0.41	24/100
Cancer	−0.57	7/100
Infant Mortality (Colorado)		
All Areas	9.8	133/301
Blacks	16.4	249/301
Other	11.6	186/301

Rural	8.8	71/301
Urban Places	10.3	153/301
Whites	9.5	112/301

 While homicide and robbery rates are extremely low, Colorado Springs has one of the highest rates of suicide.

Incidence per 1,000 Pop.	Number	Rank
Homicides (1989)	0.04	14/111
Robberies (1989)	0.94	14/111
Suicides	0.18	94/100
Accidents	0.38	80/100

$ Colorado Springs' 1988 metro population was 394,000—89th out of 113 metro areas. Its economic health at the end of 1990 was below average, ranking 72nd of 113 metro areas. Its unemployment rate ranks 64th, change in unemployment 9th (employment grew faster than the labor force) and its enterprise 110th. Contact: Mayor Robert M. Issac, City of Colorado Springs, PO Box 1575, Colorado Springs, CO 80901.

↑ **Air Quality:** There has been a decrease in the number of total suspended particles and carbon monoxide exceedances in the city's air quality. Contact: John James, El Paso County Health Department, 501 North Foote, Colorado Springs, CO 80909.

Weather: The average daily temperature is slightly below average at 48.9. Precipitation is on the low side at 15.4 inches annually.

Average Daily Temperature (degrees F)	48.9
High	62.1
Low	35.6
Average Humidity	
Morning (percent)	62
Afternoon (percent)	40
Normal Precipitation (inches)	15.4
Average Total Snowfall (inches)	43.0
Ozone, Days over 0.12 (1 hour, 1988)	0

℞ One interesting new program is the midwife program sponsored by the Health Department and a nonprofit neighborhood clinic. The city is particularly concerned with combatting drug use, alcohol abuse, teen pregnancy and child abuse. All common health-education programs are provided by the city with the exception of CPR training. The city has an extensive network of emergency hotlines. Smoking is prohibited on public transportation and partially restricted in restaurants, public offices and private offices. Contact: Dr. John Muth, El Paso County Health Department, 501 North Foote, Colorado Springs, CO 80909.

Health Resources per 1,000 Pop.	Number	Rank
Hospital beds, community hospitals, city	4.67	73/98
Doctors, metro area	1.35	111/113

The city did not respond to the recreational-facilities survey.

There are 5 different school districts within the city area. To serve 11,079 students in public school district #20 are 3 nurses and 8 psychologists. A part-time nurse is available in all of the schools. All common health-education programs are offered to students in grades K-12. Medical and psychiatric treatment are provided only for students in the special-education area. Contact: Larry Perkins, Academy District #20, 7610 North Union Blvd., Colorado Springs, CO 80920 (719) 598-2566.

Columbia, SC

Columbia's (Richland County) age-adjusted mortality rate ranks a moderate 58th. South Carolina has high infant-mortality rates for minorities and in both rural and urban areas. Contact: Michael D. Jarrett, Commissioner, Department of Health and Environmental Control, 2600 Bull Street, Columbia, SC 29201.

	Number	Rank
Age-Adjusted Death Rate	0.19	58/100
Heart Attacks	0.10	65/100
Cancer	0.04	53/100

Columbia has one of the highest rates for accidents. Suicide rates for the city are low, while homicide and robbery rates are above average for the metro areas.

Incidence per 1,000 Pop.	Number	Rank
Homicides (1989)	0.10	71/111
Robberies (1989)	2.28	66/111
Suicides	0.11	25/100
Accidents	0.47	97/100

$ Columbia's 1988 metro population was 456,000—82nd out of 113 metro areas. Its economic health at the end of 1990 was good, ranking 39th of 113 metro areas. Its unemployment rate ranks 25th, change in unemployment 81st (the labor force grew by 1.4 percent by employment by only 0.2 percent) and its enterprise 29th. Contact: Mayor T.P. Adams, City of Columbia, City Hall, Columbia, SC 29201.

↑ **Air Quality:** In 1978, Columbia was a nonattainment area for ozone and carbon monoxide. By 1985, the EPA had reclassified the city to "attainment" for both pollutants. Columbia officials do not consider 1988 a representative year since 37 cities on the East Coast experienced ozone exceedances, i.e., ozone levels exceeding Federal limits. The ozone problem was not repeated in 1989. Contact: Michael D. Jarrett, previously listed.

Hazardous Waste: Columbia has two hazardous-waste sites on the EPA's National Priorities List for "Superfund," Palmetto Recycling, Inc. and SCR&D Bluff Road Site. Palmetto Recycling, Inc. is a battery-recycling operation; it stores the acid in a below-ground dump and ships the lead plates out-of-state for recycling. SCR&D Bluff Road Site is a large drum storage facility for all types of waste. Approximately 3,495 tons of hazardous waste are generated in Richland County, most of which is disposed of out-of-state as Richland County has only three on-site facilities (primarily storage) and one off-site facility (recycling). Throughout the county, emphasis is being placed on recycling and waste minimization. Contact: Michael D. Jarrett, previously listed.

Water Quality: All of Columbia's drinking water is supplied by surface water, e.g. reservoirs. Contact: Michael D. Jarrett, previously listed.

Weather: Columbia is a warm city with an average high temperature of 75.3. Humidity and precipitation are very high, with very little snowfall.

Average Daily Temperature (degrees F)	63.3
High	75.3
Low	51.2
Average Humidity	
Morning (percent)	87
Afternoon (percent)	51

Normal Precipitation (inches)   49.1
Average Total Snowfall (inches)   1.8
Ozone, Days over 0.12 ppm (1 hour, 1988)   2

℞ In an attempt to make health care more accessible, Richland has initiated home care/services for AIDS patients and home visits for high-risk mothers and newborns. The city sponsors five health-awareness campaigns addressing prenatal care, cholesterol, high blood pressure, physical activity/exercise and drugs and alcohol. Through the governor's office there has been an increased emphasis on the importance of prenatal care. The city also sponsors a restaurant and grocery store nutrition-education program. Other important programs include Richland County's free pregnancy testing, newborn screening for hemoglobinopathy and HIV and expanded screening for HIV among high-risk groups. All common public health-education programs are provided by the city, with the exception of an anti-drug program. The city also provides emergency hotlines for suicide, alcoholism, drug abuse and AIDS information. Columbia's anti-smoking legislation prohibits smoking in public offices and on public transportation. It partially restricts smoking in restaurants and private offices. Contact: Michael D. Jarrett, previously listed.

Among Columbia's basic sports facilities are 11 spray pools, 13 volleyball courts and 3 nature trails. Concerts in the park and softball are popular recreational activities in the city. Contact: Jack Disher, Director, Columbia Parks and Recreation Department, 1932 Calhoun Street, Columbia, SC 29201.

Parkland/Total City Area (percent)   6.6

Columbia's public school system employs 13 nurses, 18 psychologists and 7 social workers for its 27,500 students. The nurses are present part-time in all of the schools. All common health-education programs are taught to students in grades K-12. Medical and dental treatment is provided for students. Contact: Dr. John Stevenson, Superintendent, Richland School District 1, 1616 Richland Street, Columbia, SC 29201.

Columbus, GA

🪦 (RIP)	♿	$	🌲	℞	🚶	👫	?
X	X	X	X	X	✓	✓	✔

Columbus (Muscogee County) has a high age-adjusted death rate, 13th highest of 100 metro areas. Its cancer and heart attack rates are also relatively high. Georgia has a high overall infant-mortality rate of 12.7, with higher rates for minorities and urban areas.

	Number	Rank
Age-Adjusted Death Rate	1.55	88/100
Heart Attacks	0.37	79/100
Cancer	0.16	73/100

Columbus has relatively high rates of homicide, suicide and accidents. Robbery rates are about average for cities.

Incidence per 1,000 Pop.	Number	Rank
Homicides (1989)	0.12	83/111
Robberies (1989)	1.84	47/111
Suicides	0.15	77/100
Accidents	0.38	79/100

$ Columbus's 1988 metro population was 247,000—99th out of 113 metro areas. Its economic health at the end of 1990 was poor, ranking 88th of 113 metro areas. Its unemployment rate ranks 102nd, change in unemployment 74th (employment declined faster than the labor force) and its enterprise 41st. Contact: Mayor Frank Martin, City of Columbus, PO Box 1340, Columbus, GA 31902.

Water Quality: All of Columbus's drinking water comes from surface water, such as reservoirs. Contact: Billy Turner, Columbus Water Works, 1501 13th Avenue, PO Box 1600, Columbus, GA 31993.

Weather: The average high temperature is warm at 75.6. The city is humid with an average humidity of 87 percent in the morning. Precipitation is also very high at 51.1 inches annually.

Average Daily Temperature (degrees F)	64.4
High	75.6
Low	53.0
Average Humidity	
Morning (percent)	87
Afternoon (percent)	55
Normal Precipitation (inches)	51.1
Average Total Snowfall (inches)	0.5

℞ Columbus offers all common public health-education programs and emergency hotlines. The city offers Dial-A-Ride, which provides curb-to-curb service for those handicapped persons who do not live on a bus route serviced by buses designed to accommodate the handicapped. The city sponsors approximately 11 health awareness campaigns such as teen pregnancy, substance abuse, AIDS and other sexually transmitted diseases, prenatal, infant mortality, WIC (Women, Infants and Children), nutrition, hypertension and child abuse. The city's anti-smoking law partially restricts smoking in restaurants, public offices and private offices and on public transportation. Contact: Dr. Craig Lichtenwalner, District Health Director, 1958 8th Street, PO Box 2299, Columbus, GA 31993.

Health Resources per 1,000 Pop.	Number	Rank
Hospital beds, community hospitals, city	5.93	56/92
Nurses, community hospitals, city	7.69	42/90
Doctors, metro area	1.48	107/113

Columbus also contributes to its citizens' general physical and mental health through its cultural arts studio, therapeutic programs for the handicapped, Special Olympics competition and senior citizen aid programs. The city has a variety of sports fields and facilities. Water facilities include a riverfront beach, a marina, fishing areas and backwater properties. The city has many sports leagues, primarily for softball, baseball, football, soccer and basketball. Columbus is consolidated with Muscogee County and therefore covers 220 square miles. Thus its 1,500 acres of parkland looks small but actually is a lot of parkland per capita. Contact: Rick Gordon, Director, Department of Parks and Recreation, PO Box 1340, Columbus, GA 31993.

Parkland/Total City Area (percent)	1.3
Aerobics classes	yes
Arts and craft classes	yes
Hiking or exploration groups	yes
Other Activities: adventure programs.	

The Columbus school system employs one nurse, 11 psychologists and one vision and hearing technician for the 29,261 students in its school system. All common health-education programs are taught to students in grades K-9. Each student must take 30 hours of alcohol education and drug education before they may apply for their driver's license, and all students and staff are required to take AIDS education. The Drug Free Schools Program implemented the D.A.R.E. project. Medical treatment is provided for students.

Columbus, OH

Columbus (Franklin County) ranks a moderate 47th in the age-adjusted mortality rate. Ohio has high infant-mortality rates among minorities and low rates among whites and in rural communities. Contact: Teresa Long, M.D., Assistant Health Commissioner, Columbus Health Department, 181 South Washington Blvd., Columbus, OH 43215.

	Number	Rank
Age-Adjusted Death Rate	−0.21	47/100
Heart Attacks	−0.11	43/100
Cancer	0.04	54/100

Columbus has the 6th lowest accident rate and the 14th lowest suicide rate among the surveyed cities. Homicide and robbery rates are slightly above average.

Incidence per 1,000 Pop.	Number	Rank
Homicides (1989)	0.08	59/111
Robberies (1989)	2.80	78/111
Suicides	0.09	14/100
Accidents	0.23	6/100

Columbus Ohio's 1988 metro population was 1,334,000—34th out of 113 metro areas. Its economic health at the end of 1990 was excellent, ranking 3rd of 113 metro areas. Its unemployment rate ranks

21st, change in unemployment 19th (employment grew by 3.5 percent, substantially faster than the labor force, which grew by 2.6 percent) and its enterprise 17th. Contact: Mayor Dana G. Rinehart, City of Columbus, 90 West Broad Street, Columbus, OH 43215.

Air Quality: Columbus had 7 days of ozone exceedances in 1988. Contact: Michael J. Pompili, Assistant Health Commissioner, Columbus Health Department, 181 South Washington Blvd., Columbus, OH 43215.

Hazardous Waste: Columbus has a hazardous waste site on the EPA's National Priorities List for "Superfund." It is the Marble Cliff Quarries Dump. Columbus is working to encourage waste minimization techniques. Contact: Michael J. Pompili, Assistant Health Commissioner, Columbus Health Department, 181 South Washington Blvd., Columbus, OH 43215.

Water Quality: 87 percent of the drinking water in Columbus comes from surface water (reservoirs) and 13 percent comes from ground water (wells). Late winter and spring runoff results in a higher level of agricultural contaminants. Contact: Michael J. Pompili, Assistant Health Commissioner, Columbus Health Department, 181 South Washington Blvd., Columbus, OH 43215.

Weather: The weather is varied, with cold winters. The area averages about one week of zero-degree days, and well over 100 freezing (32 degrees or less) days each winter. The summers, however, are generally comfortable, with about two weeks of 90-degree days.

Average Daily Temperature (degrees F)	51.7
High	102
Low	41.8
Average Humidity	
Morning (percent)	80
Afternoon (percent)	59
Normal Precipitation (inches)	37.0
Average Total Snowfall (inches)	28.5
Ozone, Days over 0.12 ppm (1 hour, 1988)	7

R̸ The city provides all major public health-education programs. Emergency hotlines for suicide, drug abuse, AIDS information and sexually transmitted disease are available. The city provides special vans for the handicapped through the public transit system under Project Main Stream. A task force exists to address indigent care for the uninsured and the under-insured. The McKinney Act funds a health-care project for the homeless. The RWJ project offers community treatment teams for the severely mentally disabled. The city addresses health issues such as smoking, drug abuse, AIDS, child care and health and injury prevention. Columbus has taken a voluntary, but active approach to non-smoking areas. Over 60 percent of workers are in smoke-free environments. Smoking is partially restricted in restaurants, public offices and private offices. Contact: Teresa Long, M.D., Assistant Health Commissioner, Columbus Health Department, 181 South Washington Blvd., Columbus, OH 43215.

Health Resources per 1,000 Pop.	Number	Rank
Hospital beds, community hospitals, city	7.26	42/92
Nurses, community hospitals, city	7.69	42/90
Doctors, metro area	2.18	71/113

Columbus has recently added 2 new community recreation centers. The city also has 100 baseball fields, 63 football/soccer fields, 47 basketball courts, 37 tennis courts, 10 swimming pools and 6 golf courses. Softball is the most popular sport with 235 sports leagues. The city also has recreational programming for preschool children. Contact: James Barney, Director, Columbus Recreation and Parks Department, 90 West Broad Street, Columbus, OH 43215.

Parkland/Total City Area (percent)   9.7

For 65,000 students enrolled in its school system, Columbus employs 56 nurses, one physician and three psychologists. A nurse is present full-time in 10 percent of the schools and part-time in 90 percent of the schools. The Columbus school system is contracting with the city health department for services of a physician, as well as for consulting services. All common health-education programs are offered to students in grades K-12. No medical, dental, or psychiatric treatment is provided for students. Contact: Damon Asbury, Associate Superintendent, Columbus Public Schools, 270 East State Street, Columbus, OH 43215.

Corpus Christi, TX

🪦	🏃	$	🌲	℞	🏃	👫	?
✔	✓	✓	✗	?	✗	✗	✓

 Corpus Christi (Nueces County) ranks an average 49th in its age-adjusted mortality rate. Infant-mortality rates in Texas are high among minorities and low among whites and in rural areas.

	Number	Rank
Age-Adjusted Death Rate	−0.15	49/100
Heart Attacks	1.21	33/100
Cancer	1.56	49/100
Infant Mortality (Texas)		
All Areas	9.1	90/301
Blacks	15.1	235/301
Other	13.5	220/301
Rural	7.9	24/301
Urban Places	9.7	125/301
Whites	8.3	46/301

 Corpus Christi has relatively low rates for homicide, robbery, suicide and accidents.

Incidence per 1,000 Pop.	Number	Rank
Homicides (1989)	0.07	43/111
Robberies (1989)	1.66	36/111
Suicides	0.32	32/100
Accidents	−0.28	33/100

$ Corpus Christi's 1988 metro population was 358,000—93rd out of 113 metro areas. Its economic health at the end of 1990 was poor, ranking 106th of 113 metro areas. Its unemployment rate ranks 108th, change in unemployment 58th (the labor force grew faster than employment) and its enterprise 107th. Contact: Mayor Mary Rhodes, City of Corpus Christi, PO Box 9277, Corpus Christi, TX 78469; 512-880-3800.

↟ **Air Quality:** Air quality in Corpus Christi has improved over the last five years despite an increase in petroleum refining activity.

Weather: The city is hot, with an average high temperature of 81.6. Humidity is also high at 90 percent in the morning. Precipitation is above average at 30.2 inches annually.

Average Daily Temperature (degrees F)	72.1
High	81.6
Low	62.5
Average Humidity	
Morning (percent)	90
Afternoon (percent)	63
Normal Precipitation (inches)	30.2
Average Total Snowfall (inches)	0.1
Ozone, Days over 0.12 ppm (1 hour, 1988)	0

℞ Corpus Christi sponsors several hundred health awareness campaigns each year addressing issues such as AIDS and other sexually transmitted diseases, cancer, diabetes, heart disease, mosquito control, animal control, communicable diseases, rat control, immunizations, drug and alcohol abuse, child abuse and family planning. All common health education programs and emergency hotlines are provided by the city. The city has anti-smoking legislation that prohibits smoking on public transportation and in grocery stores and department stores; smoking is partially restricted in restaurants, shopping malls, public offices and private offices. Contact: Dr. Nina Sisley, M.P.H., Director of Public Health, Corpus Christi City/County Health Department, 1702 Horne Road, Corpus Christi, TX 78416.

Health Resources per 1,000 Pop.	Number	Rank
Nurses, community hospitals, city	5.59	67/92
Doctors, metro area	1.71	99/113

⛹ Corpus Christi has a variety of sports facilities including 55 tennis courts, 10 football/soccer fields, 42 basketball courts, 36 baseball fields, 9 swimming pools, 11 recreation centers, 7 senior centers, and 2 golf courses. Tennis is a popular sport with 23 tennis leagues. Also popular are volleyball, softball, water aerobics and swimming programs. A gymnasium, outdoor amphitheatre, and multicultural center house many recreational and cultural events. Contact: Juan Garza, City Manager, City of Corpus Christi, PO Box 9277, Corpus Christi, TX 78469.

Parkland/Total City Area (percent)	2.0
Aerobics classes	yes
Arts and craft classes	yes

Hiking or exploration groups no
Other Activities: cultural, latchkey
(after-school) and senior programs.

The Corpus Christi public-school system employs 26 nurses, 1
physician, 1 special-education nurse practitioner and 15 licensed
practical nurses for its 40,437 students. The nurses work full-time in 3
percent of the schools and part-time in the rest. All common health-
education programs are offered to students in grades K-12. No medical,
dental or psychiatric treatment is provided for students. Contact: Charles
Benson, Superintendent, City of Corpus Christi Public Schools, c/o Office
of the Mayor, City Hall, PO Box 9277, Corpus Christi, TX 78469.

Dallas, TX

🪦	🏃	$	⬆	℞	🚶	👫	?
✔	X	✓	X	✓	✓	✔	✔

Consolidated Dallas (Dallas County) includes Forth Worth and Arlington, TX (population 1,269,000). Texas has a high infant-
mortality rate among minorities and a low rate among whites and in rural
areas. Dallas' age-adjusted mortality rate ranks 16th. Contact: Adela N.
Gonzales, Director, City of Dallas, Department of Health and Human
Services, 1500 Marilla, Dallas, TX 75201.

	Number	Rank
Age-Adjusted Death Rate	−1.47	16/100
Heart Attacks	−0.62	13/100
Cancer	−0.41	12/100

Dallas lives up to its cowboy image by having one of the ten highest
robbery and homicide rates. But its suicide and accident rates are
closer to the national average.

Incidence per 1,000 Pop.	Number	Rank
Homicides (1989)	0.17	103/111
Robberies (1989)	4.53	103/111

Suicides	0.13	52/100
Accidents	0.34	61/100

$ Dallas' 1988 metro population was 2,475,000—11th out of 113 metro areas. Its economic health at the end of 1990 was below average, ranking 67th of 113 metro areas. Its unemployment rate ranks 81st, change in unemployment 58th (the labor force grew slightly while employment shrank slightly) and its enterprise 60th. Contact: Mayor Annette Strauss, City of Dallas, City Hall, Dallas, TX 75201.

Air Quality: In the past five years there has been a decrease in the number of days that the ozone standard has been violated. Contact: Vittorio K. Argento, Chair, City of Dallas Environmental Health Advisory Commission, 1226 North Cedar Ridge Drive, Duncanville, TX 75116.

Hazardous Waste: Hazardous waste in Dallas is transported outside the county for disposal. Dallas has one inactive hazardous waste site on the EPA's National Priorities List. The site was cleaned up and closed in June 1988. It is in a 30-year post-closure maintenance period. Contact: Vittorio K. Argento, City of Dallas Environmental Health Advisory Commission, 1226 North Cedar Ridge Drive, Duncanville, TX 75116.

Water Quality: All of the drinking water for Dallas is surface water, such as reservoirs. Contact: Vittorio K. Argento, City of Dallas Environmental Health Advisory Commission, 1226 North Cedar Ridge Drive, Duncanville, TX 75116.

Weather: The Dallas-Fort Worth area has a warm, moderately humid climate. The temperature reaches 90 degrees and above an average of 95 days a year. It dips to 32 degrees or less around 40 days a year.

Average Daily Temperature (degrees F)	66.0
High	76.9
Low	55.0
Average Humidity	
Morning (percent)	82
Afternoon (percent)	56
Normal Precipitation (inches)	29.5
Average Total Snowfall (inches)	3.0
Ozone, Days over 0.12 ppm (1 hour, 1988)	5

℞ Special health-care services include a low-birth-weight program targeting infants weighing less than three-and-a-half pounds from low-income families and a program providing health-care, mental health, dental and substance-abuse services to homeless persons in the areas where they congregate. The city provides all common public health-education programs. Emergency hotlines are available for child abuse, suicide, alcoholism, drug abuse, AIDS information, family violence and runaways. Other services provided by the city are crisis counseling, elderly concerns and landlord-tenant relations. Contact: Adela N. Gonzales, Director, City of Dallas Department of Health and Human Services, 1500 Marilla, Dallas, TX.

Health Resources per 1,000 Pop.	Number	Rank
Hospital beds, community hospitals, city	5.64	60/92
Nurses, community hospitals, city	6.01	58/90
Doctors, metro area	2.07	78/113

The city has 262 tennis courts, 213 football/soccer fields, 125 basketball courts, 119 softball fields and 102 swimming pools among its sports facilities. Dallas also has a large recreational center with an indoor pool and a moveable floor for use by the handicapped and others with special programming needs. A turn-of-the-century working farm provides youth programs centered on crafts and services of the period as well as overnight camping and fishing. Old City Park is a turn-of-the-century village with authentic buildings from this period. The Dallas State Fair Grounds contains one of the largest collections of art deco buildings in the U.S. Contact: Frank Wise, Director, Parks and Recreation Department, 1500 Marilla, City Hall 6FN, Dallas, TX 75201.

Parkland/Total City Area (percent)	8.3

The Dallas public school system employs 130 nurses, 1 physician, 40 psychologists, 12 occupational therapists, 2 audiologists and 3 physician's assistants. 50 percent of the schools have a nurse present full-time and all the schools have a nurse part-time. 80 percent of the Dallas school system nursing staff have nurse-practitioner certification. All common health-education programs are offered to students in grades K-12. The city also has an AIDS education program. No medical, dental, or psychiatric treatment is provided for students. Contact: Dr. Richard Adams, Director of School Health Services, Dallas Independent School District, 3700 Ross Avenue, Dallas, TX 75204.

Dayton, OH

🪦	🏃	$	🌲	℞	🏃	👥	?
✓	✓	✓	✓	X	✔	X	✔

 Dayton (Montgomery County) has an average age-adjusted death rate. The state's infant-mortality rate is low in rural areas and average in urban areas. The rate for whites is very low, while the rate for blacks and other minorities is high (231st and 238th out of 301 cities); most of the state's minorities live in the cities.

	Number	Rank
Age-Adjusted Death Rate	−0.07	51/100
Heart Attacks	0.09	64/100
Cancer	0.05	57/100

Dayton's homicide and robbery rates are average for U.S. metro areas. Its suicide and accident rates are very low.

Incidence per 1,000 Pop.	Number	Rank
Homicides (1989)	0.08	56/111
Robberies (1989)	2.25	65/111
Suicides	0.07	5/100
Accidents	0.27	11/100

$ Dayton's 1988 metro population was 948,000—51st out of 113 metro areas. Statistics for metro Dayton include the neighboring city of Springfield, OH. Dayton's economic health at the end of 1990 was below average, ranking 64th of 113 metro areas. Its unemployment rate ranks 56th, change in unemployment 58th (the labor force grew by 2.1 percent, faster than employment, which grew by 1.7 percent) and its enterprise 62nd. Contact: Mayor Clay Dixon, City of Dayton, 101 West Third Street, Dayton, OH 45402.

Air Quality: During 1988, the Miami Valley went from "borderline" ozone attainment into a definitely nonattainment situation (meaning one in which they violated federal standards). For the period of 1983–87 no monitor was found to be in violation of the ozone standard. Due to the high temperatures in 1988, however, 10 days of unhealthy air were recorded for ozone in the Miami Valley. Contact: Dr. Morton Nelson, Health Commissioner, Montgomery County Combined General Health District, 451 West Third Street, Dayton, OH 45422.

Water Quality: Dayton's total drinking water supply comes from ground water sources. The pH of the drinking water was 8.5 in 1989. Contact: William B. Zilli, Director, City of Dayton, Department of Water, Box 22, 101 West Third Street, Dayton, OH 45401.

Weather: The average high temperature is slightly below average at 61.5. Humidity and precipitation are both slightly above average.

Average Daily Temperature (degrees F)	
High	61.5
Low	42.3
Average Humidity	
Morning (percent)	80
Afternoon (percent)	60
Normal Precipitation (inches)	34.7
Average Total Snowfall (inches)	28.6
Ozone, Days over 0.12 ppm (1 hour, 1988)	10

℞ Smoking is prohibited on public transportation and in public offices and partially restricted in restaurants and private offices. The city has all the common health-education programs and emergency hotlines. Contact: Dr. Morton Nelson, Health Commissioner, Montgomery County Combined General Health District, 451 West Third Street, Dayton, OH 45422.

Health Resources per 1,000 Pop.	**Number**	**Rank**
Hospital beds, community hospitals, city	13.93	5/92
Nurses, community hospitals, city	16.10	4/90
Doctors, metro area	1.84	94/113

The city offers aerobics, arts and crafts, tumbling and other classes and walking programs along with numerous other recreational activities. Dayton's sports facilities include 88 tennis courts, 85 baseball fields, 66 basketball courts, 23 football/soccer fields, 13 swimming pools, 6 golf courses and 5 running tracks. There are 80 softball, 24 basketball and 11 volleyball leagues. A special playground for the disabled was dedicated in 1989. A wheelchair softball team was formed last year and participated in a national tournament. Contact: Michael Alexinas, Superintendent, City of Dayton, Division of Recreation and Parks, Box 22, 101 West Third Street, Dayton, OH 45401.

Parkland/Total City Area (percent)   6.2
Aerobics classes   yes
Arts and craft classes   yes
Hiking or exploration groups   no

The 28,000 students in the public school system are served by one physician. A full-time nurse is available in 12 percent of the schools and a part-time nurse available in the rest of the schools. All common health-education programs are offered to students in grades K-12. The major emphasis of the school health education program is in sexual education, specifically sexually transmitted diseases and AIDS. Dental treatment is provided for students. Contact: Betty Holton, Supervisor, Health Services, Dayton Public Schools, 348 West First Street, Dayton, OH 45402-3079.

Denver, CO

The city and county of Denver, with a population of nearly 500,000, is the urban hub of a six-county consolidated metropolitan area with a population of approximately 1.9 million. The five other counties that make up Denver's consolidated metropolitan area are Adams, Arapahoe, Douglas, Jefferson and Boulder. Aurora, which is part of Denver County (the primary metro area), is one of many suburban jurisdictions adjacent to Denver. Denver (Denver county) has the third-best age-adjusted death rate of 100 metro areas we ranked. Denver has the lowest cancer rate and the 4th lowest rate of heart attacks. The state's infant-mortality rate is about average, though it is low for rural areas and high for blacks. This is because most of the state's minorities live in the cities.

	Number	Rank
Age-Adjusted Death Rate	−3.00	3/100
Heart Attacks	−0.90	4/100
Cancer	−0.80	1/100

Denver-Aurora has the 3rd lowest robbery rate of the surveyed cities. Rates for homicide and accidents are also relatively low. The number of suicides is high.

Incidence per 1,000 Pop.	Number	Rank
Homicides (1989)	0.05	29/111
Robberies (1989)	1.35	28/111
Suicides	0.16	88/100
Accidents	0.29	21/100

$ The Denver-Aurora (Denver County) 1988 primary metro population was 1,640,000—26th out of 113 metro areas. The consolidated Denver metro area includes all of the six counties listed above. Denver's economic health at the end of 1990 was excellent, ranking 17th of 113 metro areas. Its unemployment rate ranks 21st, change in unemployment 6th (employment grew faster than the labor force) and its enterprise 69th. Contact: Mayor's Office, City of Denver, 1437 Bannock Street, Room 350, Denver, CO 80202.

Weather: Denver averages about 300 sunny days a year, which is more than Miami or San Diego. The relative humidity is low at 40 percent and the average temperature is 50.1 degrees. The weather is marred only by the persistent haze.

Air Quality: Carbon monoxide levels in Denver are going down significantly. However, visibility is getting worse year-round. In Aurora, levels of carbon monoxide, particulates, ozone and nitrogen dioxide have all maintained concentrations below the EPA standards over the past five years. There is no significant trend toward improvement or degeneration. Contact: Tommy Massuro, Office of Environmental Affairs, 303 West Colfax, Suite 1600, Denver, CO 80202. Or: Mayor's Office, City and County of Denver Room 350, 1437 Bannock Street, Denver, CO 80202.

Water Quality: Denver's total drinking water supply comes from surface water sources. Drinking water in Aurora comes from surface water (95 percent) and ground water (5 percent). Overall presence of its few contaminants remains consistent from year to year. Contact: Stephen Work, Denver Water Board, 1600 West 12th Avenue, Denver, CO 80254. Or: Roger Knight, Water Quality Control, City of Aurora, 18301 East Quincey Avenue, Aurora, CO 80015.

Average Daily Temperature (degrees F)	50.3
High	64.3
Low	36.2
Average Humidity	
Morning (percent)	67
Afternoon (percent)	40

Normal Precipitation (inches)   15.3
Average Total Snowfall (inches)   60.3

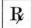 No public-health questionnaire was returned.

Health Resources per 1,000 Pop.	Number	Rank
Denver		
Hospital beds, community hospitals, city	7.76	35/92
Nurses, community hospitals, city	7.90	40/90
Doctors, metro area	2.76	38/113
Aurora		
Hospital beds, community hospitals, city	1.45	91/92
Nurses, community hospitals, city	1.61	88/90
Doctors, metro area	2.76	38/113

 Denver passed a $59.6 million bond to cover 337 capital improvement projects in the Parks and Recreation Department. The city has a variety of sports facilities including 150 basketball courts, 143 tennis courts, 132 baseball fields, 119 football/soccer fields, 23 swimming pools, 8 golf courses and 1 marina. Softball is a popular sport with 150 sports leagues. Basketball and tennis are also popular. Classes in aerobics, arts and crafts and hiking/exploration are provided by the city. Contact: Carolyn Etter, Manager, Denver Parks and Recreation Department, City of Denver, 2300 15th Street, Suite 150, Denver, CO 80202.

Aurora offers classes in aerobics, arts and crafts, outdoor recreation, swimming, gymnastics, dance and therapeutics. The city offers a variety of youth programs in sports and recreation. Also popular are programs for senior citizens. Aurora has 74 tennis courts, 59 basketball courts, 41 baseball fields, 38 football/soccer fields, 4 golf courses, 9 swimming pools, and 11 recreation centers. Softball, volleyball, basketball and tennis are the most popular sports. Contact: Lori Daniel, Manager, Aurora Parks and Recreation Department, 1470 South Havana Street, #518, Aurora, CO 80012.

Parkland/Total City Area (percent)
Denver   5.6
Aurora   7.8

No school-health questionnaire was returned.

Des Moines, IA

🪦	🏃	$	⬆	℞	🖼	👥	?
✔	✔	✔	✓	X	✔	✔	✔

🪦 Des Moines' (Polk County) age-adjusted mortality rate ranks 16th. Iowa has a high infant-mortality rate among minorities and in urban areas.

	Number	Rank
Age-Adjusted Death Rate	−1.21	19/100
Heart Attacks	−0.83	6/100
Cancer	−0.17	30/100

🏃 Des Moines has the 2nd lowest robbery rate of the 101 metro areas surveyed. Homicide and accident rates are also low.

Incidence per 1,000 Pop.	Number	Rank
Homicides (1989)	0.05	21/111
Robberies (1989)	1.04	17/111
Suicides	0.12	44/100
Accidents	0.28	15/100

$ Des Moines' 1988 metro population was 392,000—90th out of 113 metro areas. Its economic health at the end of 1990 was excellent, ranking 9th of 113 metro areas. Its unemployment rate ranks 11th, change in unemployment 27th (the labor force declined faster than employment) and its enterprise 40th. Contact: Mayor John P. Dourian, City of Des Moines, East First and Locust Streets, Des Moines, IA 50307.

⬆ **Hazardous Waste:** Polk county has no hazardous-waste disposal sites. Development of hazardous-waste facilities throughout the state is being proposed. Contact: Des Moines Metropolitan Area Solid Waste Agency, 617 East 2nd Street, Des Moines, IA 50309.

Weather: The city's average temperature is cool at 49.7. Precipitation is above average at 34.4 inches annually.

Average Daily Temperature (degrees F)	49.7
High	59.3
Low	40.0
Average Humidity	
Morning (percent)	79
Afternoon (percent)	60
Normal Precipitation (inches)	30.8
Average Total Snowfall (inches)	34.4

℞ Smoking is prohibited in public offices and on public transportation and partially prohibited in restaurants and in private offices. All common health-education programs and emergency hotlines are provided by the city. Contact: Dr. Julius Conner, Public Health Director, Polk County Health Department, 1915 Hickman Road, Des Moines, IA 50314.

Health Resources per 1,000 Pop.	Number	Rank
Hospital beds, community hospitals, city	10.78	18/92
Nurses, community hospitals, city	10.88	20/90
Doctors, metro area	1.76	97/113

The city's sports facilities include 86 tennis courts, 80 baseball/softball fields, 27 football/soccer fields, 10 basketball courts, 6 swimming pools, 3 golf courses, 1 marina and 1 beach. Softball, volleyball, basketball, water aerobics and fitness instruction are popular recreation activities. Recently there have been improvements on swimming pools and softball facilities. Contact: Donald Tripp, Director, Des Moines Park and Recreation Department, 3226 University, Des Moines, IA 50311.

Parkland/Total City Area (percent)	5.4

To serve 30,000 students (grades K-12) in the public school system are 36 nurses, 1 physician, 18 psychologists, 19 social workers and 86 "counselors". All common health-education programs are offered to students in grades K-12. No medical, dental or psychiatric treatment is provided for students. Contact: Mardelle Dallager, Supervisor, Health Services, Des Moines Public Schools, 1800 Grand Avenue, Des Moines, IA 50307.

Detroit, MI

RIP	⤵	$	↑	℞	🏃	👥	?
X	X	X	X	✓	?	✔	✓

The Detroit primary metro area includes Warren. Detroit's (Wayne and Macomb counties) age-adjusted mortality rate ranks a moderate 68th. The infant-mortality rate in Michigan is extremely high among minorities. Lower infant-mortality rates are found among whites and in rural areas. Contact: Dr. Mesa, Medical Director, Detroit Health Department, 1151 Taylor, Detroit, MI 48202.

	Number	Rank
Age-Adjusted Death Rate	0.48	68/100
Heart Attacks	0.56	83/100
Cancer	0.11	68/100

While robbery and accident rates are relatively low in Detroit, the city had the 7th highest rate for homicides in 1989.

Incidence per 1,000 Pop.	Number	Rank
Homicides (1989)	0.18	103/111
Robberies (1989)	3.56	93/111
Suicides	0.12	39/100
Accidents	0.28	16/100

Detroit's 1988 metro population was 4,352,000—5th out of 113 metro areas. Consolidated Detroit includes the Ann Arbor, Mich. primary metro area (population 268,000). Its economic health at the end of 1990 was poor, ranking 97th of 113 metro areas. Its unemployment rate ranks 103rd, change in unemployment 58th (employment declined faster than the labor force) and its enterprise 79th. Contact: Mayor Coleman Young, City of Detroit, 1126 City-County Building, Detroit, MI 48226.

Air Quality: Detroit's air quality is in the bottom fifth of rated cities, despite a strong environmental stance by the State of Michigan. The city had 6 days of ozone exceedances in 1988, 1 in 1989 and 0 in 1990. Its particulate pollution from cars and residences remains relatively high. Contact: Laura DeGuire, Environmental Quality Analyst, Michigan

Department of Natural Resources, Air Quality Division, PO Box 30028, Lansing, MI 48909. The air quality of suburban Warren rated better than Detroit's.

Weather: In spite of its northern location, Detroit's climate is relatively mild, due to the moderating effects of the Great Lakes. The winters are cloudy, with daily highs of 32 degrees and lows of 17 degrees. The summers are warm, sunny and fairly humid, with average morning lows of 61 degrees and afternoon highs of 84 degrees. The area gets about 40 inches of snow a year.

Average Daily Temperature (degrees F)	48.6
High	58.2
Low	38.9
Average Humidity	
Morning (percent)	81
Afternoon (percent)	60
Normal Precipitation (inches)	31.0
Average Total Snowfall (inches)	42.0
Ozone, Days over 0.12 ppm (1 hour, 1988)	6

℞ No public-health questionnaire was available.

Health Resources per 1,000 Pop.	Number	Rank
Hospital beds, community hospitals, city	6.08	54/92
Nurses, community hospitals, city	7.32	48/90
Doctors, metro area	2.10	75/113

 A recreation-facilities survey was not returned.

 The Detroit public-school system does not employ nurses for its 170,757 students; the Detroit Health Department supplies nurses, physicians and psychologists. There are no nurses present in any of the schools, but the school system does employ 80 psychologists. In addition to all common health-education programs, Detroit also offers curriculum on safety/first aid, family health, community health, personal health practices, disease prevention and mental health. Health education is taught to students in grades K-12. There are three supplemental school-health programs: (1) School-health centers at two high schools, (2) Teen Stop I program and (3) Teen Stop II program. Dental and psychiatric treatment are provided for students. Contact: Roy Allen, Jr., Director, Health, Physical

Education and Safety Department, Detroit Public Schools Center, 5057 Woodward, Detroit, MI 48202.

El Paso, TX

🪦	🏃	$	🌲	℞	🏃	🛌	?
✔	✓	X	✓	X	?	?	X

 El Paso (El Paso County) ranks 24th in its age-adjusted mortality rate. Infant-mortality rates in Texas are high among minorities and low among whites and in rural areas.

	Number	Rank
Age-Adjusted Death Rate	−1.10	24/100
Heart Attacks	−0.24	36/100
Cancer	−0.31	19/100

🏃 Suicide and accident rates are low in El Paso. The city has average rates for homicide and robbery.

Incidence per 1,000 Pop.	Number	Rank
Homicides (1989)	0.08	54/111
Robberies (1989)	1.98	54/111
Suicides	0.09	10/100
Accidents	0.30	22/100

$ El Paso's 1988 metro population was 586,000—71st out of 113 metro areas. Its economic health at the end of 1990 was poor, ranking 94th of 113 metro areas. Its unemployment rate ranks 109th, change in unemployment 101st (the labor force grew by 4.4 percent, much faster than employment, 2.2 percent) and its enterprise 24th. Contact: Mayor Suzie Azar, City of El Paso, 2 Civic Center Plaza, 10th Floor, El Paso, TX 79901.

 Water Quality: 80 percent of El Paso's water supply consists of ground water and 20 percent of surface water.

Weather: El Paso has the typical climate of dry areas, with abundant sunshine, low humidity and little rainfall. Temperatures average 43 degrees in January and 82.3 degrees in July.

Average Daily Temperature (degrees F)	63.4
High	77.5
Low	49.2
Average Humidity	
Morning (percent)	56
Afternoon (percent)	27
Normal Precipitation (inches)	7.8
Average Total Snowfall (inches)	5.8

 The city did not return its public-health questionnaire.

Health Resources per 1,000 Pop.	Number	Rank
Hospital beds, community hospitals, city	3.49	85/92
Nurses, community hospitals, city	2.56	87/90
Doctors, metro area	1.38	110/113

 The city did not return a recreational-facilities questionnaire.

 The city did not return a school-health questionnaire.

Flint, MI

🪦 RIP	🗳	$	🌲	℞	🚶	👫	?
X	X	X	✔	X	✔	✔	✔

Flint (Genesee county) ranks an unhealthy 96th with its age-adjusted mortality rate. Flint also has extremely high cancer and heart attack rates. Infant-mortality rates in Michigan are extremely high among minorities and low among whites and in rural areas.

	Number	Rank
Age-Adjusted Death Rate	2.72	96/100
Heart Attacks	1.11	97/100
Cancer	0.62	94/100
Infant Mortality (Michigan)		
All Areas	10.7	171/301
Blacks	21.4	298/301
Other	20.1	294/301
Rural	8.2	38/301
Urban Places	12.5	205/301
Whites	8.4	53/301

 Flint has relatively high homicide, robbery and accident rates.

Incidence per 1,000 Pop.	Number	Rank
Homicides (1989)	0.15	97/111
Robberies (1989)	3.24	89/111
Suicides	0.14	69/100
Accidents	0.40	86/100

 Flint's 1988 metro population was 431,000—86th out of 113 metro areas. Its economic health at the end of 1990 was very poor, ranking 111th of 113 metro areas. Its unemployment rate ranks 110th, change in unemployment 95th (employment fell by over 3 percent, faster than the labor force, which fell by 1.9 percent) and its enterprise 109th. Contact: Mayor Matthew Collier, City of Flint, City Hall, Flint, MI 48502.

 Weather: The average high temperature is slightly low at 56.1. Humidity and precipitation are both slightly above average.

Average Daily Temperature (degrees F)	46.8
High	56.1
Low	37.4
Average Humidity	
Morning (percent)	81
Afternoon (percent)	62
Normal Precipitation (inches)	29.2
Average Total Snowfall (inches)	45.4
Ozone, Days over 0.12 ppm (1 hour, 1988)	1

Flint offers all common public health-education programs. Emergency hotlines are provided for child abuse, suicide, alcoholism, drug abuse and AIDS information. The city also offers treatment for sexually transmitted diseases. The state of Michigan has an anti-smoking law that partially restricts smoking in restaurants and public offices. Contact: Sue Weidman, Safety Coordinator, City of Flint, 1101 South Saginaw Street, Flint, MI 48502.

Flint community schools offer numerous recreational classes ranging from dance instruction to dog obedience to card games and self-defense. Flint has an extensive senior citizen program which includes job placement and new skill instruction. Sports facilities include 93 basketball courts, 66 tennis courts, 61 baseball fields, 16 football/soccer fields, 5 golf courses, 5 running tracks and 1 swimming pool. Popular sports leagues include volleyball, basketball, baseball and soccer. Contact: Richard Daly, City of Flint Community Schools, 923 East Kearsley, Flint, MI 48502.

Parkland/Total City Area (percent)	10.1
Aerobics classes	yes
Arts and craft classes	yes
Hiking or exploration groups	yes

The Flint public school system employs six nurses, one physician on a contractual/consulting basis, nine psychologists serving the special education students only, one dental hygienist who works one day per week and one full-time vision/hearing technician. There are three nurses present in 7 percent of the schools full-time and three nurses present in the rest percent of the schools part time. All common health-education programs are offered to students in grades K-12. Medical and dental treatment are provided for students. Contact: Eleanor Poole, Coordinator, Flint Community School Health Services, 3501 Minnesota, Flint, MI 48502.

Fort Lauderdale, FL

⚰️ RIP	🏊	$	🌲	℞	🏃	👪	?
✓	✓	X	✓	✓	✓	✓	✓

Fort Lauderdale (Broward County) ranks a moderate 44th with its age-adjusted mortality rate. Florida has high infant-mortality rates among minorities and low rates among whites. Infant-mortality rates are higher in rural areas.

	Number	Rank
Age-Adjusted Death Rate	−0.26	44/100
Heart Attacks	0.52	82/100
Cancer	0.00	50/100

 Broward County has extremely high robbery and suicide rates. The frequencies of homicides and accidents are also above average.

Incidence per 1,000 Pop.	Number	Rank
Homicides (1989)	0.09	68/111
Robberies (1989)	4.28	100/111
Suicides	0.17	90/100
Accidents	0.38	81/100

$ Fort Lauderdale's 1988 metro population was 1.19 million—41st out of 113 metro areas. Its economic health at the end of 1990 was below average, ranking 79th of 113 metro areas. Its unemployment rate ranks 76th, change in unemployment 91st (the labor force grew faster than employment) and its enterprise 25th. Contact: Mayor Jim Naugle, City of Fort Lauderdale, City Hall, Fort Lauderdale, FL 33301.

♠ Air Quality: Despite a slight increase during the latter half of the 1980s in the number of days in which the ozone NAAQS (0.12 ppm) is being exceeded, Fort Lauderdale ranked 15th cleanest in 1990 out of 194 reporting areas with respect to ozone levels. No area of comparable size reported lower average ozone levels except Miami, Palm Beach and Honolulu. Contact: A.A. Linero, Chief, Air Section, Office of Natural Resource Protection, 621 S. Andrews Ave., Fort Lauderdale, FL 33301.

Hazardous Waste: Fort Lauderdale has six hazardous-waste sites on the EPA's National Priorities List for "Superfund." Ammonia, lead, iron and chlorinated compounds are deposited at the Broward County Landfill, solvents at Hollingsworth Solderless, petroleum hydrocarbons, acid, heavy metals and chlorinated hydrocarbons at Petroleum Products, petroleum hydrocarbons and lead at Wingate Road Incinerator and petroleum hydrocarbons at Wilson Concepts. The last site is called Chemforms. The wastes are disposed of outside Broward County as it is not permissible to dispose of hazardous waste within the county. Contact: Mira Barer, Office of Natural Resource Protection, 500 E Broward Blvd., #104, Fort Lauderdale, FL 33353.

Water Quality: The entire water supply in Fort Lauderdale is supplied by ground water. Contact: Patrick Brian, Water operations manager, City of Fort Lauderdale Utilities Department, PO Box Drawer 14250, Fort Lauderdale, FL 33301.

Weather: See Miami, Florida.

Ozone, Days over 0.12 ppm (1 hour, 1988)   2

℞ Fort Lauderdale has legislation prohibiting smoking on public transportation and partially restricting it in restaurants, public offices and private offices. All common health-education programs and emergency hotlines are provided by the city. The county has initiated several AIDS-education campaigns and programs. Contact: David Roach, Broward County Health Unit, 2421 S.W. 6th Avenue, Fort Lauderdale, FL 33315.

The city is currently developing new parks and sports facilities. There are 48 baseball fields, 65 tennis courts, 22 football/soccer fields, 62 basketball courts and 5 running tracks. Fort Lauderdale is famous for its 6.5 miles of beaches. Several marinas offer boat rentals and fishing areas. Fort Lauderdale has several youth programs and a summer camp program. Contact: Tom Tapp, Director, City of Fort Lauderdale Parks and Recreation Department, 301 N. Andrews Avenue, Fort Lauderdale, FL 33301.

Parkland/Total City Area (percent)	4.7
Aerobics classes	yes
Arts and craft classes	yes
Hiking or exploration groups	yes

Broward County employs 10 nurses and 83 psychologists for the 150,000 students in its school system. The nurses work full-time in ESE centers and a non-school board nurse works four hours a week in all the schools. All common health-education programs are offered to students in grades K-12. The school system has a model policy for communicable disease, family life and human sexuality. Medical, dental and psychiatric treatment is provided for students. Contact: Sam Morgan, Superintendent, Broward County Public Schools, 1320 SW 4th Street, Fort Lauderdale, FL 33302.

Fort Wayne, IN

RIP	⛏	$	▲	℞	[⛹]	👫	?
X	✓	✔	X	X	✓	X	✔

RIP Fort Wayne (Allen County) ranks 80th with its age-adjusted mortality rate. Indiana has high infant-mortality rates among minorities and low rates among whites and in rural areas.

	Number	Rank
Age-Adjusted Death Rate	0.80	80/100
Heart Attacks	0.69	90/100
Cancer	0.12	70/100

 The city has low to average rates of homicide, robbery, suicide and accidents.

Incidence per 1,000 Pop.	Number	Rank
Homicides (1989)	0.06	38/111
Robberies (1989)	1.70	37/111
Suicides	0.11	26/100
Accidents	0.34	57/100

$ Fort Wayne's 1988 metro population was 367,000—91st out of 113 metro areas. Its economic health at the end of 1990 was excellent, ranking 5th of 113 metro areas. Its unemployment rate ranks 56th, change in unemployment 52nd (the labor force grew faster than employment) and its enterprise 72nd. Contact: Mayor Paul Helmke, City of Fort Wayne, City-County Building, 1 Main Street, Fort Wayne, IN 46802.

↑ **Water Quality:** The Safe Drinking Water Act will require the city to make some water treatment improvements, even though current quality is considered exceptionally high. Contact: John McLane, Filtration Plant Manager, City-County Building, 1 Main Street, Fort Wayne, IN 46802.

Weather: The average temperature is cool at 49.7. Humidity and precipitation are slightly above average.

Average Daily Temperature (degrees F)	49.7
High	59.3
Low	40.0
Average Humidity	
Morning (percent)	82
Afternoon (percent)	62
Normal Precipitation (inches)	34.4
Average Total Snowfall (inches)	33.1

℞ No public health services questionnaire was available.

Health Resources per 1,000 Pop.	Number	Rank
Hospital beds, community hospitals, city	8.17	30/92

| Nurses, community hospitals, city | 8.64 | 34/90 |
| Doctors, metro area | 1.62 | 103/113 |

The most popular recreational facility is the children's zoo and the botanical conservatory. The city has 56 tennis courts, 53 basketball courts, 52 baseball fields, 36 horseshoe courts, 15 football/soccer fields, 4 swimming pools and 3 golf courses for its sports facilities. Other recreational facilities include an ice arena, the outdoor theatre, recreation centers, senior centers and a day camp for children. Contact: Katherine Beatty, Marketing Manager, Parks and Recreation Department, 705 East State Blvd., Fort Wayne, IN 46805.

Parkland/Total City Area (percent)   4.5

For a total of 31,942 students in the public school system (grades K-12), there are 11 nurses. Each nurse must service five to six schools, which means that a part-time nurse is available in high schools and middle schools for one and a half days per week and in the elementary schools only for one-half day. The city is working hard to increase the nursing staff. The city has recently adopted some interesting new programs. AIDS presentations are made to all of the staff each year and stress-reduction services are available to those schools that request it. The school system offers health-education programs in nutrition, hygiene, illnesses, smoking and drugs to students in grades K-5 and 7-9. Medical treatment is provided for the students. Contact: Myra Fill, Director, Health Services, 1230 South Clinton Street, Fort Wayne, IN 46802.

Fort Worth, TX

⚰	🏃	$	⬆	℞	🎿	👪	?
✔	X	X	✓	X	✓	✔	✔

Fort Worth (Tarrant County) ranks a good 15th with its age-adjusted mortality rate. Infant-mortality rates in Texas are high among minorities and low among whites and in rural areas.

	Number	**Rank**
Age-Adjusted Death Rate	−1.47	15/100
Heart Attacks	1.21	22/100
Cancer	1.36	16/100

The homicide rate is high in metro Fort Worth (30th highest); robberies are above-average in frequency. Suicide and accident rates, which are for the consolidated Dallas-Fort Worth metro, are also above average.

Incidence per 1,000 Pop.	Number	Rank
Homicides (1989)	0.12	82/111
Robberies (1989)	2.63	71/111
Suicides	0.14	72/100
Accidents	0.34	61/100

$ Fort Worth's 1988 metro population was 1.29 million—38th out of 113 metro areas. Its economic health at the end of 1990 was below average, ranking 82nd of 113 metro areas. Its unemployment rate ranks 88th, change in unemployment 74th (the labor force grew by 2.4 percent, employment by 1.7 percent) and its enterprise 42nd. Contact: Mayor Bob Bolen, City of Fort Worth, 100 Throckmorton Street, Fort Worth, TX 76102.

Air Quality: The general air quality is improving, but at a slower rate than in previous years. The number of ozone days has decreased and the highest levels are also lower. Contact: Health Planning & Promotion Unit Manager, City of Fort Worth Public Health Department, 1800 University Drive, Room 217, Fort Worth, TX 76107.

Water Quality: The city plans to use ozone in the water-purification process to insure the highest possible water quality. A storm-drain pollution-control program is now operating to reduce pollution problems in area creeks, rivers, and lakes. Contact: John Humphreys, Public Information Specialist, Public Health Department, 1800 University Drive, Fort Worth, TX 76107.

Weather: The Dallas-Fort Worth area has a warm, moderately humid climate. The temperature reaches 90 degrees and above an average of 95 days a year. It dips to 32 degrees or less around 40 days a year. (For more data on weather, see Dallas; the weather information is collected at the airport for both cities.)

Ozone, Days over 0.12 ppm (1 hour, 1988)   4

℞ Mobility Impaired Transit provides public transportation for the handicapped. There are plans to add wheelchair lifts to some buses. Smoking is properly a major health concern in the city and is prohibited in public offices and on public transportation and partially restricted in

restaurants and private offices. Two physicians work in the sexually transmitted disease clinics and maternity and child health clinics. All common
health-education programs are provided by the city. The city provides
most basic emergency hotlines. Contact: Mary Steinhausen, M.S., Health
Planning & Promotion Unit Manager, City of Fort Worth Public Health
Department, 1800 University Drive, Room 217, Fort Worth, TX 76107.

Health Resources per 1,000 Pop.	**Number**	**Rank**
Hospital beds, community hospitals, city	5.69	59/92
Nurses, community hospitals, city	7.50	45/90
Doctors, metro area	1.33	113/113

The Fort Worth area has 86 tennis courts, 76 baseball fields, 38
football/soccer fields, 12 basketball courts, 9 golf courses and 4
swimming pools among its sports facilities. Softball, basketball, volleyball
and tennis are popular sports. Contact: Ralph Emerson, Director, Parks &
Recreation Department, 100 North University Drive, Fort Worth, TX
76107.

Parkland/Total City Area (percent)	6.4
Aerobics classes	yes
Arts and craft classes	yes
Hiking or exploration groups	yes

For a total of 68,000 students in the public school system (grades
K-12) there are 64 nurses, 2 pediatric consultants, 24 psychologists
and 3 nurse's aides. There are 26 full-time nurses working in 41 percent of
the schools and 37 part-time nurses working in the rest of the schools. All
common health-education programs are offered to students in grades K-12.
Medical, dental and psychiatric treatment is provided for students. Contact: Polly Stringfield, Program Director, Health Education, Fort Worth
Independent School District, 3210 West Lancaster, Fort Worth, TX 76107.

Fresno, CA

⚰️RIP	✈	$	🌲	℞	🏃	👫	?
✓	X	X	X	X	X	X	✔

Fresno (Fresno County) ranks a moderate 59th with its age-adjusted
mortality rate. California has high infant-mortality rates among
blacks and low rates among whites and in rural areas.

	Number	Rank
Age-Adjusted Death Rate	0.24	59/100
Heart Attacks	0.20	70/100
Cancer	−0.07	43/100

Fresno has relatively high homicide and robbery rates; both are 32nd highest of 111 metro areas. Suicide and accident rates are above the average for 100 metro areas.

Incidence per 1,000 Pop.	Number	Rank
Homicides (1989)	0.11	80/111
Robberies (1989)	2.85	80/111
Suicides	0.12	43/100
Accidents	0.32	40/100

$ Fresno's 1988 metro population was 615,000—69th out of 113 metro areas. Its economic health at the end of 1990 was very poor, ranking 112th of 113 metro areas. Its unemployment rate ranks 111th, change in unemployment 97th (the labor force rose faster than employment) and its enterprise 99th. Contact: Mayor Karen Humphrey, City of Fresno, 2326 Fresno Street, Fresno, CA 93721.

Air Quality: Fresno had 43 days of ozone exceedances and 3 days of carbon-monoxide exceedances in 1988. Contact: Katie Bearden, Air Quality Planner, County of Fresno, Department of Health, Air Pollution Control District, 1221 Fulton Mall, PO Box 11867, Fresno, CA 93775.

Water Quality: Fresno's total drinking water supply comes from ground water sources. The pH of the drinking water averages 7.7. Recently there has been an intrusion of agricultural chemicals into the metropolitan water supply. Contact: William E. Burmeister, Water Systems Manager, Public Works Department, Water Division, 1910 East University Street, Fresno, CA 93703-2988.

Weather: The average temperature is slightly above average at 62.5. The average annual precipitation is low at 10.52 inches.

Average Daily Temperature (degrees F)	62.5
High	76.1
Low	49.0
Average Humidity	
Morning (percent)	78
Afternoon (percent)	41

Annual Precipitation (inches)   10.5
Average Total Snowfall (inches)   0.1
Ozone, Days over 0.12 ppm (1 hour, 1988)   43

℞ The county offers all common public health-education programs and emergency hotlines. The county health department has initiated a prenatal care program, an AIDS testing program and a cancer-awareness and reduction-through-education program. The county health department offers several community and home-based services for senior citizens. The county provides all common preventive-health and treatment programs. Contact: George Bleth, Director of Health, County of Fresno Department of Health, PO Box 11867, Fresno, CA 93774.

Health Resources per 1,000 Pop.	Number	Rank
Hospital beds, community hospitals, city	4.45	78/92
Nurses, community hospitals, city	6.40	56/90
Doctors, metro area	1.88	89/113

Fresno has recently acquired new regional park property and has constructed a new neighborhood center. Also new is a community center swimming pool and several cultural activities at the Downtown Mall. The Fresno Zoo is very popular. The city has 32 baseball fields, 31 tennis courts, 27 basketball courts, 24 soccer fields, 11 swimming pools, 9 volleyball courts and 3 golf courses among its sports facilities. Contact: Joe Wingfield, Acting Director, City of Fresno Parks & Recreation Department, 1900 Mariposa Mall, Suite 202, Fresno, CA 93721.

Parkland/Total City Area (percent)   1.5

The public-school system employs 39 nurses for its 65,000 students. A nurse is present part-time in all of the schools. All common health-education programs are offered to students in grades K-8 and grade 12. The school system provides all common screens and tests except for immunizations, mental-health exams and speech therapy. Emergency first aid is provided for ill or injured children. Contact: Anna Phillips, Director of Health Services, Fresno Unified School District, Department of Health Services, 6235 North Brawley Avenue, Fresno, CA 93722.

Grand Rapids, MI

🪦	♈	$	⬆	℞	🔫	🏊	?
✓	✔	✓	✔	X	✓	X	✔

Grand Rapids (Kent County) has an average age-adjusted mortality rate. Infant-mortality rates in Michigan are extremely high among minorities. Lower infant-mortality rates are found among whites and in rural areas. Contact: Jorge Rayon, Epidemiologist, Kent County Health Department, 700 Fuller Avenue N.E., Grand Rapids, MI 49503.

	Number	Rank
Age-Adjusted Death Rate	−0.11	50/100
Heart Attacks	−0.03	52/100
Cancer	−0.01	48/100

Grand Rapids has relatively low homicide (9th lowest of 111 metro areas), robbery and suicide rates. Its accident rate is, however, well above average.

Incidence per 1,000 Pop.	Number	Rank
Homicides (1989)	0.03	9/111
Robberies (1989)	1.14	19/111
Suicides	0.09	16/100
Accidents	0.35	62/100

Grand Rapids' 1988 metro population was 665,000—61st out of 113 metro areas. Its economic health at the end of 1990 was below average, ranking 65th of 113 metro areas. Its unemployment rate ranks 76th, change in unemployment 74th (the labor force grew faster than employment) and its enterprise 27th. Contact: Mayor Gerald Helmholt, City of Grand Rapids, 300 Monroe Avenue N.W., Grand Rapids, MI 49503.

Air Quality: Grand Rapids had 7 ozone exceedances in 1988.

Hazardous Waste: Grand Rapids has a hazardous-waste site on EPA's National Priorities List for Superfund, Butterworth Landfill, where household and industrial waste were deposited. Contact: James Biener, Director of Public Utilities, City of Grand Rapids, 1101 Monroe N.W., Grand Rapids, MI 49503.

Water Quality: All of the water in Grand Rapids is supplied by surface water (e.g., reservoirs). Contact: Monroe Filtration Plant, 1930 Monroe Avenue N.W., Grand Rapids, MI 49503.

Weather: Grand Rapids is a cool city with an average temperature of 47.5. Precipitation and humidity are slightly above average.

Average Daily Temperature (degrees F)	47.5
High	57.2
Low	37.7
Average Humidity	
Morning (percent)	83
Afternoon (percent)	62
Annual Precipitation (inches)	34.4
Average Total Snowfall (inches)	71.6
Ozone, Days over 0.12 ppm (1 hour, 1988)	7

℞ A considerable number of outreach/access programs have been recently established especially for street people, inner-city populations and people with AIDS. Numerous urgent care centers have also been created. The city has merged its health responsibilities with the County of Kent. The county offers all common health-education programs and emergency hotlines. Numerous public-awareness campaigns are backed by the County Health Department and by private nonprofit groups. The county provides all common preventive-health programs (emergency food is provided by private nonprofit groups) and treatment programs. Smoking is prohibited on public transportation and partially restricted in restaurants and in public and private offices. Contact: Phillip Van Heest, Director, Alliance for Health, 72 Monroe N.W., Grand Rapids, MI 49503.

Health Resources per 1,000 Pop.	Number	Rank
Hospital beds, community hospitals, city	10.48	19/92
Nurses, community hospitals, city	12.45	14/90
Doctors, metro area	1.79	96/113

Grand Rapids is currently working on a user preference park and recreation master plan. The city has many tennis and basketball courts, but relatively few football/soccer and baseball fields. Contact: Harry Burns, Recreation Director, City of Grand Rapids, 201 Market Avenue S.W., Grand Rapids, MI 49503.

Parkland/Total City Area (percent)   8.1

For a total of 22,000 students (grades K-12), there are 13 nurses. 60 percent of the schools have a part-time nurse and 5 percent have a full-time nurse. All common health-education programs are offered to students in grades K-9. The school system provides all common screens and tests except for immunizations, mental-health exams, well-child physical exams, speech therapy and learning disabilities. The school system does not offer any treatment programs. Contact: Mel Karnhem, Director of Health, Grand Rapids Public Schools, 143 Bostwick N.E., Grand Rapids, MI 49503.

Greensboro, NC

[RIP]	⛲	$	🌲	℞	🏃	👥	?
X	✓	✓	✔	✓	✔	✓	✔

The Greensboro metro area includes Winston-Salem. Greensboro (Guilford County) ranks 70th for age-adjusted mortality. Infant-mortality rates for North Carolina are high among minorities and in urban communities.

	Number	Rank
Age-Adjusted Death Rate	0.55	70/100
Heart Attacks	0.34	77/100
Cancer	0.12	69/100

Greensboro has above-average homicide and suicide rates. Accident rates for the city are extremely high—9th highest of 100 metro areas. The robbery rate is below average.

Incidence per 1,000 Pop.	Number	Rank
Homicides (1989)	0.09	67/111
Robberies (1989)	1.82	44/111
Suicides	0.14	67/100
Accidents	0.44	92/100

$ Greensboro-Winston-Salem's 1988 metro population was 925,000—52nd out of 113 metro areas. Its economic health at the end of 1990 was average, ranking 58th of 113 metro areas. Its unemployment rate ranks 40th, change in unemployment 90th (employment dropped by over 5 percent, while the labor force fell only 4 percent) and its enterprise 37th. Contact: Mayor V.M. Nussbaum, Jr., City of Greensboro, PO Drawer W2, Greensboro, NC 27402.

Water Quality: The city's drinking-water supply comes entirely from surface-water sources. The pH of the drinking water averaged 8.0 in 1989. Contact: R. E. Shaw, Assistant Public Works Director, City of Greensboro, Drawer W2, Greensboro, NC 27402.

Weather: Greensboro is pleasant and mild all year round, partly as a result of the city's positioning, blocked from westerly air flows by the Blue Ridge and Brushy mountains. While temperatures do fall to freezing on more than half of all winter days, sub-zero temperatures are almost unheard of in the area.

Average Daily Temperature (degrees F)	57.9
High	68.7
Low	46.9
Average Humidity	
Morning (percent)	83
Afternoon (percent)	55
Annual Precipitation (inches)	42.5
Average Total Snowfall (inches)	9.0

R Greensboro did not return a public-health questionnaire.

Health Resources per 1,000 Pop.	Number	Rank
Hospital beds, community hospitals, city	5.59	61/92
Nurses, community hospitals, city	6.92	52/90
Doctors, metro area	2.16	72/113

Of special interest is the A.H.O.Y. (Add Health to Our Years) for senior citizens. For sports facilities Greensboro has 112 tennis courts, 78 basketball courts, 23 football/soccer fields, 22 baseball fields, 9 swimming pools and 4 golf courses. Contact: Roger Brown, Parks and Recreation Director, City of Greensboro, P.O. Box 3136, Greensboro, NC 27402-3136.

Parkland/Total City Area (percent)	5.0
Aerobics classes	yes

Hiking or exploration groups   yes
Other Activities: martial arts (several
types), boxing, weight training, aerobics.

For a total of 22,000 students (grades K-12) in the public-school system, there are 12 nurses and 7 psychologists. There is a full-time
nurse available in 14 percent of the schools and a part-time nurse is available
in the rest of the schools. All common health-education programs are offered to students in grades K-12. The school system also has an AIDS-
education program. The school system provides all common screens and
tests except mental-health exams and well-child physical exams. Medical
treatment is provided for students. Contact: John A. Eberhart, Superintendent of Schools, Greensboro City Schools, Drawer V, Greensboro, NC 27402.

Hartford, CT

RIP	🗡	$	🌲	℞	🖼	👥	?
✓	✔	X	✓	✔	✓	✔	✔

The Hartford metro area includes New Britain. Hartford (Hartford
County) has an age-adjusted mortality rate that is average for the
large metro areas we have surveyed. Infant-mortality rates for Connecticut
are high among minorities and low among whites and in urban areas.

	Number	Rank
Age-Adjusted Death Rate	−0.20	48/100
Heart Attacks	0.07	59/100
Cancer	0.08	63/100

Hartford has the second lowest accidental-death rate in the country,
possibly reflecting the risk-avoiding temperament of the insurance
industry, Hartford's largest private employer. Homicide and suicide rates
are also lower than average.

Incidence per 1,000 Pop.	Number	Rank
Homicides (1989)	0.06	34/111
Robberies (1989)	2.62	70/111
Suicides	0.11	25/100
Accidental Deaths	0.16	2/100

$ Hartford's 1988 metro population was 755,000—57th out of 113 metro areas. Its economic health at the end of 1990 was poor, ranking 91st of 113 metro areas. Its unemployment rate ranks 31st, change in unemployment 91st (the labor force grew faster than employment) and its enterprise 102nd. Contact: Mayor Carrie Saxon Perry, City of Hartford, 550 Main Street, Hartford, CT 06103.

Air Quality: Hartford had 10 days of ozone exceedances in 1988. In 1989 the second-daily maximum 1-hour concentration was 0.14, well above the 0.12 EPA NAAQS maximum. But carbon monoxide exceedances and lead levels decreased in the latter half of the 1980s. Contact: Leslie Carouthers, Commissioner, Connecticut Department of Environmental Protection, 165 Capitol Avenue, Hartford, CT 06106.

Hazardous Waste: There are no hazardous-waste disposal or treatment facilities located in Hartford County. Programs for waste minimization and pollution prevention have been strengthened in recent years. Contact: Leslie Carouthers, Commissioner, Connecticut Department of Environmental Protection, 165 Capitol Avenue, Hartford, CT 06106.

Weather: Hartford is a cool city with an average temperature of 49.8. Average annual precipitation is high at 44.39 inches.

Average Daily Temperature (degrees F)	49.8
High	60.1
Low	39.5
Average Humidity	
Morning (percent)	77
Afternoon (percent)	52
Annual Precipitation (inches)	44.4
Average Total Snowfall (inches)	48.8

R̶ All common health-education programs are provided by the city. The city also provides emergency hotlines for child abuse, AIDS information and sexually transmitted diseases. Hartford sponsors several public health-awareness campaigns. The city provides all common preventive-health programs except emergency food for the needy, blood-pressure testing and cholesterol testing. It provides common treatment programs except for drug abuse and alcoholism. Contact: Director, Hartford Health Department, c/o Office of the Mayor, Hartford City Hall, 550 Main Street, Hartford, CT 06103.

Health Resources per 1,000 Pop.	Number	Rank
Doctors	4.47	7/113

[🏌] Hartford's sports facilities include 44 baseball fields, 35 basketball courts, 20 tennis courts, 10 football/soccer fields, 9 swimming pools, 2 golf courses and 2 running tracks. Softball and basketball are the most popular sports. The city offers classes in aerobics and arts and crafts. Contact: Harold Morgan, City of Hartford Parks & Recreation, 25 Stonington Street, Hartford, CT 06114.

[👥] To serve 26,000 students are 43 nurses, half of whom are nurse practitioners, 12 part-time physicians, 22 psychologists, 12 nurse-aides, 10 dental hygienists, 1 dental assistant, 6 part-time dentists, 2 occupational therapists and 2 physical therapists. Mental-health workers are available for counseling. The Hartford school system has been approved for Medicaid since 1978. The school system is the largest provider of pediatric ambulatory care in the city. 20 out of 40 schools provide primary diagnostic treatment and services via nurse practitioners. The system also operates five dental clinics and all K-6 students receive annual dental screening. Medical treatment, occupational and physical therapy is also provided for students. All common health-education programs, including AIDS education, are offered to students in grades K-12. The school system provides all common screens and tests except for learning disabilities; it also provides urinalysis, pregnancy, blood and strep tests. Contact: Hernan La Fontaine, Superintendent of Schools, Board of Education, 49 High Street, Hartford, CT 06103.

Honolulu, HI

RIP	🛫	$	↑	℞	[🏌]	👥	?
✔	✔	✔	✔	✓	✓	✓	✔

[RIP] Honolulu (Oahu County) has the top ranking out of 100 metro areas for age-adjusted mortality. Honolulu also has the 2nd lowest heart attack rate and the 3rd lowest cancer rate. Infant-mortality rates in Hawaii are high among blacks and relatively low among other minorities and in urban areas.

	Number	Rank
Age-Adjusted Death Rate	−3.42	1/100
Heart Attacks	−1.11	2/100
Cancer	−0.78	3/100

Honolulu is in among the lowest quartile among cities in robberies and suicides and is at the bottom of the quartile in homicides. Its accident rate is extremely low—fourth lowest of 100 metro areas.

Incidence per 1,000 Pop.	Number	Rank
Homicides (1989)	0.05	30/111
Robberies (1989)	0.96	15/111
Suicides	0.10	22/100
Accidental Deaths	0.22	4/100

$ Honolulu's 1988 metro population was 838,000—56th out of 113 metro areas. Its economic health at the end of 1990 was excellent, ranking 6th of 113 metro areas. Its unemployment rate ranks 3rd, change in unemployment 43rd (employment grew 4.8 percent, slightly faster than the labor force) and its enterprise 22nd. Contact: Mayor Frank F. Fasi, City of Honolulu, 530 South King Street, Honolulu, HI 96813.

Air Quality: Concentrations of particulates in the air over Honolulu have remained consistently low in the 1985–90 period. Ozone is perhaps the most serious pollutant and its highest second-daily maximum 1-hour concentration in 1989 was 0.05, less than half the EPA NAAQS ceiling. Contact: Bruce Anderson, Ph.D., Deputy Director, Environmental Protection & Health Services, State Department of Health, 1250 Punchbowl Street, Honolulu, HI 96813.

Hazardous Waste: Most of Honolulu's hazardous waste continues to be disposed of in other states. The amount of waste generated is declining as in-plant improvements and recycling increase. Contact: Bruce Anderson, Ph.D., Deputy Director, Environmental Protection & Health Services, State Department of Health, 1250 Punchbowl Street, Honolulu, HI 96813.

Water Quality: Almost all (99 percent) of Honolulu's drinking water comes from groundwater (wells); the remaining 2 percent is supplied equally by surface water and natural springs. Contact: Kazu Hayashida, Manager & Chief Engineer, Board of Water Supply, City and County of Honolulu, 630 South Beretania Street, Honolulu, HI 96843.

Weather: Honolulu is a warm city, with an average temperature of 77. Precipitation is about average at 23.5 inches annually.

Average Daily Temperature (degrees F)	77.0
High	84.2
Low	69.7

Average Humidity
    Morning (percent)   72
    Afternoon (percent)   56
Annual Precipitation (inches)   23.5
Average Total Snowfall (inches)   0.0
Ozone, Days over 0.12 ppm (one hour in   0
    1988)

℞ The state is implementing a "gap group" health-insurance plan that will make health insurance accessible to virtually all Hawaii residents, after having already moved in 1990 toward full health coverage by extending Medicaid eligibility to 11,000 previously excluded uninsured individuals, nearly half of them children. The state sponsors health-awareness campaigns addressing AIDS, family abuse, drug-abuse prevention, physical fitness, litter control and a Project LEAN. Honolulu sponsors an environmental-awareness campaign. Smoking is prohibited on public transportation and in restrooms, elevators, taxis, museums, libraries and theaters. It is partially restricted in restaurants, public offices, health-care facilities and public and private savings and loans and banks. Honolulu implemented the Hawaii Seroprevalence AIDS medical-management program, which provides physician visits and testing biannually to persons seropositive for the HIV virus. All common health-education programs and emergency hotlines are provided by the State Department of Health and private agencies. The state provides all common preventive-health and treatment programs plus body-fat screening, diabetes testing and screening for psychosocial risk. Honolulu also emphasizes worksite wellness programs, incorporating nutrition and exercise. Contact: John C. Lewin, M.D., Director (or: Peter Sybinsky), Department of Health, State of Hawaii, 1250 Punchbowl Street, Honolulu, HI 96813; (808) 548-3263.

Health Resources per 1,000 Pop.	Number	Rank
Hospital Beds	4.50	74/92
Nurses	5.48	69/90
Doctors	2.41	62/113

Honolulu's beach parks are considered the most important recreation area. The city has 53 beaches and 11 community garden sites among its natural attractions. To facilitate other leisure activities the city has 200 baseball fields, 174 tennis courts, 169 basketball courts, 21 football/soccer fields, 17 swimming pools and 5 golf courses. The City Parks Department is focusing more funds on community-wide programs and facilities which serve the greatest number of people. Contact: Walter Ozawa, Director, Department of Parks & Recreation, City and County of Honolulu, 650 South King Street, Honolulu, HI 96813.

Parkland/Total City Area (percent)   2.5

 The nurses for the Honolulu school system are employed by the Department of Health. Health aides are present in all of the schools on a part-time basis. The school system employs 40 school psychologists and psychological examiners. All common health-education programs are offered to students in grades K-12. Additional health-education programs include AIDS education, growth and development, community health, consumer health, fitness and health careers. The school system provides all common screens and tests except for mental-health exams and tests for scoliosis. All entering students at age 5 are required to have vaccinations; in Hawaii all insurers must provide vaccination as a benefit. Children not covered by insurance are vaccinated by the Health Department. Some dental treatment is provided for students. Contact: Lynda Asato, Health Specialist, Office of Instructional Services, State Department of Education, 595 Pepeekeo Street, Honolulu, HI 96825.

Houston, TX

RIP	🚮	$	🌲	℞	🏃	👥	?
✔	X	✓	X	✓	X	X	✓

Houston (Harris County) ranks 20th with its age-adjusted mortality rate. Infant-mortality rates for Texas are high among minorities and low among whites and in rural areas. Contact: Janeen Pappas, Acting Chief of Epidemiology, Department of Health and Human Services, 8000 North Stadium Drive, Houston, TX 77054.

	Number	Rank
Age-Adjusted Death Rate	−1.20	20/100
Heart Attacks	−0.46	21/100
Cancer	−0.26	23/100

Houston has high homicide and robbery rates. Rates for suicide and accidents are slightly above average.

Incidence per 1,000 Pop.	Number	Rank
Homicides (1989)	0.17	104/111
Robberies (1989)	3.60	94/111
Suicides	0.14	62/100
Accidental Deaths	0.34	55/100

| $ | Houston's 1988 metro population was 3,247,000—7th out of 113 metro areas. Its economic health at the end of 1990 was good, ranking 42nd of 113 metro areas. Its unemployment rate ranks 76th, change in unemployment 40th (employment grew by 3.1 percent, slightly faster than the labor force at 3.0 percent) and its enterprise 31st. Contact: Mayor Kathryn Whitmire, City of Houston, PO Box 1562, Houston, TX 77251.

| ↑ | **Air Quality:** Houston's Pollutant Standards Index (PSI) in 1988 exceeded the EPA NAAQS limit of 100 on 25 days; in 1989 it exceeded 100 on 12 days. Better, but still one of the worst polluted cities. The ozone index in 1989 was 0.23 ppm, well above the NAAQS maximum of 0.12 ppm.

Weather: Although Houston's climate is humid, its location on the Gulf Coast results in moderate temperatures. It has an average of fewer than 23 days a year with temperatures of 32 degrees or less. On about 92 days a year the temperature reaches 90 degrees or more. The average high in winter is 65 degrees and in summer 92 degrees.

Average Daily Temperature (degrees F)	68.3
High	79.1
Low	57.4
Average Humidity	
Morning (percent)	90
Afternoon (percent)	60
Annual Precipitation (inches)	44.8
Average Total Snowfall (inches)	0.4
PSI, Days over 100, 1988	25
PSI, Days over 100, 1989	12

| ℞ | A new medical-center clinic for sexually transmitted diseases has been opened, the STD/Chest Clinic has been reopened and a Southwest Health Center is being developed. The City of Houston has a number of interesting new programs. One such program is the Baby Buddy Program, which is a support group for pregnant teens. The Maternity Record System has been improved in order to facilitate the inter-agency transfer of prenatal data between the Department of Health and Human Services and the Harris County Hospital District. All common health-education programs and emergency hotlines are provided by the city, along with all common preventive-health programs except emergency food for the needy (other than the WIC supplemental food program for women). The city provides treatment for sexually transmitted diseases, but not for drug abuse, alcoholism or mental illness. Contact: Dr. Arradondo, Director, Department of Health and Human Services, 8000 North Stadium Drive, Houston, TX 77054.

Health Resources per 1,000 Pop.	Number	Rank
Nurses	5.82	62/90
Doctors	2.39	63/113

The 50-mile Hike and Bike Trails are especially popular. Also, portions of the Harris County Flood Control District right of way are often used as jogging routes. The city is in the midst of a $67.5 million bond program to acquire new parks and to renovate older parks. During the past decade the size of the parks system has more than doubled. The city's abundant sports facilities include 224 tennis courts, 212 baseball fields, 168 basketball courts, 126 football/soccer fields, 46 swimming pools and 8 golf courses. Popular recreational activities include the Alkeck velodrome, the Houston Zoo, 2 nature centers and 60 recreation centers. Contact: Don Olson, Director, Parks and Recreation Department, 2999 South Wayside, Houston, TX 77023.

Parkland/Total City Area (percent)   7.8

For a total of 190,000 students in the public-school system there are 201 nurses, 15 psychologists, 1 audiologist and 4 dental hygienists. School-health policies and procedures are reviewed and updated annually. The Health Education Curricula are being updated with Project ACCESS. All common health-education programs are offered to students in grades K-10. The school system provides all common screens and tests except for mental-health exams and well-child physical exams. Emergency and dental services are provided for students. Contact: Dr. Matty Glass, Houston Independent School District, 3830 Richmond Avenue, Houston, TX 77027.

Indianapolis, IN

Indianapolis (Marion County) has an average age-adjusted death rate. Indiana has high infant-mortality rates among minorities and low rates among whites and in rural communities.

	Number	Rank
Age-Adjusted Death Rate	0.38	62/100
Heart Attacks	0.09	63/100
Cancer	0.19	76/100

Indianapolis' rates of homicide, robbery, accidents and suicide are average for the cities in our survey. Homicides are relatively low, suicides relatively high, which is the West Coast rather than the East Coast pattern.

Incidence per 1,000 Pop.	Number	Rank
Homicides (1989)	0.06	41/111
Robberies (1989)	1.94	53/111
Suicides	0.14	60/100
Accidental Deaths	0.33	52/100

$ Indianapolis' 1988 metro population was 1.2 million—39th out of 113 metro areas. Its economic health at the end of 1990 was excellent, ranking 6th of 113 metro areas. Its unemployment rate ranks 17th, change in unemployment 15th (the labor force declined faster than employment) and its enterprise 36th. Contact: Mayor William H. Hudnut III, 2501 City-County Building, Indianapolis, IN 46204.

Air Quality: In the 1985–90 period, the city attained NAAQS levels for carbon monoxide. But ozone in 1989 was borderline at 0.12 ppm. Contact: David Jordan, Administrator, Department of Public Works, Air Pollution Division, Administration Building, 2700 South Belmont Avenue, Indianapolis, IN 46221.

Hazardous Waste: Marion County has two hazardous-waste sites. The county holds a biennial Tox-a-Way-Day, for free disposal of household hazardous waste, and in 1991 planned a permanent drop-off location for the public. Contact: Robert Holm, Administrator, Department of Public Works, Water and Land Division, Administration Building, 2700 South Belmont Avenue, Indianapolis, IN 46221.

Weather: The climate is characterized by very warm summers and no dry season. The temperature hits 90 degrees or more on a total of 17 days each year. It dips to 32 degrees or less, however, on 120 days each year and to zero degrees on nine days. The city of Indianapolis is cloudy, with clear, sunny days only about one-quarter of the time. In an average year, thunderstorms occur about once every 8 days.

Average Daily Temperature (degrees F)	52.1
High	62.0
Low	42.2
Average Humidity	
Morning (percent)	82
Afternoon (percent)	62
Annual Precipitation (inches)	39.1
Average Total Snowfall (inches)	22.9
Ozone, Days over 0.12 ppm (one hour in 1988)	5

℞ In 1989, Indianapolis set up the Campaign for Healthy Babies, to reduce infant mortality. Two recent projects are the construction of a new public-health community clinic and a new prenatal care center. The city sponsors the mayor's fitness council, which includes physical fitness and "special community events." Other sponsored projects include Healthy Cities Indianapolis and Indianapolis Alliance for Health Promotion. The city provides all common health-education programs. Emergency hotlines are available for child abuse, suicide and alcoholism. The city-county provides all common preventive-health programs and treatment programs. A Mother-Baby healthline offers assistance and referrals for pregnant women. Contact: Dr. Frank Johnson, Director, Marion County Health Department, 222 East Ohio, Indianapolis, IN 46204.

Health Resources per 1,000 Pop.	Number	Rank
Hospital Beds	5.45	66/92
Doctors	2.70	43/113

The Indianapolis-Scarborough Peace Games, held annually, is an international sports competition. About 1,000 persons from each city take part in the 16 different sports and activities. A 27-hole golf course has recently been reconstructed to include family training facilities. Other sports facilities include 145 tennis courts, 119 baseball fields, 79 basketball courts, 49 football/soccer fields, 17 swimming pools and 12 golf courses. Basketball, softball and volleyball are the most popular sports. The city offers classes in rowing, canoeing, kayaking, hiking, aerobics and arts and crafts. Contact: Arthur Strong, Director, Department of Parks and Recreation, 1426 West 29th Street, Indianapolis, IN 40208 or at (317) 924-7036.

Parkland/Total City Area (percent)	3.6

To serve 49,500 students in the public-school system are 7 nurses, 13 psychologists and 7 medical assistants. A full-time nurse is present in only 4 of the schools and a part-time nurse in all of the schools provided by the Marion County Health Department. An all-inclusive Family Life curriculum is offered to students in grades K through 12. In special education, medically fragile students attend school and receive nursing services, including catheterization, G-tube feedings, tracheostomy care, and oxygen therapy among others. All common health–education programs are offered to students in grades K-7 and 9. The school system provides all common screens and tests except for mental-health exams and well-child physical exams. No medical, dental or psychiatric treatment is provided for students, except those attending Arsenal Technical School through the Tech Teen Clinic. Contact: Pat Kiergan, Indianapolis Public Schools, 120 East Walnut, Indianapolis, IN 46204.

Jackson, MS

RIP	⛏	$	🌲	℞	🏚	👫	?
✓	✔	✔	?	✔	?	?	X

 Jackson (Hinds County) has a lower-than-average age-adjusted mortality rate. Infant-mortality rates in Mississippi are high among minorities and low among whites. Infant-mortality rates are slightly higher in cities.

	Number	Rank
Age-Adjusted Death Rate	−0.44	39/100
Heart Attacks	−0.33	27/100
Cancer	−0.18	28/100

Jackson has one of the lowest rates for suicide. Rates for robbery and accidents are average for cities.

Incidence per 1,000 Pop.	Number	Rank
Homicides (1989)	0.05	31/111
Robberies (1989)	1.86	51/111
Suicides	0.07	4/100
Accidental Deaths	0.33	51/100

$ Jackson's 1988 metro population was 396,000—88th out of 113 metro areas. Its economic health at the end of 1990 was excellent, ranking 12th of 113 metro areas. Its unemployment rate ranks 62nd, change in unemployment 7th (employment grew by 5.9 percent, substantially faster than the labor force) and its enterprise 16th. Contact: Mayor Kane Ditto, City of Jackson, City Hall, Jackson, MS.

Weather: The city's average temperature is above the national average at 64.6. Humidity is high (91 percent in the morning), as is precipitation at 52.82 inches annually.

Average Daily Temperature (degrees F)	64.6
High	76.3
Low	52.9
Average Humidity	
Morning (percent)	91
Afternoon (percent)	58
Annual Precipitation (inches)	52.8
Average Total Snowfall (inches)	1.0

Jackson did not return the health-services questionnaire.

Health Resources per 1,000 Pop.	Number	Rank
Hospital beds	11.20	17/92
Nurses	10.26	23/90
Doctors	3.12	20/113

Jackson did not return the recreational-facilities questionnaire.

Jackson did not return the public-school-health questionnaire.

Jacksonville, FL

	⛵	$	🌲	R	🏃	👥	?
✓	X	✔	✓	✔	✓	✓	✓

 Jacksonville (Duval County) has an average age-adjusted mortality rate. Florida has high infant-mortality rates among minorities and low rates among whites. Infant-mortality rates are lower in cities than in rural areas.

	Number	Rank
Age-Adjusted Death Rate	0.41	64/100
Heart Attacks	−0.05	50/100
Cancer	0.10	67/100

 Jacksonville has extremely high rates for homicide and robbery. Rates for suicide and accidents are slightly above average.

Incidence per 1,000 Pop.	Number	Rank
Homicides (1989)	0.19	107/111
Robberies (1989)	4.61	104/111
Suicides	0.14	65/100
Accidental Deaths	0.36	67/100

$ Jacksonville's 1988 metro population was 898,000—54th out of 113 metro areas. Its economic health at the end of 1990 was good, ranking 52nd of 113 metro areas. Its unemployment rate ranks 84th, change in unemployment 56th (the labor force grew faster than employment) and its enterprise 18th. Contact: Mayor Tommy Hazouri, City of Jacksonville, 220 East Bay Street, Jacksonville, FL 32202.

Air Quality: In spite of Jacksonville's tremendous growth, pollution levels have decreased and are now better than the EPA's NAAQS levels for healthy air. Ozone, however, was barely in compliance at 0.11 ppm in 1989. Contact: James L. Manning, Deputy Director, Department of Health and Welfare Bio-Environmental Services, 421 West Church Street, Jacksonville, FL 32202.

Hazardous Waste: Eight hazardous-waste disposal sites in the Jacksonville area handle PCBs, hydraulic fluid, military waste and wood preservatives. In 1987, 12 million pounds were disposed of in Duval County. In 1988, a Hazardous Materials Activity was added to the Department of Health, Welfare and Bio-Environmental Services to oversee the disposal of hazardous waste. Contact: James L. Manning, Deputy Director, Department of Health and Welfare Bio-Environmental Services, 421 West Church Street, Jacksonville, FL 32202.

Water Quality: All of the city's water comes from ground water (wells). Jacksonville has the highest lead content in its water of the over 60 cities that provided this information, 0.02 mg/l. The turbidity of Jacksonville's water is also very high, ranking 52nd of 57 cities for which we have this information. But residual chlorine and nitrates are relatively low. Contact: Chris Carter, Environmental Specialist, Sanitary Engineering Division, Duval County Public Health Unit, 515 West 6th Street, Jacksonville, FL 32206.

Weather: Situated on St. John's River on the northeast coast of Florida, Jacksonville has a humid, subtropical climate characterized by mild winters and hot, stormy summers. There are about 10 freezing days a year and about 80 days in the 90s.

Average Daily Temperature (degrees F)	68.8
High	78.7
Low	57.2
Average Humidity	
Morning (percent)	88
Afternoon (percent)	56
Annual Precipitation (inches)	52.8
Average Total Snowfall (inches)	Trace
Ozone, Days over 0.12 ppm (one hour in 1988)	1

℞ The city, in cooperation with the State Department of Health and Rehabilitative Services, has extended funding to open a Public Health Center for Women and to expand staff and services at selected clinics to address maternity and family planning needs. The new services have greatly increased access to health care and have resulted in an increased number of first-trimester visits. The City of Jacksonville cooperated with other agencies to sponsor "Jacksonville Gets Fit." A new project entitled "Jacksonville Jump Starts A Life" for CPR training is being developed. Smoking is prohibited on public transportation and in county public health units and partially prohibited in restaurants and in public and private offices. Due to the consolidated efforts of the city/county/state public health unit, a system of primary care has been created, operating through a network of Comprehensive Health Care Centers located throughout the county. The city offers all common health-education programs with the exception of prenatal care and sexually transmitted diseases. The city provides all common preventive-health programs, except providing food to the needy. The city has an extensive network of emergency hotlines. Contact: Rufus M. DeHart, M.D., Director, Department of Health, Welfare & Bio-Environmental Services, 515 West 6th Street, Jacksonville, FL 32206.

Health Resources per 1,000 Pop.	Number	Rank
Hospital Beds	4.47	75/92
Nurses	4.45	79/90
Doctors	1.98	85/113

Two miles of beaches are home to swimming, recreational boating and beachcombing. The city's sports facilities include 162 baseball fields, 119 basketball courts, 114 tennis courts, 45 football/soccer fields, 32 swimming pools, 3 running tracks and 2 golf courses. Contact: Laura D'Alisera, Director, Recreation and Parks, 851 North Market Street, Room 208, Jacksonville, FL 32202.

Parkland/Total City Area (percent)	6.3

Duval County Public Schools employs 29 school nurses, 1 school physician, 1 vision clinician, 1 dental hygienist, 1 nutritionist, 2 audiologists and 126 speech pathologists provide services to students in the county's 151 schools. Nine of the schools receive full-time nurse services. The remaining 142 schools receive nurse services on a part-time basis. The school system provides all common screens and tests except for mental-health exams; in addition, it provides growth and development screening and TB skin tests. Other services to students include identification, referral and follow-up of students at risk; nursing assessment and counseling; dental education, counseling and referral; nutrition assessment; emergency care; administration of medication; and communicable- and infectious-disease control. Other health programs include a comprehensive health education program that incorporates AIDS education for students; therapy by speech pathologists, 9 physical therapists and 11 occupational therapists for identified students; psychological evaluations by 36 school psychologists for referred students; medical examinations and treatment for eligible Chapter I students; and a Wellness Program for employees. Contact: Hodges H. Sneed, General Director, Student Services, Duval County Public Schools.

Jersey City, NJ

RIP		$		℞			?
X	✓	X	✓	✓	?	✔	✓

Jersey City (Hudson County) has an extremely high age-adjusted mortality rate. New Jersey infant-mortality rates are high among minorities and in cities.

	Number	**Rank**
Age-Adjusted Death Rate	2.53	95/100
Heart Attacks	0.76	92/100
Cancer	0.51	90/100

The Jersey City primary metro area (i.e., Hudson County) has one of the nation's highest rates for robberies. The city has relatively low rates of suicide and accidents. The homicide rate is high but just escapes being in the highest one-third.

Incidence per 1,000 Pop.	Number	Rank
Homicides (1989)	0.10	74/111
Robberies (1989)	5.51	106/111
Suicides	0.10	19/100
Accidental Deaths	0.31	27/100

Jersey City's 1988 metro population was 542,000—74th out of 113 metro areas. Metro economic health at the end of 1990 was poor, ranking 101st of 113 metro areas. Its unemployment rate ranks 104th, change in unemployment 97th (the labor force grew 2.5 percent while employment grew a bit over one-fourth this rate) and its enterprise 52nd. Contact: Mayor Gerald McCann, City of Jersey City, City Hall, 280 Grove Street, Jersey City, NJ 07302.

Hazardous Waste: Only one site in the city is on the EPA's National Priority list—the PJP Landfill, ranked 109th of 110 New Jersey sites (second least serious). Most of the hazardous wastes have already been removed. Additional investigations are underway to see whether the site should be taken off the EPA's list. No newly generated wastes are disposed of in Jersey City; the city has no commercial hazardous-waste facilities.

Water Quality: Trihalomethanes have been significantly lowered by using sodium hypochlorite.

Weather: The average temperature is close to the U.S. average at 54.2 degrees. Annual precipitation is high at 42.3 inches.

Average Daily Temperature (degrees F)	54.2
High	62.5
Low	45.9
Average Humidity	
Morning (percent)	73
Afternoon (percent)	54
Annual Precipitation (inches)	42.3
Average Total Snowfall (inches)	28.0
Ozone, Days over 0.12 ppm (one hour in 1988)	14

Public-health nursing records have recently been computerized, which permits more timely follow-ups on the home-health-aide clientele. The city offers health-education programs in CPR training, AIDS education, anti-drug, prenatal and infant care and family planning. The city does not provide any emergency hotlines, but it promotes Federal and private poison-control, substance-abuse and crisis-intervention hotlines. It provides all common preventive-health and treatment programs. Contact: Irene Hunt, Senior Program Development Specialist, 586 Newark Ave., Jersey City, NJ 07306 (201) 547-6807.

Health Resources per 1,000 Pop.	Number	Rank
Hospital beds	5.37	67/92
Nurses	4.57	78/90
Doctors	2.08	76/113

Jersey City did not return the recreational-facilities questionnaire.

Jersey City's school system was in 1990–91 temporarily being operated by the State of New Jersey. To serve 28,000 students in the public-school system are 43 nurses, 11 physicians, 2 psychiatrists, 1 neurologist, 30 psychologists and 2 audiometrists. A full-time nurse is present in all of the schools. All common health-education programs are offered to students in grades K-12. The school system provides all common screens and tests plus blood pressure, height and weight, and athletic physicals. Two school-based clinics were created and a TEMP (teen-age expectant mothers program) are among the medical treatments provided for students.

Kansas City, KS and MO

🏠RIP	☠	$	🌲	℞	🏃	👥	?
✔	X	X	✓	✓	X	✔	✔

Kansas City (KS), is located in Wyandotte County and the larger Kansas City (MO) is located in Jackson, Clay and Platte Counties. Metro Kansas City includes both of these Kansas Cities and has a relatively low age-adjusted mortality rate, i.e., it is in the top third in longevity. Infant-mortality rates for Kansas and Missouri are high among minorities and in urban areas. Kansas tends to have lower overall infant-mortality rates (although not for blacks). Kansas City, KS, is the one that tended to respond to our questionnaires.

	Number	Rank
Age-Adjusted Death Rate	−1.07	26/100
Heart Attacks	−0.33	26/100
Cancer	−0.12	36/100

 The Kansas City metro area has relatively high rates of homicide, robbery and suicide. Accident rates are below average.

Incidence per 1,000 Pop.	Number	Rank
Homicides (1989)	0.13	92/111
Robberies (1989)	3.25	90/111
Suicides	0.14	74/100
Accidental Deaths	0.30	24/100

$ Kansas City's 1988 metro population was 1.58 million—28th out of 113 metro areas. Its economic health at the end of 1990 was below average, ranking 77th of 113 metro areas. Its unemployment rate ranks 51st, change in unemployment 47th (the labor force and employment both grew by 2.5 percent) and its enterprise 92nd. Contact: Mayor Joe Steineger, City of Kansas City, Civic Center Plaza, Kansas City, KS 66101.

↑ Air Quality: In Kansas City (KS) the general trend of ambient-air-pollution concentrations is downward. The city's PSI was over 100 on three days in 1988 and two days in 1989. Ozone was barely below the NAAQS maximum in 1989, but the city had no exceedances of EPA standards in 1990. Contact: Richard S. Michael, Kansas City-Wyandotte Department of Health, 619 Ann, Kansas City, KS 66101.

Water Quality: Surface water provides Kansas City (KS) with all of its drinking water. The pH of the drinking water is 8.1. Recently disinfection-process byproducts and runoffs from farmland herbicides and insecticides have contributed to water contamination. Contact: Bill Bell, Public Information Officer, Water Pollution Control Department; 913-573-5408. Also: Board of Public Utilities, 51 Market Street, Kansas City, KS 66101; (913) 573-9345.

Hazardous Waste: Kansas City (KS) has no hazardous-waste site on the EPA's superfund list nor within Wyandotte County. Contact: Jim Grohusky, Director of Environmental Health, Kansas City-Wyandotte County Department of Health, 619 Ann, Kansas City, KS 66101.

Weather: The average Kansas City temperature, 54.1 degrees, is close to the national average. Humidity and precipitation are both higher than average.

Average Daily Temperature (degrees F)	54.1
High	63.7
Low	44.4
Average Humidity	
Morning (percent)	81
Afternoon (percent)	60
Annual Precipitation (inches)	35.2
Average Total Snowfall (inches)	20.3
Ozone, Days over 0.12 ppm (one hour in 1988)	0
PSI, Days over 100, 1988 and 1989	3, 2

R̸ Kansas City (KS) is currently working on a comprehensive neighborhood health center. Also new is the Mayor's Heart Challenge, a public health campaign sponsored by the city. Anti-smoking laws include partial restriction in restaurants, public offices and on public transportation. All common health-education programs are provided by the city. The city provides emergency hotlines for child abuse, suicide and AIDS information. The city and county provide all common preventive-health and treatment programs. Contact: Richard S. Michael, Kansas City-Wyandotte County Department of Health, 619 Ann, Kansas City, KS 66101.

Health Resources per 1,000 Pop.	Number	Rank
Hospital Beds	7.53	37/92
Nurses	6.84	54/90
Doctors	2.25	69/113

Kansas City, KS, has 44 baseball fields, 36 tennis courts, 13 basketball courts, 6 football/soccer fields, 1 swimming pool and 1 golf course. The city has a small percentage of parkland. Contact: Burt Cavin, Director, Kansas City Parks and Recreation, 75 South 23rd Street, Kansas City, KS 66101.

Parkland/Total City Area (percent)	1.7

Kansas City has developed a comprehensive drug and alcohol curriculum for grades K-12. The city also has developed a sexuality and AIDS curriculum. The school system employs 23 nurses, 22 psychologists and 24 social workers to provide for 22,607 students. Nurses are present full-time in 13 percent of the schools and part-time in the rest of the schools. All common health education programs are offered to students in grades 3-5 and 8-10. The school system provides all common screens and tests except mental-health exams. Psychiatric treatment is provided for students. Contact: Dr. Donald M. Moritz, Director of Pupil Services & Research, Kansas City, KS Public Schools, U.S.D. #500, 625 Minnesota, Kansas City, KS 66101.

Knoxville, TN

RIP	🏃	$	🌲	℞	🎭	👫	?
✓	✓	✓	✓	✓	✓	✓	✔

RIP The Knoxville (Knox County) metro area ranks 35th in the age-adjusted mortality rate. Infant-mortality rates for Tennessee are high among minorities and in urban areas.

	Number	Rank
Age-Adjusted Death Rate	−0.61	35/100
Heart Attacks	−0.30	31/100
Cancer	−0.09	42/100

🏃 Knoxville has relatively low rates of robbery, suicide and accidents. Homicide rates are average.

Incidence per 1,000 Pop.	Number	Rank
Homicides (1989)	0.07	52/111
Robberies (1989)	1.09	18/111
Suicides	0.09	13/100
Accidental Deaths	0.31	28/100

$ Knoxville's 1988 metro population was 600,000—70th out of 113 metro areas. Its economic health at the end of 1990 was good, ranking 40th of 113 metro areas. Its unemployment rate ranks 44th, change in unemployment 34th (the labor force shrunk faster than employment) and its enterprise 58th. Contact: Mayor Victor Ashe, City of Knoxville, City-County Building, Knoxville, TN 37902.

🌲 **Water Quality:** 100 percent of the water supply in Knoxville is from surface water (e.g., reservoirs). Recent years have seen a decline in the levels of trihalomethane (one of the family of organic compounds, derived from methane, where three of the four hydrogen atoms in methane are replaced by a halogen atom; possible effects include damage to liver, kidney and skin, and the ozone layer) as rainfall amounts have returned to normal. Contact: Director of Municipal Utilities, c/o Office of the Mayor, Knoxville City-County Building, 400 West Main Avenue, Knoxville, TN 37902.

Weather: The average temperature is close to the national average at 58.9 degrees. Annual precipitation is high at 47.3 inches.

Average Daily Temperature (degrees F)	58.9
High	69.0
Low	48.7
Average Humidity	
Morning (percent)	85
Afternoon (percent)	59
Annual Precipitation (inches)	47.3
Average Total Snowfall (inches)	12.5

 The city did not respond to the health-services survey.

Health Resources per 1,000 Pop.	Number	Rank
Hospital Beds	13.11	7/92
Nurses	13.98	10/90
Doctors	2.03	80/113

Knoxville's recreation department has a community band program with over 200 participants that performs 24 times a year in the city parks. The city recently completed a museum of art. The city's sports facilities include 70 baseball fields, 24 basketball courts, 18 running tracks, 16 football/soccer fields, 14 tennis courts, 4 swimming pools and 2 golf courses. Softball, baseball and basketball are popular sports. Contact: Sam Anderson, Director, City of Knoxville Parks & Recreation, PO Box 1631, Knoxville, TN 37901.

Parkland/Total City Area (percent)	3
Aerobics Classes	yes
Arts and Crafts Classes	yes
Hiking or Exploration Groups	yes
Other Activities: eight senior citizen recreation centers and 24 regular recreation centers.	

For a total of 49,974 students in the public-school system, there are 12 nurses, 1 physician, 31 psychologists, 7 physical therapists, 5 occupational therapists and 2 licensed practical nurses. A nurse is available on a part-time basis in all of the schools and on a full-time basis in 1 percent of the schools. The Developmental Center has a full-time registered nurse and two full-time licensed practical nurses. All common health-education programs are offered to students in grades K-12. The school system provides all common screens and tests. No medical, dental, or psychiatric treatment is provided for students. Contact: Aleece Stewart, Head Nurse, Knox County Schools, 101 5th Avenue, Knoxville, TN 37902.

Las Vegas, NV

🪦	🔪	$	⬆	℞	🏃	⛱	?
✓	X	✓	X	X	X	✔	✔

Las Vegas (Clark County) ranks 38th in the age-adjusted mortality rate. Infant-mortality rates in Nevada are high among blacks. Infant-mortality rates are higher in rural areas than in cities.

	Number	Rank
Age-Adjusted Death Rate	−0.57	38/100
Heart Attacks	−0.77	9/100
Cancer	0.02	51/100

Las Vegas has the highest suicide rate of 100 metro areas. Rates for homicide and robberies are also high.

Incidence per 1,000 Pop.	Number	Rank
Homicides (1989)	0.10	78/111
Robberies (1989)	3.21	88/111
Suicides	0.26	100/100
Accidental Deaths	0.34	59/100

 Las Vegas' 1988 metro population was 631,000—66th out of 113 metro areas. Its economic health at the end of 1990 was good, ranking 51st of 113 metro areas. Its unemployment rate ranks 70th, change in unemployment 81st (its labor force grew an astonishing 12 percent, while employment struggled to keep up, with a growth rate of nearly 11 percent) and its enterprise 1st (Las Vegas is the most entrepreneurial large city in the U.S.). Contact: Mayor Ron Lurie, City of Las Vegas, 400 East Stuart Avenue, Las Vegas, NV 89101.

Air Quality: In 1985–90 carbon-monoxide levels have stayed fairly constant despite increased numbers of automobiles and fuel consumed. But the level was too high at 12 ppm in 1989 versus an 8-hour NAAQS maximum of 9 ppm. In 1989 Las Vegas also exceeded the PM10 particulate standard, showing 69 $\mu g/m^3$—38 percent above the NAAQS maximum of 50 $\mu g/m^3$. Contact: Mike Naylor, Director, Clark County Health District Air Pollution Control Division, 625 Shadow Lane, PO Box 4426, Las Vegas, NV 89127.

Hazardous Waste: The city made plans in 1987 to expand its waste-water treatment facility, though there was opposition to adding more sludge beds, despite the money spent on odor control.

Water Quality: Over the past eight years, the city has seen a decrease in total dissolved solids in its drinking water. The water supply comes 80 percent from surface water (e.g., reservoirs) and 20 percent from ground water (e.g., wells). Contact: Patricia Mulroy, General Manager, Las Vegas Valley Water District, 3700 West Charleston Blvd., Las Vegas, NV 89153.

Weather: Las Vegas' climate is typical of desert areas—characterized by low humidity, sparse precipitation, warm sunshine, hot days and cool nights. During summer, daytime highs frequently reach into the 100s, while nighttime lows drop back to the 70s. Winters are mild, with daytime temperatures averaging in the 60s; Las Vegas residents are strangers to zero-degree days. Snow is rare, but in January of 1949 the city received a 17-inch snowfall (the yearly average works out to one-and-a-half inches).

Average Daily Temperature (degrees F)	66.3
High	79.6
Low	52.8
Average Humidity	
Morning (percent)	40
Afternoon (percent)	21
Normal Precipitation (inches)	4.2
Average Total Snowfall (inches)	1.3
Ozone, Days over 0.12 ppm (one hour in 1988)	1

The Las Vegas area has eight hospitals. The largest facility is Humana Hospital-Sunrise. The next largest is the county hospital, University Medical Center of Southern Nevada, which has a special burn-care unit. The city of Las Vegas has anti-smoking legislation which partially restricts smoking in restaurants and offices and on public transportation. In an attempt to make health care more accessible to its citizens, Las Vegas has instituted a sexually-transmitted-disease outreach project. It also offers a free health-care clinic to residents over 65 and a monthly clinic for children with AIDS. Las Vegas sponsors health-awareness campaigns addressing drinking and driving and the benefits of oxygenated fuels. All common health-education programs are provided by the city. The city also provides emergency hotlines for child abuse, suicide, alcoholism and AIDS information. The county provides all common preventive-health and treatment programs. Contact: Otto Ravenholt, M.D., M.P.H., Chief Health Officer, Clark County Health District, PO Box 4426, 625 Shadow Lane, Las Vegas, NV 89127.

Health Resources per 1,000 Pop.	Number	Rank
Hospital Beds	8.69	26/92
Nurses	8.60	35/90
Doctors	1.40	109/113

For those capable of recovering from the city's nightlife, daytime recreational opportunities include nearby Wet and Wild Water Park and visits to Nevada's numerous ghost towns. Las Vegas holds a corporate-challenge olympics which consists of 24 events during the month of April. For sports facilities, Las Vegas has 27 baseball fields, 24 football fields, 20 soccer fields, 20 basketball courts, 20 tennis courts, 6 swimming pools, 6 running tracks and 3 golf courses. Contact: David Kuiper, Director, City of Las Vegas, Department of Parks & Leisure Activities, 749 Veterans Memorial Drive, Las Vegas, NV 89101.

Parkland/Total City Area (percent)	2.8

To serve over 110,000 pupils in the public-school system are 55 nurses, 74 psychologists and 75 speech therapists. All schools have a nurse present on a part-time basis. All the usual health tests are conducted at these schools. Recently the school system has been revising its sex-education document. It also has made changes in its health-care services and policies for substance abuse and AIDS education. All common health-education programs are offered to students in grades 1–12. The school system provides all common screens and tests except mental-health exams. Contact: Brian Cram, Superintendent, Clark County School District, 2832 East Flamingo Road, Las Vegas, NV 89121.

Lexington, KY

🪦	🏃	$	🌲	℞	🖼	👫	?
✓	✓	✓	✓	✓	✓	✗	✓

The Lexington metro area includes the surrounding county of Fayette plus five counties surrounding Fayette. The state capital, Frankfort, is situated between the Lexington and Louisville metro areas. Lexington ranks 55th in the age-adjusted mortality rate. Infant-mortality rates for Kentucky are high among minorities and low among whites. Infant-mortality rates for rural and urban communities are the same.

	Number	Rank
Age-Adjusted Death Rate	0.03	55/100
Heart Attacks	−0.05	48/100
Cancer	0.19	77/100

 Lexington has relatively low rates for homicide and robberies, but high rates for suicide and accidents.

Incidence per 1,000 Pop.	Number	Rank
Homicides (1989)	0.05	27/111
Robberies (1989)	1.12	20/111
Suicides	0.14	73/100
Accidental Deaths	0.38	83/100

$ Lexington's 1988 metro population was 348,000—96th out of 113 metro areas. Its economic health at the end of 1990 was excellent, ranking 9th of 113 metro areas. Its unemployment rate ranks 19th, change in unemployment 40th (employment grew faster than the labor force) and its enterprise 19th. Contact: Mayor Scotty Baesler, City of Lexington, 200 East Main Street, Lexington, KY 40507.

Air Quality: Lexington's particulate pollution in 1988 was 133 μg/m³, slightly worse than Frankfort's 116 μg/m³ but in compliance with the EPA NAAQS maximum of 260 μg/m3. However, Lexington exceeded Federal ozone standards on 5 days in 1988, reaching 0.138 ppm, high for a relatively small city. In 1989 the city's maximum ozone level went to 0.11 ppm, just below the NAAQS maximum. Contact: Tommy

Flora, Deputy Commissioner, Lexington Fayette Health Dept., 650 Newtown Pike, Lexington, KY 40508; or William C. Eddins, State Division of
Air Quality, 18 Reilly Road, Frankfort, KY 40601.

Hazardous Waste: No hazardous-waste disposal sites, nor any sites on the
EPA's National Priorities List, are in Fayette County. Several counties to
the south, in Madison County, a nerve-gas incinerator has been proposed.
Contact: Caroline P. Haight, Assistant Director, State Division of Waste
Management, 18 Reilly Road, Frankfort, KY 40601.

Weather: The average temperature is about normal at 54.9. Precipitation is
high at 45.68 inches annually.

Average Daily Temperature (degrees F)	54.9
High	64.7
Low	45.0
Average Humidity	
Morning (percent)	81
Afternoon (percent)	60
Normal Precipitation (inches)	45.7
Average Total Snowfall (inches)	16.4
Ozone, Days over 0.12 ppm (one hour in 1988)	5

℞ In an attempt to make health care more accessible to its citizens,
Lexington has integrated primary care with traditional public-
health services for indigent health care. The city is involved in a health-
awareness campaign. Public-health faculty at nearby universities, the Red
Cross, the Lung Association and the Heart Association all address a variety
of health issues. The city provides all common health-education programs
and emergency hotlines. The county provides all common preventive-
health and treatment programs. The city does not have any anti-smoking
legislation; but smoking is partially restricted in restaurants and in offices.
Contact: Dr. John Poundstone, Commissioner, Lexington Fayette Health
Department, 650 Newtown Pike, Lexington, KY 40508.

Health Resources per 1,000 Pop.	Number	Rank
Hospital Beds	8.86	24/92
Nurses	9.02	28/90
Doctors	3.78	10/113

Unique to Lexington are an equestrian program for the general
public, the Bluegrass 10-kilometer race and senior games for senior
citizens. In 1989, three new swimming pools were added, and in 1990, an

18-hole championship golf course designed by Pete Dye was added. The city's sports facilities include 117 tennis courts, 55 baseball fields, 47 basketball courts, 32 football/soccer fields, 13 swimming pools and 4 golf courses. Lexington has several sports leagues for softball, basketball, baseball, volleyball, football and tennis. The city has also instituted a pilot program for a skateboard park. Contact: Shirley R. Watts, Director, City of Lexington Parks & Recreation, 545 North Upper Street, Lexington, KY 40507.

Parkland/Total City Area (percent)	2.3
Aerobics Classes	yes
Arts and Craft Classes	yes
Hiking or Exploration Groups	yes
Other Activities: aqua-aerobics and tennaerobics (tennis/aerobics) for senior citizens, clogging and jazzercize.	

The Lexington public-school system employs 14 nurses and 2 psychologists (as field-based consultants) for its 31,000 students. All schools have a part-time nurse, give most of the usual programs and have a standard health-education program. The school system requires rubella, T.B., mumps and measles vaccinations. All common health-education programs are offered to students in grades K-8 and 10. The school system provides all common screens and tests except mental-health exams and well-child physical exams. Medical treatment is provided for students. Contact: James Komara Fayette County Schools, 701 East Main Street, Lexington, KY 40507.

Lincoln, NE

🪦 (RIP)	⚕	$	⬆	℞	⚕	👥	?
✓	✔	✔	✔	X	✓	✓	✔

Lincoln (Lancaster County) ranks 41st in the age-adjusted mortality rate. Infant-mortality rates for Nebraska are high among minorities and low among whites. Infant-mortality rates are higher in urban areas of the state. Contact: Scott Holmes, Epidemiologist, Lincoln-Lancaster County Health Department, 2200 St. Mary's Avenue, Lincoln, NE 68502.

	Number	Rank
Age-Adjusted Death Rate	−0.40	41/100
Heart Attacks	−0.08	45/100
Cancer	−0.10	40/100

Lincoln is one of the safest metro areas you'll find. It has the 4th lowest homicide rate and the 5th lowest number of robberies. Accidental deaths are the 7th lowest and suicides the 9th lowest of the 100 metro areas.

Incidence per 1,000 Pop.	Number	Rank
Homicides (1989)	0.02	4/111
Robberies (1989)	0.49	5/111
Suicides	0.09	9/100
Accidental Deaths	0.24	7/100

$ Lincoln's 1988 metro population was 212,000—104th out of 113 metro areas. Its economic health at the end of 1990 was the strongest of 113 metro areas. Its unemployment rate ranks 1st (lowest), change in unemployment 11th (employment grew by 1.7 percent, faster than the 0.6 percent growth in the labor force) and its enterprise 6th. Contact: Mayor Bill Harris, City of Lincoln, 555 South 10th Street, Lincoln, NE 68508.

Air Quality: In recent years, Lincoln has seen a decrease in carbon-monoxide levels and its ozone maximum is well below the NAAQS maximum. Contact: M. Jane Ford, Director, Lincoln-Lancaster County Health Department, 2200 Saint Mary's Avenue, Lincoln, NE 68502. 402-471-8000.

Hazardous Waste: One hazardous-waste site in Lancaster County is on the EPA's National Priorities List, the Waverly Water Contamination Site, where carbon tetrachloride has been deposited. Since 1985, Lincoln and Lancaster County have held household hazardous waste collections. A pilot program is planned for curbside collection of oil. The county has a special process to keep hazardous waste out of the landfill and wastewater treatment plant. An extensive underground monitoring program has probably uncovered the majority of past contamination. Even the smallest dumping is reported to public officials due to an ongoing hazardous waste awareness program. Contact: M. Jane Ford, address cited above.

Water Quality: 100 percent of the water supply in Lincoln comes from ground water (e.g., wells). Some wells exhibit higher total solids and nitrates than others. Contact: Dick Erixson, Director, 555 South 10th Street, Rm. B318, Lincoln, NE 68508.

Weather: The average temperature is slightly below average at 50.5. Humidity is above average at 82 percent in the morning.

Average Daily Temperature (degrees F)	50.5
High	62.3
Low	38.6
Average Humidity	
Morning (percent)	82
Afternoon (percent)	59
Normal Precipitation (inches)	26.9
Average Total Snowfall (inches)	28.1
Ozone, Days over 0.12 ppm (one hour in 1988)	0

℞ The Lincoln-Lancaster County Health Department has received dozens of national awards for its programs in health education such as the Lifetime Health Program's daily talk show on the public access channel. It has a very active community-based health-education effort with numerous awareness campaigns. Lincoln has developed an indigent clinic and a medical-referral program, a public-private joint venture. It also has a trauma center. The city offers follow-ups for high-risk infants at all of its three hospitals. The city provides all common health-education programs and emergency hotlines including sexually transmitted diseases and AIDS. The city and county provide all common preventive-health (food for the needy is provided by a private organization) and treatment programs. State legislation partially restricts smoking in restaurants and offices, and on public transportation. Contact: M. Jane Ford, address cited above.

Health Resources per 1,000 Pop.	Number	Rank
Hospital Beds	4.44	79/92
Nurses	5.75	64/90
Doctors	1.83	95/113

The city's sports facilities include 65 tennis courts, 50 softball fields, 21 volleyball courts, 9 swimming pools, 7 football/soccer fields, 6 basketball courts, 5 running tracks and 4 golf courses. Other recreational facilities include ice skating areas, boating lakes, horseshoe courts, a rifle and pistol range, 6 recreational centers and 47.68 miles of hiking and biking trails. Contact: Donald J. Smith, Director, Parks and Recreation Department, 2740 "A" Street, Lincoln, NE 68502.

Parkland/Total City Area (percent)	13.8

For the 27,800 students in the public-school system, Lincoln employs 17 nurses, 3 licensed practical nurses, 19 psychologists and 42 other health personnel. The Special Education department has 12 occupational and physical therapists and 14 aides. The high schools have a nurse present on a full-time basis, and the junior high and elementary schools have a nurse present on a part-time basis. The school system has an AIDS policy for its staff and students. All common health-education programs are offered to students in grades K-12. The school system provides all common screens and tests except well-child physical exams. Medical treatment is provided for students. Contact: Dr. Dean Austin, Consultant for Physical Education and Health, Lincoln Public Schools, P.O. Box 82889, Lincoln, NE 68501.

Little Rock, AR

RIP	🏃	$	🌲	℞	🖼	👥	?
✔	X	✓	?	✓	?	?	XX

Little Rock (Pulaski County) ranks 23rd in the age-adjusted mortality rate, meaning it is in the top quartile of longevity. Infant-mortality rates for Arkansas are low among whites. But infant-mortality rates are high for blacks and other minorities. The rates are slightly higher in cities than in rural areas.

	Number	Rank
Age-Adjusted Death Rate	−1.12	23/100
Heart Attacks	−0.47	20/100
Cancer	−0.29	21/100

Homicide and robbery rates are high in the Little Rock metro area, but suicide and accident rates are below the median of the 100 metro areas we compared.

Incidence per 1,000 Pop.	Number	Rank
Homicides (1989)	0.13	90/111
Robberies (1989)	2.91	81/111
Suicides	0.12	37/100
Accidental Deaths	0.32	34/100

Little Rock's 1988 metro population was 513,000—78th out of 113 metro areas. Its economic health at the end of 1990 was average, ranking 57th of 113 metro areas. Its unemployment rate ranks 64th, change in unemployment 30th (employment rose faster than the labor force) and its enterprise 71st.

Weather: The average temperature is slightly above average at 61.9. Precipitation is high at 49.2 inches annually.

Average Daily Temperature (degrees F)	61.9
High	72.9
Low	50.8
Average Humidity	
Morning (percent)	84
Afternoon (percent)	57
Normal Precipitation (inches)	49.2
Average Total Snowfall (inches)	5.3

℞ The city did not respond to the health-services survey, although it does not lack for health-services personnel, ranking in the top quartile in every health-resource category.

Health Resources per 1,000 Pop.	Number	Rank
Hospital Beds	13.07	9/92
Nurses	15.81	5/90
Doctors	2.96	28/113

 The city did not respond to the recreational-services survey.

 The city did not respond to the school-health survey.

Los Angeles, CA

🪦	✈	$	▲	℞	🎒	👥	?
✔	✕	✕	✕	✓	✕	✔	✔

🪦 The Los Angeles (Los Angeles County) primary metro area includes the City of Los Angeles, Glendale and Long Beach; the county extends up to Lancaster. (The consolidated Los Angeles metro area adds the Riverside-San Bernardino, Anaheim-Santa Ana, and Oxnard-Ventura primary metro areas.) The Los Angeles metro area ranks 28th in the age-adjusted mortality rate. Infant-mortality rates for California are high among blacks and low among whites. Rates are higher in cities than in rural areas of the state.

	Number	Rank
Age-Adjusted Death Rate	−0.93	28/100
Heart Attacks	−0.05	49/100
Cancer	−0.32	17/100

The Los Angeles metro area has the third highest robbery rate and the 6th highest homicide rate of the 111 metro areas we surveyed. The suicide rate is also above average, the accidental-death rate slightly below average.

Incidence per 1,000 Pop.	Number	Rank
Homicides (1989)	0.18	106/111
Robberies (1989)	6.16	109/111
Suicides	0.13	57/100
Accidental Deaths	0.33	49/100

$ Los Angeles' 1988 metro population was 8,588,000—1st out of 113 metro areas (its metro area includes Long Beach). Its economic health at the end of 1990 was below average, ranking 82nd of 113 metro areas. Its unemployment rate ranks 81st, change in unemployment 88th (the labor force increased faster than employment) and its enterprise 35th. Contact (for central city): Mayor Tom Bradley, City of Los Angeles, 200 North Spring Street, Los Angeles, CA 90012.

Air Quality: Air pollution is especially bad in the South Coast Air Basin, which reported 148 days with ozone levels above the Federal maximum of 0.12 ppm (one hour) in 1988. In 1989 Los Angeles exceeded NAAQS maxima for particulates (64 ppm vs. 50 ppm), carbon monoxide (18 ppm vs. 9 ppm), nitrogen dioxide (0.057 ppm vs. 0.053 ppm) and ozone (0.33 ppm vs. 0.12 ppm). Things aren't quite as bad as they seem because the worst air pollution reportedly occurs miles from population centers. But Los Angeles doesn't seem to be getting much better—with its PSI violating EPA standards 218 days in 1988 and 206 days in 1989. Contact: John Dunlap, Public Advisor, South Coast Air Quality Management District, 9150 Flair Drive, El Monte, CA 91731.

Hazardous Waste: Glendale, a large suburb of Los Angeles, is working to establish a permanent hazardous waste storage and transfer facility. Contact: Vasken Demirjian, Hazardous Materials supervisor, City of Glendale, Fire Department, 633 East Broadway, Glendale, CA 91206.

Water Quality: Water quality is substantially better than required by state and Federal legislation, but 64 percent of the residents of the city of Los Angeles drink bottled water or use home-treatment devices for their water. Contact: Robert Yoshimura, Assistant Engineer, Water Quality Division, Department of Water and Power, 111 North Hope Street, Los Angeles, CA 90051.

Weather: The Los Angeles area generally enjoys a two-season (summer-winter) climate. Summer is characterized by morning lows of 61 degrees and afternoon highs of 81 degrees; the average winter morning low is 47 degrees, but the temperature usually rises to about 67 by afternoon. Dry weather is the rule, with relative humidity averaging slightly more than 50 percent yearly. The area average yearly rainfall of 14 inches occurs during the cooler season (November–April). Snow is a rarity, except in the outlying mountains and elevated desert regions.

Average Daily Temperature (degrees F)	65.3
High	74.7
Low	55.9
Average Humidity	
Morning (percent)	75
Afternoon (percent)	53
Normal Precipitation (inches)	14.8
Average Total Snowfall (inches)	Trace
Ozone, Days over .12 ppm (one hour in 1988)	24
PSI, Days over 100, 1988	218
PSI, Days over 100, 1989	206

℞ The quality, accessibility and variety of health care in the Los Angeles metro area is excellent, but costs are high. Well-staffed departments exist for virtually every medical specialty, including cancer treatment, cardiac rehabilitation, psychiatry and substance abuse. The county is heavily involved with public-awareness campaigns concerning measles, AIDS and other sexually transmitted diseases. All common health-education programs and emergency hotlines are provided by the city. The city provides all common preventive-health (*except* for providing food to the needy) and treatment programs. Smoking is prohibited on public transportation and partially restricted in restaurants and public offices. Contact: Robert Gates, Los Angeles County Department of Health Services, 313 North Figueroa Street, Los Angeles, CA 90012.

Health Resources per 1,000 Pop.	Number	Rank
Hospital Beds	4.16	82/92
Nurses	4.35	80/90
Doctors	2.80	36/113

The City of Los Angeles offers aerobics and Park Ranger-led hike programs. Some 3,000 teams with more than 100,000 participants operate through various departments of the Municipal Sports program for adults. Another 100,000 participants are involved in these sports in independent sports leagues not led by the city's Department of Recreation and Parks. The city has recently completed an adaptive sports facility for disabled persons. Two more are under construction. The city has multipurpose fields that are used for football, soccer and softball. Other sports facilities include 360 tennis courts, 275 basketball courts, 64 swimming pools and 13 golf courses. When measured against the large population served by these facilities, they rank 77th of 82 cities. Contact: Al Goldfarb, Public Relations Director, Department of Recreation and Parks, 200 North Main Street, City Hall East, Los Angeles, CA 90012.

Glendale, a suburb to the north of Los Angeles and enveloped by Beverly Hills, Burbank and Pasadena, has an extraordinarily vigorous recreational program with an attractive catalog of activities, although the number of facilities in 1991 was not large (it has 1 soccer field and 1 football field). It offers a special adaptive program offered to developmentally disabled people of all ages. The city plans to open a new sports facility that will combine 3 soccer fields and 2 baseball fields. The city offers several classes in fitness and the arts. The parkland figure below includes undeveloped open space. Contact: Nello Iacono, Director of Parks, Recreation & Community Services, 613 East Broadway, Glendale, CA 91206. 818-956-2000.

Parkland/Total City Area (percent)	
Los Angeles	3.6
Glendale	24.0

Los Angeles, serving a total of 610,000 students, employs 485 nurses, 45 physicians, 2 clinical psychologists, 375 educational psychologists, 25 audiometrists and 29 psychiatric social workers. A full-time nurse is present in 38 percent of the schools and a part-time nurse present in the rest of the schools. Discussions were under way in 1990 concerning the possible creation of joint programs to provide public-health services with the County Public Health System. All common health-education programs are offered to students in grades K-12. The Los Angeles school system provides all common screens and tests. Medical treatment is provided for students. Contact: Dr. Roy S. Nakawatase, Student Health Services Division, 6520 New Castle Avenue, Reseda, CA 913358.

Glendale, serving 24,495 students, employs 5 nurses, 1 physician and 6 psychologists. Contact: Glendale Unified School District Health Services, 223 North Jackson, Glendale, CA 91206.

Long Beach, serving 72,000 students, employs 63 nurses in 53 positions, 1 physician, 19 psychologists and 41 speech therapists. All common health-education programs are offered to students in grades K-12. Long Beach has a K-12 AIDS education program, and a gang-and-drug diversion program. Contact: Sandra L. Sanders, Nursing Services, Long Beach Unified School District, 701 Locust Avenue, Long Beach, CA 90813.

Louisville, KY

🪦 RIP	🔪	$	↟	℞	🖼	👥	?
✓	✓	✔	X	✔	✔	✓	✔

 Louisville (Jefferson County) ranks 36th in the age-adjusted death rate. Infant-mortality rates for Kentucky are high among minorities and low among whites. Rates are the same in cities and rural areas of the state.

	Number	Rank
Age-Adjusted Death Rate	−0.60	36/100
Heart Attacks	−0.24	37/100
Cancer	−0.02	47/100

Louisville has average suicide and accident rates and a below-average number of homicides and robberies.

Incidence per 1,000 Pop.	Number	Rank
Homicides (1989)	0.07	43/111
Robberies (1989)	1.78	43/111
Suicides	0.12	50/100
Accidental Deaths	0.33	54/100

$\boxed{\$}$ Louisville's 1988 metro population was 967,000—48th out of 113 metro areas. Its economic health at the end of 1990 was excellent, ranking 24th of 113 metro areas. Its unemployment rate ranks 40th, change in unemployment 22nd (employment grew faster than the labor force) and its enterprise 44th. But compared to a decade ago Louisville has fewer manufacturing jobs and more lower-paid, less-skilled service jobs such as sorting UPS parcels. Contact: Mayor Jerry E. Abramson, City of Louisville, 101 City Hall, Louisville, KY 40202.

$\boxed{\spadesuit}$ **Air Quality:** Louisville's ozone level went up to 0.18 ppm in 1988; the EPA's NAAQS specify a limit of 0.12 ppm. Louisville had 9 ozone exceedances in 1988, a large number for a relatively small city. It was in compliance with all other NAAQS limits. Ozone in 1989 stayed at 0.11 ppm, just below the NAAQS maximum. One problem Louisville has is geography—the air is prone to be trapped in the Ohio Valley, leading to smog inversions. Contact: Air Pollution District of Jefferson County, 914 E. Broadway, Louisville, KY 40404.

Hazardous Waste: Lee's Lane Landfill is an inactive hazardous-waste site. A Remedial Action Plan has been implemented, which is located off Lee's Lane for mixed residential and industrial waste. Locals refer to a nearby Superfund site as "the Valley of the Drums." Proposals have been made to replace the old city incinerator, which has been closed, with a modern one that would handle hazardous waste; but as of mid-1991 the city's only disposal facility is a landfill. Contact: Louisville-Jefferson County Board of Health, 400 East Gray Street, Louisville, KY 40202.

Water Quality: Louisville's water is 100 percent from surface sources. It is provided by the Louisville Water Company. The 1990 water-quality data showed the city's water to be high in chlorine and nitrates and to have a high pH. One problem with Louisville's water supply is that the infrastructure is old, having pumped its first water in 1860. The Louisville Water Company has pioneered in studies of water filtration and chlorination, but has been less successful at upgrading its distribution network sufficiently to permit a lower level of residual chlorine. Contact: Jerry R. Ford, Manager, Administrative Services, Louisville Water Company, 436 South Third Street, Louisville, KY 40402.

Weather: The average temperature is about normal at 56.2. Precipitation is high at 43.6 inches.

Average Daily Temperature (degrees F)	56.2
High	66.1
Low	46.2

Average Humidity
    Morning (percent)   81
    Afternoon (percent)   59
Normal Precipitation (inches)   43.6
Average Total Snowfall (inches)   17.3
Ozone, Days over 0.12 ppm (1 hour, 1988)   9

℞ Two outpatient medical clinics have established joint outpatient-indigent-care centers, and Louisville also has a community-based homeless project. All common health-education programs and emergency hotlines are provided by the city. Its major health-education program has been in fire safety. The city distributes smoke detectors to the indigent. The city and county provide all common preventive-health and treatment programs except food to the disabled and elderly. As of 1990 the city of Louisville had no laws restricting smoking. A local health-care resource is the headquarters of the Humana proprietary-hospital chain. Contact: Dr. David Allen, Executive Director, Louisville-Jefferson County Department of Health, 400 East Gray Street, Louisville, KY 40202.

Health Resources per 1,000 Pop.	Number	Rank
Hospital Beds	12.84	11/92
Nurses	12.21	17/90
Doctors	2.46	56/113

A 4,000-acre urban forest is situated within a 20-minute drive from downtown Louisville. The city's sports facilities include 236 tennis courts, 111 basketball courts, 109 baseball fields, 15 swimming pools, 9 football/soccer fields, 9 golf courses, 4 running tracks and 20 indoor-recreation centers. Contact: Robert Kirchdorfer, Director, Metropolitan Parks & Recreation, 1297 Trevilian Way, PO Box 37280, Louisville, KY 40233 (502) 459-0440.

Parkland/Total City Area (percent)   3.8

To serve 90,884 students are 19 nurses, 25 psychologists and a large number of physical therapists, occupational therapists, speech/language clinicians and audiologists; 14 full-time nurses are available in 3 percent of the schools and five part-time nurses serve 57 percent of the schools. In recent years school-health officials have focused on enforcing health requirements and insuring the control of communicable and infectious diseases. All common health-education programs are offered to students in grades K-12. The school system provides all common screens and tests. Medical, dental and psychiatric treatments are provided for students.

Lubbock, TX

RIP	↴	$	▲	℞	[⚡]	♙	?
✓	✓	✗	?	✓	?	✗	✗

 Lubbock (Lubbock County) ranks 67th in the age-adjusted mortal-ity rate. Infant-mortality rates for Texas are high among minorities and low among whites. Infant-mortality rates are higher in cities.

	Number	Rank
Age-Adjusted Death Rate	0.48	67/100
Heart Attacks	0.08	61/100
Cancer	−0.09	41/100

 Lubbock has high rates for suicide and accident, but below-average numbers of homicide and robberies.

Incidence per 1,000 Pop.	Number	Rank
Homicides (1989)	0.07	50/111
Robberies (1989)	1.22	26/111
Suicides	0.16	86/100
Accidental Deaths	0.40	85/100

$ Lubbock's 1988 metro population was 227,000—102nd out of 113 metro areas. Its economic health at the end of 1990 was poor, rank-ing 99th of 113 metro areas. Its unemployment rate ranks 64th, change in unemployment 74th (the labor force grew slightly, employment shrank slightly) and its enterprise 104th. Contact: Mayor B.C. McMinn, City of Lubbock, PO Box 2000, Lubbock, TX 79457.

Weather: The average temperature is about normal at 59.9. Precipi-tation is slightly below average at 17.76 inches annually.

Average Daily Temperature (degrees F)	59.9
High	73.5
Low	46.2
Average Humidity	
Morning (percent)	74
Afternoon (percent)	47

Normal Precipitation (inches)	17.8
Average Total Snowfall (inches)	10.6

℞ The city did not respond to the health-services survey.

Health Resources per 1,000 Pop.	Number	Rank
Hospital Beds	8.50	28/92
Nurses	7.71	41/90
Doctors	2.70	42/113

The city did not respond to the recreational-services survey.

 Lubbock Independent School District has 57 campuses, which include 40 elementary schools, 9 junior high schools (grades 7–9), five senior high schools (grades 10–12), and three campuses with special programs. The district employs 36 registered nurses full-time, plus one part-time nurse who works with the school-age parenting grant and one full-time nurse coordinator. Ten nurses are employed at their campuses full-time. The school system offers most of the usual vaccination programs. All common health-education programs (except sex education) are offered to students in grades K-12. The school system provides all common screens and tests except mental-health exams and well-child physical exams. No medical, dental or psychiatric treatment is provided. Contact: Jane Tustin, R.N., M.S.N., C.S.N., Coordinator, Health Services, Lubbock Independent School District, 1628 19th Street, Lubbock, TX 79401 (806) 766-1972.

Madison, WI

⚰️ RIP	🏃	$	⬆	℞	🎭	👥	?
✔	✔	✔	✔	✔	✔	✗	✔

⚰️ RIP The Madison (Dane County) metro area ranks 32nd in the age-adjusted mortality rate. Infant-mortality rates for Wisconsin are high among minorities and low among whites. Infant-mortality rates are higher in cities.

	Number	Rank
Age-Adjusted Death Rate	−0.75	32/100
Heart Attacks	0.23	71/100
Cancer	−0.14	32/100

Madison has the 5th lowest accident rate and the 9th lowest number of robberies. Homicide and suicide rates are also below average.

Incidence per 1,000 Pop.	Number	Rank
Homicides (1989)	0.04	14/111
Robberies (1989)	0.64	9/111
Suicides	0.11	29/100
Accidental Deaths	0.23	5/100

$ Madison's 1988 metro population was 353,000—95th out of 113 metro areas. Its economic health at the end of 1990 was excellent, ranking 13th of 113 metro areas. Madison has a cushion during recessions, because its major employers include a large university and the state government, both relatively recession-proof. Its unemployment rate ranks 3rd, change in unemployment 47th (employment grew 1.4 percent, the labor force 1.3 percent) and its enterprise 38th. Contact: Mayor Paul R. Soglin, City of Madison, 210 Martin Luther King Blvd., Madison, WI 53710.

Air Quality: Average pollutant levels have been fairly stable over the 1985–90 period, but 1990 maximum particulate levels reported to us by the city were a surprisingly high 239 µg/m³—very close to the maximum value in New York City! The difference is that New York's *average* particulate level was over three times that of Madison's. Sulfur-dioxide levels in Madison were also high in 1988, but carbon monoxide and ozone levels were fairly low. In 1989, ozone remained at 0.10, below the NAAQS maximum of 0.12 ppm.

Hazardous Waste: A combination of programs exist to address disposal of hazardous waste and solid waste. The Clean Sweep program for disposal of household hazardous waste was initiated seven years ago. The program has grown each year. A special collection site for paint disposal has recently been developed. This supplements the regular hazardous-materials drop-off program. Drop-off stations are also available throughout the city for waste oil. Recently, the city initiated a city-wide recycling program. This program expanded the newspaper/paperboard pickup to include plastics, glass and metal containers. Contact: Patricia Natzke, M.P.H., Director, Department of Public Health, 210 Martin Luther King, Jr. Blvd., Madison, WI 53710.

Water Quality: One hundred percent of the city's drinking water comes from the ground (i.e., wells). Recently, average chloride levels have been increasing gradually. A couple of active wells have very low levels of VOC's (volatile organic compounds).

Weather: The average temperature in Madison is well below the national average low at 45.2 degrees. Humidity and precipitation are slightly above average.

Average Daily Temperature (degrees F)	45.2
High	56.1
Low	34.3
Average Humidity	
Morning (percent)	84
Afternoon (percent)	62
Normal Precipitation (inches)	30.8
Average Total Snowfall (inches)	42.3
Ozone, Days over 0.12 ppm (one hour in 1988)	0

℞ Madison sponsors health-awareness campaigns on the issues of AIDS, influenza, WIC (women and infant children) and prenatal care. Madison has recently added a community relations position in the Health Department. The city provides all common health-education programs and emergency hotlines, and all common preventive-health programs *except* provision of food to the needy, disabled or elderly. It provides treatment for sexually transmitted diseases but not for drug abuse, alcoholism or mental illness. Anti-smoking laws in Madison include partial restriction in restaurants and full restriction in public offices and on public transportation. Contact: Patricia J. Natzke, M.P.H., Director, Madison Department of Public Health, 210 Martin Luther King, Jr. Blvd, Madison, WI 53710.

Health Resources per 1,000 Pop.	Number	Rank
Hospital Beds	8.09	32/92
Nurses	8.75	33/90
Doctors	4.58	6/113

Adult-league teams and open-play sports are immensely popular, with up to 1,000 organized teams in softball alone. Madison residents in large numbers engage in bicycling, canoeing, boating, cross-country skiing, ice skating and hockey. Thousands of fitness enthusiasts enjoy running, weightlifting and exercise/aerobic classes. Madison also has several full-service sports-medicine facilities and in 1991 was considering a marina development on Lake Monona. Sports facilities are extensive for such a relatively small city and include 84 tennis courts, 67 basketball courts, 35 football/soccer fields, 16 running tracks, 4 baseball fields and 4 golf courses. Water facilities include 13 beaches and 11 boat-launch areas. Contact: Robert Humke, Director, Madison Schools & Community Recreation Department, 1045 East Dayton Street, Madison, WI 53703.

Parkland/Total City Area (percent)　　　　　14.6

The public-school system has a total of 22,600 students and employs 20 nurses; a nurse is present full-time in 15 percent of the schools and part-time in 85 percent. This school-health personnel input is in the bottom third of cities for which we have this information; possibly Madison doesn't have the same school-health needs as larger inner-city school systems. All common health-education programs are offered to students in grades K-12 and medical treatment is provided for students. The school system provides all common screens and tests except mental-health exams and well-child physical exams. Contact: Mary Gulbrandsen, Program Coordinator, Health Services, 545 West Dayton Street, Madison, WI 53703.

Memphis, TN

RIP	⤵	$	⬆	℞	🏃	👥	?
X	X	✓	?	✓	X	?	X

Memphis (Shelby County) ranks a high 83rd in the age-adjusted mortality rate. Infant-mortality rates for Tennessee are high among minorities and low among whites. Rates are much higher in cities than in rural areas of the state.

	Number	Rank
Age-Adjusted Death Rate	0.93	83/100
Heart Attacks	−0.04	51/100
Cancer	0.17	74/100

Memphis has extremely high rates of homicide, robberies and accidents. The suicide rate is below average.

Incidence per 1,000 Pop.	Number	Rank
Homicides (1989)	0.17	101/111
Robberies (1989)	4.26	99/111
Suicides	0.11	30/100
Accidental Deaths	0.44	93/100

$ Memphis' 1988 metro population was 979,000—45th out of 113 metro areas. Its economic health at the end of 1990 was good, ranking 43rd of 113 metro areas. Its unemployment rate ranks 51st, change in unemployment 52nd (the labor force grew slightly faster than employment) and its enterprise 45th. Contact: Mayor Richard Hackett, City of Memphis, 125 North Mid-America Mall, Memphis, TN 38103.

↑ **Weather:** Indirectly affected by opposing airflows from both Canada and the Gulf of Mexico, Memphis has a climate characterized by capricious storms. While zero degree temperatures are all but unknown, the temperature does drop to freezing or below about 60 days a year. On the other end of the spectrum, Memphis experiences about the same number of days a year of 90-degrees-or-over weather.

Average Daily Temperature (degrees F)	61.8
High	71.6
Low	51.9
Average Humidity	
Morning (percent)	81
Afternoon (percent)	57
Normal Precipitation (inches)	51.6
Average Total Snowfall (inches)	5.7

℞ Health care in Memphis is big business. Specialized facilities exist for cardiovascular, cancer, eye, ear, and nose and throat research, as well as childhood cancer treatment, liver and kidney transplant, spinal cord injury, stroke, head trauma, substance-abuse rehabilitation and psychiatry. Recent developments include a $35 million expansion of the Regional Medical Center to include ambulatory care. Teen pregnancy, AIDS, sexually transmitted diseases, nutrition and prenatal care are major concerns in the city. Smoking is partially restricted in restaurants, public transportation and in public offices and private offices. All common health-education programs and emergency hotlines are provided by the city. The city and county provide all common preventive-health and treatment programs. Contact: Richard Swiggart, Director, Memphis/Shelby County Health Department, Memphis, TN 38103.

Health Resources per 1,000 Pop.	Number	Rank
Hospital Beds	7.42	39/92
Nurses	7.10	50/90
Doctors	2.52	49/113

 Memphis sports facilities include 133 tennis courts, 109 baseball fields, 60 basketball courts, 16 swimming pools, 15 running tracks,

15 football/soccer fields, 8 golf courses and 2 rugby fields. Softball, basketball and golf are especially popular. A new 18-hole golf course and a new softball complex are in the planning stages. Contact: Bob Brame, Director, Memphis Park Commission, 2599 Avery Avenue, Memphis, TN 38112.

Parkland/Total City Area (percent)	2.9

 The city did not respond to the school-health survey.

Miami, FL

⚰️RIP	🏃	$	↑	R	🏃	👫	?
✔	X	X	✔	✔	X	✔	✔

The Miami (Dade County) metro area includes Hialeah. Miami ranks a healthy 9th in the age-adjusted mortality rate. Infant-mortality rates for Florida are high among minorities and low among whites. Rates are higher in rural areas than in cities.

	Number	Rank
Age-Adjusted Death Rate	−2.04	9/100
Heart Attacks	−0.43	22/100
Cancer	−0.65	4/100

Miami can be a dangerous place. It has the highest number of robberies and the 3rd highest number of homicides. Suicide and accident rates are also above average.

Incidence per 1,000 Pop.	Number	Rank
Homicides (1989)	0.22	109/111
Robberies (1989)	11.08	111/111
Suicides	0.17	89/100
Accidental Deaths	0.37	77/100

Miami's 1988 metro population was 1,814,000—25th out of 113 metro areas. Its economic health at the end of 1990 was poor, ranking 89th of 113 metro areas. Its unemployment rate ranks 100th, change in unemployment 85th (the labor force grew faster than employment) and its enterprise 33rd. Contact: Mayor Xavier L. Suarez, City of Miami, 3500 Pan American Drive, Miami, FL 33133.

 Hazardous Waste: The city has no hazardous-waste sites. Encapsulation of heavy metals has been used at a former wood-treatment site.

Weather: Miami's subtropical climate has essentially no seasons, except that during summer months it rains a lot, and during the winter it's dry. The temperature almost never goes down to freezing, and there's about a month of 90-degree days each year.

Average Daily Temperature (degrees F)	75.6
High	82.6
Low	68.7
Average Humidity	
Morning (percent)	84
Afternoon (percent)	61
Normal Precipitation (inches)	57.5
Average Total Snowfall (inches)	0.0

℞ Health care in the Miami area is good but expensive. The area boasts 37 licensed hospitals, including 3 teaching hospitals, 7 cardiac rehabilitation centers and 1 cancer treatment center.

Health Resources per 1,000 Pop.	Number	Rank
Hospital Beds	13.08	8/92
Nurses	15.25	7/90
Doctors	3.62	13/113

Miami has a rowing and sailing program. Tennis facilities were increased by 22 courts between 1989 and 1991, at the expense of basketball, baseball and football facilities, which were reduced. Sports facilities in mid-1991 include 76 tennis courts, 42 basketball courts, 30 baseball fields, 10 football/soccer fields, 10 swimming pools and 2 golf courses. A strong feature is the summer camps program established for the convenience of working parents. Activities include tennis classes, learn-to-swim, educational and recreational field trips, exposure to arts and cultural experience and sports. Contact: Albert Ruder, Director, City of Miami Parks and Recreation, 1390 NW 7th Street, Miami, FL 33125.

Parkland/Total City Area (percent)	2.9

For a total of 273,500 students in the public-school system, there are 101 psychologists, 100 therapists and 100 speech-hearing specialists. High-risk schools (approximately 40 percent) have weekly visits from a specified school nurse. The other 60 percent have a nurse on call. All common health-education programs are offered to students in grades K-10. The school system provides all common screens and tests except mental-health exams. Medical, dental and psychiatric treatments are provided for students. Contact: Robert Adams, Health Department, Dade County Public Schools, 1450 NE 2nd Avenue, Miami, FL 33132.

Milwaukee, WI

RIP	⌁	$	▲	Rx	[👤]	👥	?
X	✓	✓	✔	✓	✓	?	✓

Milwaukee (Milwaukee County) ranks a high 84th in the age-adjusted mortality rate. Cancer and heart attack rates are also high. Infant-mortality rates for Wisconsin are high among minorities and low among whites. Rates are higher in cities than in rural areas.

	Number	Rank
Age-Adjusted Death Rate	1.00	84/100
Heart Attacks	0.68	88/100
Cancer	0.28	85/100

Milwaukee has above-average suicide and homicide rates. Accident rates are below average.

Incidence per 1,000 Pop.	Number	Rank
Homicides (1989)	0.08	62/111
Robberies (1989)	1.92	52/111
Suicides	0.15	79/100
Accidental Deaths	0.29	18/100

 Milwaukee's 1988 metro population was 1.4 million—31st out of 113 metro areas. Its economic health at the end of 1990 was good, ranking 46th of 113 metro areas. Its unemployment rate ranks 6th, change in unemployment 43rd (employment grew slightly faster than the labor force) and its enterprise 101st. Contact: Mayor John O. Norquist, City of Milwaukee, 200 East Wells Street, Milwaukee, WI 53202.

Water Quality: Milwaukee's water supply comes 99 percent from surface-water sources and 1 percent from groundwater sources. The drinking water is contaminated with an above-average level of trihalomethanes. Contact: Paul Biedrzychi, M.P.H., Manager of Technical Services, City of Milwaukee Health Department, 841 North Broadway, Milwaukee, WI 53202.

Weather: Milwaukee is a cold city with an average temperature of 46.1. Precipitation is slightly above average at 30.9 inches annually.

Average Daily Temperature (degrees F)	46.1
High	54.6
Low	37.6
Average Humidity	
Morning (percent)	80
Afternoon (percent)	64
Average Total Snowfall (inches)	46.7

The city did not respond to the health-services survey.

Health Resources per 1,000 Pop.	Number	Rank
Hospital Beds	6.47	51/92
Nurses	7.42	47/90
Doctors	2.62	45/113

The city offers aerobics, arts and crafts classes, hiking and exploration groups, slow-pitch softball, water aerobics, lifetime-skills programs for exceptional students, instructional swimming and wheelchair sports. Recently the city has placed resilient surfaces under all play equipment, except for those located on turf. The city's sports facilities include 256 basketball courts, 152 tennis courts, 105 baseball fields, 48 football/soccer fields, 27 swimming pools, 15 running tracks and 6 golf courses. Softball is a very popular sport with 28,000 participants in organized leagues. Basketball, volleyball, football and soccer are also popular. Contact: Gary Coplien, Director, Department of Municipal Recreation and Community Education, 5225 West Vliet Street, Box 461, Milwaukee, WI 53201-0461.

Parkland/Total City Area (percent)	9.3

The city did not respond to the school-health survey.

Minneapolis—Saint Paul, MN

🪦	🏃	$	🌲	℞	🏃	🏃	?
✔	✔	✔	✔	✔	✔	✔	✔

Minneapolis (Hennepin County) and Saint Paul (Ramsey County) rank 14th in the age-adjusted mortality rate. Cancer and heart-attack rates for Minneapolis-Saint Paul are relatively low. Infant-mortality rates for Minnesota are high among blacks and low among whites and in rural areas of the state.

	Number	Rank
Age-Adjusted Death Rate	−1.61	14/100
Heart Attacks	1.54	23/100
Cancer	1.57	14/100

The Minneapolis-Saint Paul metro area has relatively low rates of homicide, robberies and accidents. But suicide rates are above average.

Incidence per 1,000 Pop.	Number	Rank
Homicides (1989)	0.04	14/111
Robberies (1989)	1.64	35/111
Suicides	0.14	72/100
Accidental Deaths	0.31	26/100

$ Minneapolis-Saint Paul's 1988 metro population was 2.39 million—13th out of 113 metro areas. Its economic health at the end of 1990 was excellent, ranking 27th of 113 metro areas. Its unemployment rate ranks 10th, change in unemployment 58th (the labor force grew slightly faster than employment) and its enterprise 48th. Contact: Mayor Donald Fraser, City of Minneapolis, 350 5th Street, Room 127, Minneapolis, MN 55415. Or: Mayor James Scheibel, City of Saint Paul, 15 West Kellogg Blvd., Room 347, Saint Paul, MN 55102.

Air Quality: The 1985–90 period saw a decrease in the level of lead in the air, in part because less leaded gasoline was in use. Ozone is not monitored in Saint Paul. The city is in attainment of EPA's NAAQS standards for all pollutants *except* for carbon monoxide; in 1989 the metro area had a carbon-monoxide level of 11 ppm, well above the NAAQS limit. The whole of the Twin Cities Seven County Metropolitan Area was non-attainment for carbon monoxide as of mid-1991. Contact: Gary Eckhardt, Supervisor, Minnesota State Pollution Control Agency, Air Monitoring Unit, Air Quality Division, 520 Lafayette Road, Saint Paul, MN 55155-6300.

Hazardous Waste: Minneapolis reports that it has no hazardous-waste landfills. All Superfund Sites are handled by the Minnesota Pollution Control Agency. Contact: Glenn Kiecker, Supervisor, Environmental Review, Department of Inspections, 300 Public Health Building, 250 South 4th Street, Minneapolis, MN 55415.

Weather: Minneapolis-Saint Paul is the second-coldest U.S. metro area, after Anchorage. One-tenth of the year (35 days) the mercury stays below zero all day. But Twin Cities architecture copes with the cold, with many "skyways" (second-floor enclosed pedestrian bridges) to connect buildings. Average temperature for the Twin Cities is 44 degrees. In the 1986–1987 winter, no snow fell at all, and locals argue that it is easier to cope with snowless below-zero weather than with mushy, slushy 30s characteristic of more southerly winters. The rain falls mainly in the spring. The summers are cool and dry. Some days the temperature climbs over 100 degrees, but also whole summers have occurred when the temperature hasn't gone above 90.

Average Daily Temperature (degrees F)	44.7
High	54.2
Low	35.2
Average Humidity	
Morning (percent)	79
Afternoon (percent)	60
Annual Precipitation (inches)	26.4
Average Total Snowfall (inches)	49.1

℞ *Minneapolis* has expanded its lead-poisoning-prevention program. Smoking is prohibited on public transportation and partially prohibited in restaurants and in private and public offices. Minneapolis offers AIDS risk assessment and counseling for women concerning family planning and prenatal care. All common health-education programs and emergency hotlines are provided by the city. The city provides all common preventive-health programs except food to the needy disabled and elderly. It provides treatment for sexually transmitted diseases but not for drug abuse, alcoholism or mental illness. Contact: David Lurie, Commissioner, Health Department, PHC Bldg., 250 South 4th Street, Minneapolis, MN

55415. *Saint Paul* did not respond to the health-services questionnaire, so that all information about public-health programs is from Minneapolis.

Health Resources per 1,000 Pop.	Number	Rank
Hospital Beds		
Minneapolis	11.43	15/92
Saint Paul	5.14	68/92
Nurses		
Minneapolis	14.16	9/90
Saint Paul	5.89	59/90
Doctors (Minneapolis-Saint Paul)	2.62	60/113

Minneapolis has 44 full-time professionally staffed recreation centers. There are numerous parklands and park facilities. The parks also provide cultural opportunities with numerous facilities for concerts, plays, movies and art. The Mississippi Riverfront offers many amenities. Parks have become a focal point in many neighborhoods. Minneapolis and Saint Paul have always impressed me with their commitment to making its social programs work as efficiently and effectively as possible. They are working hard to bridge gaps in government programs in health, law enforcement, drug education, childcare and crime prevention. Minneapolis sports facilities include 183 tennis courts, 96 football/soccer fields, 71 basketball courts, 41 baseball fields and 5 golf courses. Contact: David L. Fischer, Superintendent of Parks, Minneapolis Park and Recreation Board, 310 4th Avenue South—second floor, Minneapolis, MN 55415.

Minneapolis Parkland/Total City Area (percent)	6

Saint Paul has responded to the popularity of cross-country skiing by expanding its cross-country ski program to Como Park. Saint Paul has several adult and youth athletic leagues. Sports facilities include 127 softball fields, 68 tennis courts, 65 basketball courts, 40 football/soccer fields, 36 baseball fields, 5 ski areas and 3 golf courses. Water facilities include beaches, marinas and lakeside activities centers. Contact: Robert Piram, Superintendent, Division of Parks and Recreation, 25 West 4th Street, 3rd Floor City Hall Annex, Saint Paul, MN 55102.

Saint Paul Parkland/Total City Area (percent)	9.9
Aerobics class	yes
Arts and craft classes	yes
Hiking or exploration groups	yes
Other Activities: Lessons in downhill and cross-country skiing, canoeing, rowing, and windsurfing.	

Saint Paul public schools employ 41 nurses, 16 psychologists and 4 dental hygienists for 34,586 students. Nurses are present on a full-time basis in 24 percent of the schools and on a part-time basis in the remainder. The school system provides daycare and case management for adolescent women who are parents. All common health-education programs (including AIDS education) are offered to students in grades K-7 and 10. The school system provides all common screens and tests except mental-health exams, speech therapy and learning disabilities. Medical and dental treatments are provided for students. Contact: Wanda Miller, Supervisor, Health Department, Saint Paul Public Schools, 360 Colborne, Saint Paul, MN 55102. *Minneapolis* did not respond to the school-health questionnaire, so that all data below on school-health programs is for Saint Paul.

Mobile, AL

A RIP	🏃	$	↑	℞	🎿	👥	?
X	X	✔	✔	X	✓	X	✔

Mobile (Mobile County) ranks a high 78th in the age-adjusted mortality rate. Cancer rates are also very high in the city. Infant-mortality rates for Alabama are high among minorities and low among whites. Infant-mortality rates are higher in cities than in rural areas of the state.

	Number	Rank
Age-Adjusted Death Rate	0.76	78/100
Heart Attacks	-0.07	46/100
Cancer	0.33	86/100

Mobile has the 9th highest accident rate of the 100 metro areas. Homicide rates are also high. Suicide rates are below average.

Incidence per 1,000 Pop.	Number	Rank
Homicides (1989)	0.12	86/111
Robberies (1989)	2.21	63/111
Suicides	0.10	20/100
Accidental Deaths	0.43	91/100

| $ | Mobile's 1988 metro population was 486,000—80th out of 113 metro areas. Its economic health at the end of 1990 was good, ranking 37th of 113 metro areas. Its unemployment rate ranks 96th, change in unemployment 4th (employment rose four times as fast as the labor force) and its enterprise 32nd. Contact: Mayor Michael Dow, City of Mobile, PO Box 1827, Mobile, AL 36633.

Air Quality: Monitoring has been discontinued for carbon monoxide, nitrogen and lead. Past levels were very low. The low level of nitrogen is due to the relatively few automobiles in Mobile. Levels of ozone, particulates and sulfur dioxide are all better than the EPA's national air quality standards. Contact: Catherine G. Lamar, Public Affairs Officer, Alabama Department of Environmental Management, 2204 Perimeter Road, Mobile, AL 36615.

Hazardous Waste: Hazardous waste is not disposed of in Mobile County. Contact: Alabama Department of Environmental Management, 2204 Perimeter Road, Mobile, AL 36615.

Water Quality: 100 percent of the water supply in Mobile is from surface water (e.g., reservoirs). Water quality has remained uniform over the 1985–90 period. Lead and nitrate levels are low, pH is average and residual chlorine is relatively high. Contact: John Von Sprecken, Superintendent, Mobile Water Service System, 207 North Catherines Street, Mobile, AL 36604.

Weather: The average temperature is high at 67.5. Precipitation is extremely high at 64.64 inches annually.

Average Daily Temperature (degrees F)	67.5
High	77.4
Low	57.6
Average Humidity	
Morning (percent)	86
Afternoon (percent)	57
Normal Precipitation (inches)	64.6
Average Total Snowfall (inches)	0.3

The city did not respond to the health-services survey.

Health Resources per 1,000 Pop.	Number	Rank
Hospital Beds	8.32	29/92
Nurses	11.02	18/90
Doctors	1.95	86/113

Mobile offers community-activity programs including ceramics and other arts and crafts classes. The city's sports facilities include 84 tennis courts, 40 baseball fields, 28 basketball courts, 17 football/soccer fields, 6 swimming pools, 4 running tracks and 3 golf courses. Gymnastics and racquetball are also popular. Contact: Richmond Brown, Superintendent of Recreation, 2301 Airport Blvd., Mobile, AL 36606.

Parkland/Total City Area (percent)   2.6

The Mobile school system employs 19 nurses and 1 audiologist for its 67,000 students. A nurse is present full-time in 3 schools and part-time in 48 schools. Health education is taught to students in grades K-10. The school system provides all common screens and tests except for immunizations, mental-health exams, well-child physical exams and learning disabilities; it also provides psychological testing on referred students. The school system passed an AIDS policy in 1987. No medical, dental or psychiatric treatment is provided for students. Contact: Elaine Maxime, Supervisor of Health Services, Mobile County Public Schools, 504 Government Street, Mobile, AL 36602.

Nashville, TN

⚰️ RIP	🏃	$	🌲	℞	🎨	👥	?
✓	✓	✔	✓	✓	✗	✓	✔

Nashville (Davidson County) ranks 42nd in the age-adjusted mortality rate. Infant-mortality rates for Tennessee are extremely high among minorities and relatively low among whites. Infant-mortality rates are higher in cities than in rural areas of the state.

	Number	Rank
Age-Adjusted Death Rate	−0.29	42/100
Heart Attacks	−0.19	38/100
Cancer	−0.04	46/100

 Nashville has an extremely high accident rate. Homicide and suicide rates are slightly above average.

Incidence per 1,000 Pop.	Number	Rank
Homicides (1989)	0.10	69/111
Robberies (1989)	1.84	46/111
Suicides	0.14	66/100
Accidental Deaths	0.42	90/100

$ Nashville's 1988 metro population was 972,000—46th out of 113 metro areas. Its economic health at the end of 1990 was excellent, ranking 15th of 113 metro areas. Its unemployment rate ranks 25th, change in unemployment 58th (the labor force grew by 0.5 percent, employment by 0.1 percent) and its enterprise 10th. Contact: Mayor William Boner, City of Nashville, Rm. 107, Metro Courthouse, Nashville, TN 37201.

Air Quality: The number of days of excessive carbon monoxide was reduced from 21 in 1983 to zero in 1987 and 1988. But Nashville's ozone in 1989 was still 0.14 ppm, above the NAAQS ceiling of 0.12 ppm. Contact: Paul Bontrager, Metropolitan Health Department, 311 23rd Avenue North, Nashville, TN 37203 (615) 327-9313.

Water Quality: Surface water (reservoirs) provides 100 percent of Nashville's drinking water supply. The pH of the drinking water is a good 7.5. Contact: Joseph F. Roesler, Superintendent of Laboratories, Department of Water and Sewage Services, 1600 Second Avenue North, Nashville, TN 37208 (615) 259-6597.

Weather: Nashville is cloudy and it rains often, but extremes in temperature seldom occur. There are about 70 days a year with temperatures of 32 degrees or below, and only 30 days with temperatures of 90 or above.

Average Daily Temperature (degrees F)	59.2
High	69.8
Low	48.5
Average Humidity	
Morning (percent)	84
Afternoon (percent)	57
Annual Precipitation (inches)	48.5
Average Total Snowfall (inches)	0
Ozone, Days over 0.12 ppm (one hour)	3

℞ Nashville has a strong commitment to health care, and it is relatively low in cost. No fewer than 18 hospitals serve the Nashville metro area. In numbers of beds and personnel relative to population, Nashville outranks Memphis; the two metro areas are about the same size, about 1 million population, but Nashville grew twice as fast in the 1980s.

Four Nashville hospitals are teaching facilities, two are cardiac-rehabilitation programs and one is a psychiatric facility. Contact: Dr. Frieda Wadley, Director of Health, Metropolitan Department of Health, 311 23rd Avenue North, Nashville, TN 37203 (615) 327-9313.

Health Resources per 1,000 Pop.	Number	Rank
Hospital beds, community hospitals, city	7.84	34/92
Nurses, community hospitals, city	9.62	24/90
Doctors, metro	2.72	40/113

Nashville has 37 sports facilities per 100,000 residents, ranking 74th out of 82 metro areas. The city has a number of pay-per-use facilities, including a wave-action pool, ice rink, indoor pools, a fitness center and a tennis complex. Nashville has extensive sports facilities including over 100 tennis courts, 50 baseball fields, 20 basketball courts, 15 swimming pools, 10 football/soccer fields and 7 golf courses. Other recreational facilities include 26 community centers, 43 playgrounds, 3 water slides and 1 steeplechase. Contact: Jim Fyke, Director of Parks and Recreation, Board of Parks and Recreation, Centennial Park Office, Nashville, TN 37201 (615) 259-6400.

Parkland/Total City Area (percent) 1.9

For a total of 66,000 students in the public-school system, there are 3 nurses and 35 psychologists. A part-time nurse is available in 4 percent of the schools. Students are provided with all common health-education programs and nursing assessments, and referrals. The school system provides all common screens and tests. No dental or psychiatric treatment is offered. A family life and AIDS curriculum is taught in grades K-8 and in grade 10. Two new clinics are based in schools. Contact: Department of Health, Division of School Health, 311 23rd Avenue North, Nashville, TN 37203.

New Orleans, LA

⚰️	🏊	$	🌲	℞	🏃	👫	?
✓	X	✓	✓	✓	X	✓	✓

New Orleans (Orleans County) ranks 57th of 101 metro areas in terms of age-adjusted death rate. Louisiana has high infant-mortality rates among minorities and in urban areas. Infant-mortality rates among whites are relatively low.

	Number	Rank
Age-Adjusted Death Rate	0.13	57/100
Heart Attacks	−0.16	39/100
Cancer	0.05	55/100

New Orleans' 1989 homicide rate was the highest of the 111 metro areas surveyed; its 1989 robbery rate was 7th highest, 105th out of 111. Suicides and accidental deaths are also somewhat above average.

Incidence per 1,000 Pop.	Number	Rank
Homicides (1989)	0.25	111/111
Robberies (1989)	5.50	105/111
Suicides	0.14	71/100
Accidental Deaths	0.34	60/100

$ New Orleans' 1988 metro population was 1,307,000—36th out of 113 metro areas. Its economic health at the end of 1990 was below average, ranking 60th of 113 metro areas. Its unemployment rate ranks 70th, change in unemployment 1st (like Baton Rouge, its employment increased while its labor force declined, yielding a drop in unemployment from 8.4 percent to 5.4 percent) and its enterprise 97th. Contact: Mayor Sidney Barthelemy, City of New Orleans, 1300 Perdido, New Orleans, LA 70112.

Air Quality: New Orleans did not return our air-quality questionnaire, but EPA data for 1989 indicate that the city is in compliance with all NAAQS ceilings on pollutant levels. However, it is close to the NAAQS ceilings for carbon monoxide, ozone and particulates.

Weather: The temperature is higher than the national average, at 68.2 degrees. Humidity is high as is precipitation (59.74 inches annually).

Average Daily Temperature (degrees F)	68.2
High	77.7
Low	58.7
Average Humidity	
Morning (percent)	87
Afternoon (percent)	63
Annual Precipitation (inches)	59.7
Average Total Snowfall (inches)	0.2

℞ New Orleans did not respond to the health-services survey.

Health Resources per 1,000 Pop.	Number	Rank
Hospital beds, community hospitals, city	7.91	33/92
Nurses, community hospitals, city	7.14	49/90
Doctors, metro	3.22	19/113

New Orleans has 51 sports facilities per 100,000 residents, ranking 64th out of 82 cities. Cabbageball, an adaptation of baseball, is very popular in New Orleans. Many of the Parks & Recreation Department's facilities have been improved through extensive renovations. The city's sports facilities include 71 baseball fields, 55 football fields, 29 soccer fields, 54 basketball courts, 64 tennis courts, 15 swimming pools and 9 golf courses. The city offers classes in aerobics, hiking/exploration, canoeing and sailing. Contact: Dolores T. Aaron, Director, New Orleans Recreation Department, 2400 Canal Street, Room 211, New Orleans, LA 70119.

To serve 85,000 students in the public-school system are 61 nurses, 1 medical director, 46 part-time physicians, 30 psychologists, 2 part-time psychiatrists and 64 social workers. There is a part-time nurse in all schools. An assessment of the student's medical history, along with physical examinations in the first grade, provide a basis for remediation of undiagnosed illnesses. Students are offered all essential health-education programs in grades K-12. The school system provides all common screens and tests. No medical, dental or psychiatric treatment is offered. Contact: Dr. Joseph A. Labat, Associate Director, New Orleans Public Schools, Medical and Health Services Unit, 703 Carondelet Street, New Orleans, LA 70130.

New York, NY

🪦	🗑	$	🌲	℞	🏌	👥	?
X	X	X	X	✔	X	✓	✓

The primary New York metro area, which is our focus, covers the city itself and three counties to the north of it (the five boroughs plus Putnam, Rockland and Westchester counties, the last of which includes Yonkers; Yonkers is a large city that has its own entry below). Metro

New York ranks poorly overall as a healthy city, 89th out of 100 on the age-adjusted death rate—i.e., in the bottom dozen metro areas. The major factor seems to be its high age-adjusted heart-attack rate, third highest. Its age-adjusted cancer rate escapes being in the bottom quartile. The state's infant-mortality rankings show less difference between blacks and whites (257th vs. 84th out of 301 state rankings) than between urban and rural residents (201st vs. 16th), suggesting that the problems of urban living transcend those of race.

	Number	Rank
Age-Adjusted Death Rate	1.57	89/100
Heart Attacks	1.18	98/100
Cancer	0.13	72/100

New York ranks second highest on both homicides and robberies. Yet it has the lowest suicide rate of 100 metro areas. A possible explanation is that in an environment where survival is a battle, suicide is likely to be perceived as a superfluous act of despair and failure; in other parts of the country where life is less of a daily challenge, suicide may have more honor attached to it. New York's accident rate is in the third quartile—high-rise apartments are less accident-prone than single-family homes and congested streets are less prone to fatal accidents (adjusted for population size) than less busy ones.

Incidence per 1,000 Pop.	Number	Rank
Homicides (1989)	0.23	110/111
Robberies (1989)	11.08	110/111
Suicides	0.04	1/100
Accidental Deaths	0.35	63/100

The primary *New York* metro area population was 8.6 million in 1988—2nd out of 113 metro areas, after Los Angeles. The consolidated Los Angeles metro area remains smaller in population than New York's. The consolidated New York metro area includes several metro areas in northern New Jersey (see the Jersey City, Newark and Paterson entries in this book), Long Island and Connecticut (see the Bridgeport entry in this book). The primary New York metro area's economic health at the end of 1990 was ailing, ranking 104th of 113 metro areas. Its unemployment rate ranks 96th, change in unemployment 102nd (unemployment went from 4.5 percent to 6.7 percent, as employment grew by only 0.2 percent while the labor force grew by 2.5 percent) and its enterprise 73rd.

In truth, the city was an economic loser right through the 1987–91 period. A major source of the city's prosperity in the 1980s was the financial sector, which was heavily hit by the stock market crash of October 19, 1987—as I predicted it would be in a *New York Times* Op-Ed five days after the crash ("What the Market Crash Says About New York City," p. 31). The pain on Wall Street was shared with other New York mainstays—travel and tourism, professional services, fashion, communications and entertainment. The draining of blood out of the city continued into 1991. During the summer of 1990, New York City lost 34,000 jobs, more than half in the private sector, according to the Bureau of Labor Statistics, as cited by Richard Levine, "New York Lost 34,000 Jobs Over Summer," *The New York Times*, October 19, 1990, p. B1.

The *Long Island* 1988 primary metro population (Nassau and Suffolk counties) was 2.6 million—10th out of 113 metro areas. Its economic health at the end of 1990 was good, ranking 54th of 113 metro areas. Its unemployment rate ranks 13th, change in unemployment 50th (employment fell by 4.5 percent, slightly faster than the drop in the labor force) and its enterprise 98th. Defense-procurement cuts in mid-1991 are slicing off jobs at Grumman and other defense contractors.

Air Quality: Overall, New York City's air quality seems to be improving. The Pollutant Standards Index (PSI) exceeded the 100 level on 119 days in 1980 and this was down to 35 days in 1988 and 9 in 1989. But ozone levels are defying reduction. Having dropped from a high of 29 days of exceedances in 1981 to 18 in the mid-1980s, by 1990 the figure had risen back to 28, suggesting virtually no net improvement. Carbon monoxide levels, though substantially lower than in the 1970s, are also on the rise, reflecting the growing number of cars in the city. In 1989 carbon monoxide levels reached 12 ppm, well above the NAAQS maximum of 9 ppm. Particulate levels reached 66 $\mu g/m^3$, well above the NAAQS maximum of 50 $\mu g/m^3$. The ozone problem on *Long Island* (Nassau and Suffolk Counties) is even worse; their peak ozone level in 1989 was 0.15 ppm, compared to New York's 0.13 and the NAAQS ozone maximum of 0.12 ppm.

Hazardous Waste: The Radium Chemical site is located at 600–06 27th Avenue, Woodside, Queens. No active commercial disposal sites remain in New York City, but several storage sites are used prior to shipment to commercial facilities in other parts of the state or out of state. A citywide mandatory recycling law went into effect in 1990 and is making slow headway.

Water Quality: New York has long been known for its high-quality drinking water. New development near the upstate reservoirs, which supply the New York City area, threatens the purity of the water. The city may end up having to spend several billion dollars to install filtration systems. The problems are described by Robert F. Kennedy Jr. in "New York City's Water: Down the Drain," *The New York Times*, August 22, 1989, p. A23.

Weather: With about 80 days a year during which the temperature dips to freezing or below, and only about two weeks a year of 90-degree temperatures, New York's climate is fairly mild. Proximity to the Atlantic Ocean, however, makes Gotham vulnerable to capricious storms during winter, summer and fall; hurricanes and heavy snowfalls are not unknown.

Average Daily Temperature (degrees F)	54.5
High	62.2
Low	46.9
Average Humidity	
Morning (percent)	72
Afternoon (percent)	56
Annual Precipitation (inches)	44.1
Average Total Snowfall (inches)	28.6
PSI, Days over 100, 1988	35
PSI, Days over 100, 1989	9

℞ New York's mix of health-care facilities is unmatched anywhere in the world. The city has long adhered to a compassionate but costly policy of providing medical care to all who need it, regardless of their ability to pay. The Federal, state and city governments combined pay more than 55 percent of the costs of the city's voluntary hospitals and cover nearly 90 percent of costs in over a dozen municipal hospitals. In addition to supporting the hospital system, the city contributes 23 percent of all Medicaid services for low-income people—a very high share, unmatched by any city or county outside of New York State. The quality of specialized health care in New York is broadly considered the highest in the nation, but, unfortunately, is also the nation's most expensive.

We did not receive a response to our health-services survey from the New York City Department of Health.

Health Resources per 1,000 Pop.	Number	Rank
Hospital beds, community hospitals, city	4.70	72/92
Nurses, community hospitals, city	4.93	71/90
Doctors, metro	3.99	9/113

New York City has only 19 sports facilities per 100,000 residents, ranking it on the bottom (82nd out of 82 cities). New York City has 366 baseball fields, 46 football/soccer fields, 444 basketball courts, 532 tennis courts, 12 golf courses, 25 running tracks, 34 swimming pools, 6 beaches and 3 marinas. Triathlons and biathlons at the beaches, in Central Park and other sites are especially popular. The city has recently refurbished citywide track facilities, highlighted by Downing Stadium, which has a fully equipped track and field facility. The city also boasts 100 boccie courts.

Parkland/Total City Area (percent)   13

Despite efforts to obtain information from the Board of Education and Department of Health, the author was unable to elicit a response to the School Health portion of the survey. However, from earlier research done under the author's direction (*Public School Health Programs in 35 U.S. Cities: No Standards, No Systems*) published by the Council on Municipal Performance, 1979), it may be said that as of the mid-1970s New York City's preventive-health programs in its elementary schools were extensive—not as extensive as its upstate sisters Buffalo and Rochester, but ahead of nearby cities like Newark (which has since then greatly strengthened its school-health program; see below under Newark). Its detection and follow-up procedures were very extensive. New York City's school-health programs are administered jointly by the Board of Education and the Department of Health. Unfortunately these programs were mentioned as places that beleaguered Mayor David Dinkins' ax might fall during the summer of 1991.

DISTRIBUTION OF MORTALITY BY BOROUGHS

New York City is unique among American cities in that it consists of more than one county. Its five counties ("boroughs") are Manhattan, Brooklyn, the Bronx, Queens and Staten Island. As already mentioned, the New York primary metro area includes, in addition to the City, three counties to the north: Putnam, Rockland and Westchester. The other counties that are added to make up the consolidated metro area are, to the east, Nassau and Suffolk counties, N.Y. (i.e., Long Island); Bergen, Essex, Morris, Passaic, Somerset and Union Counties, N.J.; and the Town of Fairfield in Connecticut (a Connecticut town is equivalent to a county in non-New England states).

The information below shows as wide a variability in health patterns within New York City as occurs nationwide. New York City has the best and worst of facilities. It has some of the safest neighborhoods and some of the most dangerous. Your health in New York City depends a lot on where, when and how you spend your time.

Brooklyn: Kings County. Population 2.3 million (December 1988), down from 2.4 million in the mid-1970s; 223 doctors and 634 hospital beds per 100,000 residents. The age-adjusted death rate (1980) is 6.7, a tiny bit better than the Bronx, but worse than the other three boroughs.

The Bronx: Population 1.2 million (December 1988); 225 doctors and 610 hospital beds per 100,000 residents. The age-adjusted death rate of 6.8 is the worst of the five New York City boroughs. It is interesting to note that the poor neighborhoods in the Bronx have *lower* mortality rates for heart disease. For example, in the three wealthiest neighborhoods in the Bronx, the 1986 death rates from heart disease are 479,469 and 444 per 100,000 population; in the three poorer neighborhoods, the rates are 269, 231 and 182.

Why should people die in larger numbers if they are wealthier? Answer: For the same reason that some very poor cities in India have the lowest cancer mortality rates in the world—people die of other diseases before they are old enough to get cancer (in India) or heart disease (in New York). In the Bronx, the poor areas have a staggeringly high incidence of homicide, suicide (one-fifth the rate of homicide, whereas nationwide the suicide rate is higher than the homicide rate) and deaths related to cirrhosis of the liver, drugs and AIDS (increasingly, AIDS in poorer areas is related to drug use as much as homosexual activity) and "injuries of undetermined cause."

The affluent neighborhoods in the Bronx have matching health indicators. Fordham-Riverside has a low age-adjusted death rate of 6.0; a low 1986 AIDS death rate of 25.1 per 100,000 population, a low drug-dependence death rate of 8.5; a fairly low homicide rate of 26.8. Morrisania's age-adjusted death rate is high, 8.8. Its AIDS death rate is a high 61.0; its drug-dependence death rate is a high 21.6; its homicide rate a high 45.4. Similarly, Mott Haven has a high age-adjusted death rate of 7.9 and AIDS death rate of 52.4; a drug-dependence death rate of 23.4; a homicide rate of 54.8. Pelham Bay has the lowest age-adjusted death rate of all the neighborhoods in the Bronx, 5.0; the second lowest AIDS death rate of 23.7; by far the lowest drug-dependence death rate of 3.6; and by far the lowest homicide rate of 14.6. Tremont has a high age-adjusted death rate of 8.0; a high AIDS death rate of 57.2; a high drug-dependence death rate of 20.8; a high homicide rate of 53.3. Westchester has a low age-adjusted death rate of 6.3; a low AIDS death rate of 20.7; a low drug-dependence death rate of 9.2; a fairly low homicide rate of 21.9.

Manhattan: New York County. Population 1.5 million (Dec. 1988), up from 1.4 million in the mid-1970s; 846 doctors and 1,710 hospital beds per 100,000 residents. Age-adjusted death rate is 6.6, slightly better than

Brooklyn. See Table 9-1 for health district data on death rates. Exclamation marks in the table below are the author's.

The death rate for black men in Harlem is higher than that of Bangladesh (see Chapter 1 for other foreign death rates). Harlem has a death rate twice the national average for whites and 50 percent higher than the national average for blacks.

Queens: Population 2.0 million, unchanged since the mid-1970s; 201 doctors and 387 hospital beds per 100,000 residents. Age-adjusted death rate is 5.6, far better than the other boroughs.

Staten Island: Richmond County. Population 385,000, up from 325,000 in the mid-1970s; 188 doctors and 706 hospital beds per 100,000 residents. Its age-adjusted death rate is 6.0, second only to Queens among the five boroughs.

TABLE 9–1
MANHATTAN HEALTH DISTRICT DEATH RATES

	Death Rates per 100,000 Pop.				
	Age-Adjusted	Heart Disease	AIDS	Drugs	Homicide
Central Harlem	12.2	482	84.4	42.6	66.4!
East Harlem	7.9	338	66.5	20.8	36.9
Kips Bay-Yorkville	4.6	352	36.7	2.2!	3.0!
Lower East Side	6.7	345	80.6	15.7	17.4
Lower West Side (Clinton-Vill.)	6.2	363	138.6!	6.6	14.0
Riverside (West Side)	6.3	202	71.6	11.1	15.5
Washington Heights	6.2	309	28.1	9.9	39.3

DISTRIBUTION OF MORTALITY BY COMMUNITY DISTRICTS

New York City is divided up for administrative and land-use planning purposes into 59 community districts, each one of which has a district manager, who reports to the Community Board, which in turn is composed of people who are appointed jointly by the elected Council Members and Borough President. Table 9-2 shows the mortality rates for each community district when AIDS deaths are subtracted from total deaths. Borough Park, Brooklyn, has the lowest age-adjusted death rate, followed by

TABLE 9–2
COMMUNITY DISTRICT DEATH RATES

	Community District	AIDS-Adjusted Death Rate*	Age-Adjusted Residual		Community District	AIDS-Adjusted Death Rate*	Age-Adjusted Residual
1 B12	Borough Park	8.6	-2.72	31 B5	East New York	8.1	-0.17
2 M2	Greenwich Village	6.0	-2.17	32 B6	Park Slope/Red Hook	8.4	-0.13
3 Q1	Astoria/LIC	7.9	-1.85	33 B18	Canarsie	8.9	-0.10
4 Q9	Woodhaven Richmond Hill	8.7	-1.78	34 Q4	Elmhurst/Corona	6.6	-0.09
5 Q13	Queensville/Laurelton	6.3	-1.64	35 S1	St. George	9.4	0.09
6 B4	Bushwick	6.8	-1.58	36 B11	Bensonhurst	11.0	0.18
7 M12	Washington Heights	8.3	-1.56	37 Q5	Ridgewood/Glendale	10.9	0.25
8 Q11	Bayside/Douglaston	7.6	-1.55	38 Bx8	Riverdale	11.6	0.28
9 B14	Flatbush/Midwood	8.8	-1.55	39 Bx12	Williamsbridge	9.8	0.34
10 Bx5	Morris Heights/Mt. Hope	5.8	-1.50	40 M9	Manhattanville	9.5	0.39
11 S2	Willowbrook	6.6	-1.47	41 Bx2	Hunts Point/Longwood	8.3	0.53
12 Q3	Jackson Heights	8.0	-1.44	42 Bx1	Melrose/Mott Haven	8.7	0.54
13 Q8	Pomonok/Jamaica Hills	8.9	-1.43	43 Bx4	Concourse/Highbridge	8.4	0.57
14 Q2	Sunnyside/Woodside	8.6	-1.35	44 B9	East Flatbush	7.6	0.68
15 Bx7	Fordham/Bedford Park	10.2	-1.34	45 B10	Bay Ridge	12.2	1.04
16 B7	Windsor Terr./Sunset Pk.	8.3	-1.30	46 B15	Sheepshead Bay	11.9	1.05

17 M4	Chelsea & Clinton	8.1	−1.25
18 M8	Upper East Side	7.7	−1.12
19 B1	Greenpoint/Williamsburg	8.2	−1.07
20 Q6	Rego Pk./Forest Hills	10.1	−1.06
21 B17	Rugby/Farragut	5.8	−0.92
22 Bx6	Belmont/E. Tremont	8.1	−0.66
23 M6	Murray Hill/Tudor City	8.2	−0.60
24 Bx9	Parkchester/Soundview	8.7	−0.55
25 M7	Upper West Side	8.2	−0.55
26 M5	Midtown	8.6	−0.55
27 Q10	Ozone Park/Howard Beach	8.4	−0.41
28 Q7	Flushing	9.3	−0.35
29 M1	Tribeca, Soho	6.2	−0.27
30 M3	Lower East Side	9.0	−0.24
47 B2	Bklyn. Heights/Ft. Greene	8.9	1.21
48 M11	East Harlem	10.1	1.27
49 Q12	Jamaica/Hollis	9.7	1.29
50 Bx3	Morrisania/Claremont	10.0	1.41
51 Bx10	Coop City/Throgs Neck	11.8	1.61
52 B16	Brownsville	10.0	1.97
53 B8	Crown Heights	9.7	1.97
54 B13	Coney Island/Brighton	14.3	2.12
55 Q14	Rockaways	14.4	2.64
56 Bx11	Pelham Bay	14.3	2.72
57 S3	Great Kills	9.2	2.73
58 B3	Bedford-Stuyvesant	11.2	3.08
59 M10	Central Harlem	16.2	6.37

* AIDS-related deaths are subtracted from total deaths to obtain a picture of how healthy each Community District is, independent of the incidence of AIDS. The AIDS death rate is shown in the next table, Table 9-3.

SOURCES: Information on Community Districts from New York City Department of City Planning, *Community District Statistics*, 1984. Death rates by Community District from the Bureau of Health Statistics and Analysis, City of New York, *New York City Community District Vital Statistics Data Book*, 1988. (For this table the following adjustments were made to the data: To allow for a general comparison of all NYC Community Boards we first eliminated AIDS deaths from our data, and show them separately in Table 9-3. The remaining death rate was used as the dependent variable in a linear multiple regression with median age and the percentage of the population over 60 years old as independent variables. The regression yielded an R-squared of almost 45 percent. The remaining unexplained variance in city-wide death rates is shown in the residual column in Table 9-1. This can be interpreted as an indicator of the relative healthiness of the neighborhoods that were compared.)

Greenwich Village. Central Harlem and Bedford-Stuyvesant have the highest age-adjusted death rate. For the method of calculating these death rates, see the notes to Table 1-1 in Chapter 1.

DISTRIBUTION OF AIDS-RELATED DEATHS
BY COMMUNITY DISTRICT

The AIDS-related deaths omitted from Table 9-2 are shown in Table 9-3. The lowest AIDS rate is in Bayside/Douglaston, Community District 11 in Queens, 10 per 100,000 residents (8 males, 2 females per 100,000 residents), followed by Willowbrook, Community District 2 in Staten Island, with 11 per 100,000.

At the other end of the spectrum, Chelsea-Clinton, Manhattan Community Board 4, has the highest AIDS death rate in New York City—an incredibly high 412 AIDS deaths per 100,000 population (4 per thousand residents), followed by Greenwich Village, Community District 2 in Manhattan, with 376 AIDS deaths per 100,000. More people die each year of AIDS in Chelsea-Clinton than die from all causes in Anchorage. Among men in Chelsea-Clinton, the death rate from AIDS is over twice the death rate for all residents in Anchorage.

NEW YORK CITY'S SUBURBAN AREAS

For those who want to work in Manhattan but not to live there, a wide range of suburban communities will be glad—eager, given the 1991 real-estate market—to offer you a home. If you work in Manhattan and will have to travel at rush hours, take the stress test of using the relevant transportation system(s) at peak hours before you make any irrevocable decisions.

Upstate and Out-Island Suburban Areas. The New York primary metro area includes, in addition to the city, three counties to the north: Putnam, Rockland and Westchester counties.

Nassau and Suffolk counties in New York make up the second-largest primary metro area in Greater New York. The two-county area to the east of New York City makes up the rest of Long Island (Queens and Brooklyn take up the western tip of the island).

New Jersey Suburban Areas. The City of Newark is located in Essex County. The Newark primary metro area includes suburban Morris, Somerset and Union Counties, N.J. See entry under Newark.

Bergen-Passaic, N.J.: These neighboring northernmost metro area New Jersey counties include the large city of Paterson. See entry under Paterson.

Middlesex-Hunterdon, N.J. includes the two noncontiguous (separated by Somerset) suburban counties of Middlesex (major city: New Brunswick) and Hunterdon (major city: Flemington). The other two counties are Hudson County, N.J. (see entry under Jersey City) and Orange County, N.Y.

Connecticut Suburban Areas. The Town of Fairfield (equivalent to a county) includes four primary metro areas: Bridgeport-Milford, the northeastern end of the Town of Fairfield; Stamford, the southwestern end of the Town of Fairfield; Danbury, the northern end of the Town of Fairfield and Norwalk, the middle of the southern end of the Town of Fairfield. See entry under Bridgeport.

IS NEW YORK CITY HEALTHY?

The good quality in 1991 of New York City's water, its high standards of health care for most of the population, coupled with the sprawling metro area's prime if often inconvenient or costly recreational facilities, low-to-moderate air pollution and relatively low mortality rates in most neighborhoods suggest that for those willing to make the effort, New York City and its suburban areas can provide a surprisingly healthy environment. Within the city itself, some neighborhoods are quiet and peaceful. Indeed, for the affluent individual and family, the greatest risk may well be work-related stress; the big city is stimulating and the bonus-and-commission incentives and pressures driving the city's producers can be over-stimulating on the job. The fact is, New York has an extremely high incidence of stress-related diseases—in contrast, for example, to Washington, D.C., where the IRS collects the taxes and workers are mostly on salary—and relatively few people die of stress-related diseases. The reason for New York's low ranking on overall mortality is its large population of poor people in poor neighborhoods. The poor bear not only the burden of higher death rates from drugs and homicides, they also suffer more than wealthier neighborhoods from stress-related diseases. Only AIDS, a major killer in New York, strikes its (mostly young and male) victims with relatively equal force, both rich and poor.

TABLE 9–3
NEIGHBORHOOD AIDS DEATHS

	Community Board	AIDS Deaths per 100,000 pop. Males	Females		Community Board	AIDS Deaths per 100,000 pop. Males	Females
1 Q11	Bayside/Douglaston	8	2	31 B9	East Flatbush	65	19
2 S2	Willowbrook	11	0	32 B1	Greenpoint/Williamsburg	78	19
3 S3	Great Kills	14	6	33 Bx7	Fordham/Bedford Park	79	19
4 B10	Bay Ridge	19	3	34 B5	East New York	85	18
5 Q7	Flushing	23	4	35 B7	Windsor Terr./Sunset Pk.	94	15
6 Q8	Pomonok/Jamaica Hills	19	11	36 Q12	Jamaica/Hollis	96	20
7 B15	Sheepshead Bay	27	3	37 B6	Park Slope/Red Hook	106	17
8 Q6	Rego Pk./Forest Hills	34	0	38 M1	Tribeca, Soho	110	15
9 B12	Borough Park	31	4	39 Bx9	Parkchester/Soundview	99	26
10 B18	Canarsie	29	9	40 M9	Manhattanville	112	26
11 Q5	Ridgewood/Glendale	39	5	41 Bx6	Belmont/E. Tremont	114	32
12 Q9	Woodhaven/Richmond Hill	41	4	42 B4	Bushwick	116	31
13 Bx8	Riverdale	40	6	43 B2	Bklyn. Heights/Ft. Greene	147	21

Rank	District	Neighborhood		
14	Q13	Queensville/Laurelton	32	16
15	B11	Bensonhurst	42	7
16	Bx10	Coop City/Throgs Neck	41	9
17	B13	Coney Island/Brighton	49	6
18	S1	St. George	41	15
19	Bx11	Pelham Bay	49	9
20	Q14	Rockaways	47	14
21	Q10	Ozone Park/Howard Beach	40	22
22	M12	Washington Heights	58	4
23	Q4	Elmhurst/Corona	54	10
24	Q1	Astoria/LIC	55	11
25	B14	Flatbush/Midwood	60	10
26	Bx12	Williamsbridge	57	13
27	M8	Upper East Side	70	1
28	B17	Rugby/Farragut	54	18
29	Q3	Jackson Heights	73	2
30	Q2	Sunnyside/Woodside	73	11
44	Bx5	Morris Heights/Mt. Hope	137	33
45	B8	Crown Heights	156	28
46	Bx2	Hunts Point/Longwood	125	71
47	M6	Murray Hill/Tudor City	190	7
48	Bx3	Morrisania/Claremont	159	40
49	M7	Upper West Side	188	11
50	Bx1	Melrose/Mott Haven	152	49
51	Bx4	Concourse/Highbridge	161	41
52	B3	Bedford Stuyvesant	153	56
53	B16	Brownsville	136	75
54	M11	East Harlem	176	49
55	M3	Lower East Side	194	38
56	M5	Midtown	213	21
57	M10	Central Harlem	196	55
58	M2	Greenwich Village	371	5
59	M4	Chelsea & Clinton	404	18

SOURCE: The neighborhoods were ranked according to *total* AIDS deaths per 100,000 residents.

SOURCE: Bureau of Health Statistics and Analysis, City of New York, *New York City Community District Vital Statistics Data Book*, 1988.

Newark, NJ

🪦	🏃	$	🌲	℞	🏃	👫	?
X	✓	X	✓	✓	?	✔	✓

Newark (Essex County) gets bottom rankings for its age-adjusted death, heart attack and cancer rates. Cities like Newark and Trenton account for the high statewide black infant-mortality rate, 273rd out of 301 metro areas, and starkly contrasts with the very low figure for whites. Contact: Denise Clark, Epidemiologist, Department of Health and Human Services, 110 William Street, Newark, NJ 07102.

	Number	Rank
Age-Adjusted Death Rate	2.71	97/100
Heart Attacks	0.97	96/100
Cancer	0.70	95/100

Newark's homicide rate is higher than average, 69th out of 111 metro areas, while its suicide rate is among the country's lowest. But the city's robbery rate puts it near-bottom, 107th of 111.

Incidence per 1,000 Pop.	Number	Rank
Homicides (1989)	0.10	69/111
Robberies (1989)	5.52	107/111
Suicides	0.08	8/100
Accidental Deaths	0.32	41/100

Newark's 1988 metro population was 1,886,000—22nd out of 113 metro areas. Its economic health at the end of 1990 was poor, ranking 86th of 113 metro areas. Its unemployment rate ranks 64th, change in unemployment 97th (the labor force grew by 3.8 percent, nearly twice the rate of growth of employment) and its enterprise 52nd. Contact: Mayor Sharpe James, City of Newark, 920 Broad Street, Newark, NJ 07102.

Air Quality: Maximum lead concentrations in Newark in 1988 were 55 percent of the NAAQS, down from 60 percent in 1987; maximum ozone concentrations were 174 percent of the NAAQS, down from 199 percent in 1987. Newark's air quality complied with all NAAQS maxima in 1989 except for ozone, which reached 0.13 ppm, above the NAAQS maximum. Contact: Joseph P. McGinley, Director, Division of Environmental Health, 94 William Street, Newark, NJ 07102 (201) 733-3719.

Hazardous Waste: In 1991, Newark's Mayor Sharpe James received the EPA's Administrator's Award for local government. The award recognizes the city's recycling program as the best sponsored by an American municipality. The program has several innovative aspects which include requiring the recycling of ozone-depleting compounds, deputizing youth as special recycling assistants to the Mayor, and "precycling" by purchasing recycled and recyclable goods. Contact: Frank Sudol, 201-733-4356.

Water Quality: Newark's entire water supply comes from surface water. A $44.5-million water filtration plant came on line in 1990. Contact: Daniel Berardinelli, Manager, Division of Water/Sewer Utility, 1294 McBride Avenue, Little Falls, NJ 07424; 201-256-4965.

Weather: Newark's temperature is close to the national average. Precipitation is above average at 42.3 inches annually.

Average Daily Temperature (degrees F)	54.2
High	62.5
Low	45.9
Average Humidity	
Morning (percent)	73
Afternoon (percent)	54
Annual Precipitation	42.3
Average Total Snowfall (inches)	28.0

 Newark did not respond to the health-services survey.

Health Resources per 1,000 Pop.	Number	Rank
Hospital beds, community hospitals, city	7.01	43/92
Nurses, community hospitals, city	7.93	39/90
Doctors, metro	2.97	26/113

 Newark did not respond to the recreational-facilities survey.

Newark has a total of 48,451 students in its public-school system. Employed by the school system are 100 nurses, 20 physicians, 42 psychologists, 2 psychiatrists, 70 social workers, 42 learning consultants, and 1 cardiac consultant. Nurses are present full-time in all schools. Nurses in Newark's public schools work in conjunction with crisis centers for assistance in helping with problems such as suicide, drugs and emotionally disturbed children. Children entering Newark public schools for the first time are assessed by the school nurse prior to admission. Children lacking immunization have a comprehensive follow-up. The schools provide all essential health-education programs to grades K-12. In response to the AIDS crisis, Newark public schools have recently included an AIDS admissibility policy, handling of bodily fluids policy, an upgrade in the health-education curriculum to include AIDS education and an upgrade of the immunization policy. The school system provides all common screens and tests except immunization and mental-health exams. No dental or psychiatric treatment is offered. First Aid and dental treatment are provided for students. Contact: Theresa Garcin, Assistant Director, Division of Health Education and Service, 2 Cedar Street, Newark, NJ 07102 (201) 733-7150.

Newport News, VA

⚰RIP	✈	$	⬆	℞	🖼	👥	?
X	✓	✔	✓	X	✔	X	✓

Cities in Virginia are not part of the surrounding counties; they are independent entities. Metro area includes Norfolk and Virginia Beach. Newport News ranks a high 75th in the age-adjusted mortality rate. Infant-mortality rates in Virginia are high among minorities and low among whites. Infant-mortality rates are much higher in cities than in rural areas of the state. Contact: Dr. Daniel C. Warren, Health Director, Newport News Health Department, 416 J. Clyde Morris Boulevard, Newport News, VA 23606 (804) 594-7305.

	Number	Rank
Age-Adjusted Death Rate	0.70	75/100
Heart Attacks	0.17	68/100
Cancer	0.27	83/100

Newport News had a higher-than-average 1989 homicide ranking, 74th out of 111, but a slightly lower-than-average robbery rank, 50th. The city's accident and suicide ratings were also middling.

Incidence per 1,000 Pop.	Number	Rank
Homicides (1989)	0.10	74/111
Robberies (1989)	1.86	50/111
Suicides	0.13	55/100
Accidental Deaths	0.32	42/100

$\boxed{\$}$ Since Newport News is part of the same primary metro area as Norfolk and Virginia Beach, its economic-health rating is the same. Contact: Mayor Jessie M. Rattlery, City of Newport News, 2400 Washington Avenue, Newport News, VA 23607.

$\boxed{\spadesuit}$ **Air Quality:** In 1989–90 ozone has increased on the peninsula where Newport News is located. As of 1989, EPA data indicate that the Norfolk-Virginia Beach-Newport News metro area had an ozone level of 0.10, which was within NAAQS limits. Contact: Charles C. Allen, Deputy Director of Planning, Department of Planning and Development, 2400 Washington Avenue, Newport News, VA 23607 (804) 247-8728.

Hazardous Waste: Yorktown Power Plant, located in the Chrisman Creek drainage basin in York County, has contaminated surface and ground water with coal residue and refinery residue from ash pits. Newport News is not in this drainage basin. EPA-defined hazardous wastes are not accepted at the Newport News landfill, while household hazardous wastes are. Contact: Charles C. Allen, Deputy Director of Planning, Department of Planning and Development, 2400 Washington Avenue, Newport News, VA 23607.

Water Quality: All of Newport News' water supply comes from surface water sources. Newport News has had successful control of trihalomethanes in recent years. Elevated phosphorus levels in the distribution system correlate with lake turnover rate. The pH of the drinking water was a good 7.2 in 1988. Contact: Charles C. Allen, Deputy Director of Planning, Department of Planning and Development, 2400 Washington Avenue, Newport News, VA 23607.

Weather: The average daily temperature is about average at 59.5. Precipitation is high at 45.2 inches annually.

Average Daily Temperature (degrees F)	59.5
High	68.2
Low	50.7
Average Humidity	
Morning (percent)	78
Afternoon (percent)	57
Annual Precipitation (inches)	45.2
Average Total Snowfall (inches)	7.5
Ozone, Days over 0.12 ppm (1 hour, 1988)	2

$\boxed{\text{R}}$ Newport News did not respond to the health-services survey. But since it is part of the Norfolk-Virginia Beach metro area, we can comment on the fact that it is poorly supplied with physicians, i.e., in the bottom third of the metro areas.

Health Resources per 1,000 Pop.	Number	Rank
Doctors, metro	1.91	88/113

Newport News has 123 sports facilities per 100,000 residents, giving the city a good stance in that department (17 out of 82 cities). Sports Facilities in the city include 91 indoor and outdoor basketball courts, 48 free outdoor tennis courts, 44 baseball fields, 14 football/soccer fields, 6 running tracks and 2 golf courses. Water facilities include 3 beaches and 1 marina with boat-ramps, fishing piers and canoe and boat rentals. Tennis and softball are the most popular sports in Newport News. Also common are basketball, soccer, volleyball and football leagues. Contact: Ronald Burroughs, Director of Parks and Recreation, City of Newport News, 2400 Washington Avenue, Newport News, VA 23607; 804-247-8451.

Parkland/Total City Area (percent)   13.7

Recently Newport News has implemented a Family Life curriculum for grades K-10. Also added are substance abuse counseling services and Elementary School guidance counselors. A policy statement has been issued for employees and students concerning contagious and infectious disease. All major health-education programs are offered to students in grades K-10. The school system provides all common screens and tests except immunizations and well-child physical exams. No medical, dental or psychiatric treatment is provided for students. Contact: Donald S. Bruno, School Superintendent, Newport News Public Schools, 12465 Warwick Blvd., Newport News, VA 23606 (804) 599-8606.

Norfolk, VA

RIP	⛏	$	♠	℞	🏃	👪	?
X	✓	✔	✔	X	?	✔	✓

Cities in Virginia are not within counties; they are independent entities. Norfolk ranks a high 83rd in the age-adjusted mortality rate. Infant-mortality rates in Virginia are high among minorities and low among whites. Infant-mortality rates are much higher in cities than in rural areas of the state.

	Number	**Rank**
Age-Adjusted Death Rate	0.27	83/100
Heart Attacks	0.17	68/100
Cancer	0.27	83/100

Norfolk's crime, accident and suicide statistics put it solidly in the middle of cities surveyed. But its homicide rate is on the edge of being in the bottom third of cities.

Incidence per 1,000 Pop.	**Number**	**Rank**
Homicides (1989)	0.10	74/111
Robberies (1989)	1.86	50/111
Suicides	0.13	55/100
Accidental Deaths	0.32	42/100

Norfolk-Virginia Beach's 1988 metro population was 1,380,000— 33rd out of 113 metro areas. Its economic health at the end of 1990 was excellent, ranking 8th of 113 metro areas. Its unemployment rate ranks 31st, change in unemployment 22nd (employment grew by 2.9 percent, faster than the labor force, 2.3 percent) and its enterprise 20th. Contact: Mayor Joseph A. Leafe, City of Norfolk, Norfolk, VA 23508.

Water Quality: Norfolk's water supply comes from surface water. If the data for neighboring Newport News are any indication, the water is excellent. Contact: Vernon Land, Water Quality Manager, Utilities Department, City of Norfolk, 6040 Waterworks Road, Norfolk, VA 23502.

Weather: The average daily temperature is about average at 59.5. Precipitation is high at 45.22 inches annually.

Average Daily Temperature (degrees F)	59.5
High	68.2
Low	50.7
Average Humidity	
Morning (percent)	78
Afternoon (percent)	57
Annual Precipitation (inches)	45.2
Average Total Snowfall (inches)	7.5

Norfolk is well equipped with public health-education programs and emergency hotlines in all common areas. The city provides all common preventive-health and treatment programs. New programs sponsored by the city include a Healthy Mothers/Healthy Babies Campaign to fight infant mortality, AIDS Awareness Campaign focusing on minority education and City Wellness Program addressing health in the city work force. In addition, the Medical College of Hampton Roads provides primary care in free clinics two evenings per week. Contact: Valerie Stallings, M.D., Public Health Director, Department of Public Health, City of Norfolk, 401 Colley Avenue, Norfolk, VA 23507.

Health Resources per 1,000 Pop.	Number	Rank
Hospitals, community hospitals, city	7.75	35/92
Nurses, community hospitals, city	9.47	25/90
Doctors, metro	1.91	88/113

Norfolk did not respond to the recreational-services survey.

 Norfolk's 37,000 public school students are served by 42 registered nurses, 41 nursing aides, 6 nurse supervisors, 1 nurse manager and 1 pediatrician that are employed by the Norfolk Department of Public Health. The public-school system employs 22 psychologists. Nurses are present full-time in 30 percent of the schools and part-time in 70 percent. All of the schools covered part-time by a nurse are also covered full-time by a nursing aide. In addition, one high school has a health center in which the Department of Public Health provides comprehensive clinical services to students enrolled in the center. Students are provided with medical, dental and mental health screenings and referrals as appropriate. All common health-education programs are offered in grades K-12, including a course on family life. The school system provides all common screens and tests. Contact: Ms. Joyce Bollard, PHN, BSN, Assistant Director of Nursing, Department of Public Health, School and Field Nursing Branch, 401 Colley Avenue, Norfolk, VA 23507.

Oakland, CA

RIP	🏆	$	🌲	℞	🏃	👫	?
✔	✗	✓	✓	✓	?	✓	✓

Oakland (Alameda County) is considered part of the San Francisco metro area, so its age-adjusted death rate, cancer and heart attack statistics get factored in with San Francisco's. That may partly explain the high rankings in those areas. The metro area ranks 27th in the age-adjusted mortality rate. Infant-mortality rates for California are high among blacks and relatively low among whites. Infant-mortality rates are higher in cities than in rural areas of the state.

	Number	Rank
Age-Adjusted Death Rate	−0.98	27/100
Heart Attacks	−0.53	15/100
Cancer	−0.17	29/100

 Oakland has high rates of homicides, robberies and suicides.

Incidence per 1,000 Pop.	Number	Rank
Homicides (1989; Oakland only)	0.12	87/111
Robberies (1989; Oakland only)	3.20	87/111
Suicides	0.15	80/100
Accidental deaths	0.35	65/100

$ Oakland's 1988 metro population was 2.01 million—20th out of 113 metro areas. Its economic health at the end of 1990 was fairly good, ranking 49th of 113 metro areas. Its unemployment rate ranks 40th, change in unemployment 56th (the labor force increased faster than employment) and its enterprise 55th. Contact: Mayor Lionel J. Wilson, City of Oakland, 1 City Hall Plaza, Oakland, CA 94612.

↑ Air Quality: Air quality in Oakland has been good throughout the 1980s. Ozone excesses reported in the Oakland-San Francisco Metro Area are in the outlying suburbs to the south and east, and they have also decreased in the latter half of the 1980s. Contact: Ted McHugh, Director of Public Information, Bay Area Air Quality Management Control Board, 939 Ellis Street, San Francisco, CA 94109 (415) 771-6000.

Hazardous Waste: There are no hazardous-waste sites in Alameda County on the EPA's Superfund list. The county has proposed construction of three hazardous-household-waste transfer stations. Contact: Hazardous Materials Management Program, Alameda County Health, 80 Swan Way, Oakland, CA 94612 (415) 271-4320.

Water Quality: Treated-water turbidity was extremely low in 1989, far below recently tightened drinking water standards because the water-treatment process was upgraded during the decade. All of the city's drinking water comes from surface water sources. The pH of the drinking water is a high 9. Contact: Jerome Gilbert, Executive Director, East Bay Municipal Utility District (EBMUD), 2130 Adeline Street, Oakland, CA 94612 (415) 835-3000.

Weather: The average daily temperature is about average at 56.7. Humidity is high, while precipitation is low at 19.33 inches annually.

Average Daily Temperature (degrees F)	56.7
High	62.5
Low	51.0
Average Humidity	
Morning (percent)	85
Afternoon (percent)	66
Annual Precipitation (inches)	19.3
Average Total Snowfall (inches)	Trace
Ozone, Days over 0.12 ppm (1 hour, 1988)	0

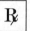 Oakland did not respond to the author's health-services survey.

Health Resources per 1,000 Pop.	Number	Rank
Hospitals	3.77	83/92
Nurses, community hospitals, city	4.65	76/90
Doctors, metro	2.59	48/113

 Oakland did not respond to the author's recreational-services survey.

The Oakland public-school system employs 38 nurses, 40 psychologists and 6 health assistants for its 51,000 students. The nurses are present on a full-time basis in some of the schools and on a part-time basis in the other schools. All common health-education programs are offered to grades K-12, including courses on self-esteem and community living. The school system is developing a comprehensive health and safety program that will focus on the needs of all students more systematically. The school system provides all common screens and tests except immunization, mental-health exams and well-child physical exams. No medical, dental or psychiatric treatment is provided for students. Alfreda Abbot, President, Oakland Public Schools Board of Education, 1025 2nd Avenue, Oakland, CA 94606 (415) 836-8402.

Oklahoma City, OK

⌂ RIP	↗	$	↟	℞	[人]	👥	?
✔	✓	X	✓	✓	X	X	✔

 If healthiness were the only issue and earning a living was not a criterion, then Oklahoma City looks good—the city ranks 29th in the age-adjusted mortality rate. Cancer and heart attack rates are below average. The problem is that the city has tied its economic fate to two industries that are fickle—farming and petroleum. Infant-mortality rates for Oklahoma are high among blacks, lower among whites and other minorities, and they are higher in cities than in rural areas of the state.

	Number	Rank
Age-Adjusted Death Rate	−0.92	29/100
Heart Attacks	−0.30	30/100
Cancer	−0.23	24/100

Oklahoma City has average rates of homicides, robberies, suicides and accidental deaths.

Incidence per 1,000 Pop.	Number	Rank
Homicides (1989)	0.08	56/111
Robberies (1989)	2.04	57/111
Suicides	0.12	48/100
Accidental Deaths	0.32	47/100

$ Oklahoma City's 1988 metro population was 964,000—49th out of 113 metro areas. Its economic health at the end of 1990 was poor. It ranks 107th of 113 metro areas. Its unemployment rate ranks 84th, change in unemployment 91st (labor force grew 3.3 percent, employment 1.7 percent) and its enterprise 105th. Contact: Mayor Ronald Norick, Oklahoma City, 200 North Walker, Oklahoma City, OK 73102.

Air Quality: Overall, a modest decrease in all criteria pollutants has been observed during the latter half of the 1980s. All pollutants were below NAAQS ceilings. Contact: Director of Environmental Air Quality Control, Department of Public Works, Oklahoma City Hall, Oklahoma City, OK 73102.

Water Quality: All of the city's drinking water is provided by surface water except 0.1 percent that is provided by ground water. The pH of the drinking water is 10.3, highest of all the cities for which we have this information. In the 1985–90 period trihalomethanes in the water supply have been reduced. The city has a high relative level of chlorine residue (1.9 mg/l). Contact: City of Oklahoma City, Water and Wastewater Utilities Department, 100 North Walker, 4th Floor, Oklahoma City, OK 73102.

Weather: Winters are mild and summers long and hot. Average precipitation is high.

Average Daily Temperature (degrees F)	59.9
High	71.2
Low	48.6
Average Humidity	
Morning (percent)	79
Afternoon (percent)	54
Annual Precipitation (inches)	30.9
Average Total Snowfall (inches)	9.3
Ozone, Days over 0.12 ppm (1 hour, 1988)	0

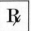 Oklahoma City did not respond to the author's health-services survey.

Health Resources per 1,000 Pop.	Number	Rank
Hospital beds, community hospitals, city	7.39	40/92
Nurses, community hospitals, city	8.51	37/90
Doctors, metro	2.41	61/113

Oklahoma City has 64 sports facilities per 100,000 residents, ranking 55th out of 82 metro areas. The summer of 1990 marked the third season that the City Parks and Recreation Department worked with Oklahoma County to open eight public swimming pools that would have otherwise remained closed due to budget cuts. Softball leagues are very popular in the city, along with basketball and volleyball. The city's sports facilities include 165 baseball fields, 12 soccer fields, 18 basketball courts, 81 tennis courts, 16 swimming pools and 6 golf courses. The city operates 3 lakes with places for boating and fishing. Contact: Ms. Jo Ann Pearce, Director, City of Oklahoma City, Parks and Recreation Department, 201 Channing Square, Oklahoma City, OK 73102.

Parkland/Total City Area (percent)	5.0

The city employs 26 nurses for the public-school system's 37,804 students. The nurses are present full-time in 1.5 percent of the schools and part-time in the rest of the schools. Nursing services are provided for handicapped students. No medical, dental, or psychiatric treatments are provided. The school system only offers health-education programs in hygiene, sex education and dental health to students in grades K-12. A drug-education specialist has been added to the district. The school system provides all common screens and tests except mental-health exams and well-child physical exams. It also provides height, weight, blood pressure and dental screening. Contact: Ms. Emmy Gleichman, Supervisor of Nurses, Oklahoma City Public Schools, 900 N. Klein, Room 301, Oklahoma City, OK 73106.

Omaha, NE

🪦 RIP	🏃	$	⬆	℞	🚶	👫	?
✓	✔	✔	✓	✓	?	✓	✓

Omaha (Douglas County) has a fairly low age-adjusted death rate, although the statistical picture of degenerative disease is unusual—the ranking for heart disease is several times worse than it is for cancer. Infant-mortality rates for Nebraska are high among minorities and low among whites. Rates are higher in cities than in rural areas of the state.

	Number	Rank
Age-Adjusted Death Rate	−0.62	34/100
Heart Attacks	0.18	69/100
Cancer	−0.21	25/100

The violent crimes of robbery and homicide, and accidental-death rates, are low in Omaha. Suicide, which is violent but not necessarily a crime, occurs relatively more frequently in Omaha than in other metro areas.

Incidence per 1,000 Pop.	Number	Rank
Homicides (1989)	0.04	20/111
Robberies (1989)	1.12	22/111
Suicides	0.12	46/100
Accidental Deaths	0.32	31/100

$ | Omaha's 1988 metro population was 622,000—67th out of 113 metro areas. Its economic health at the end of 1990 was excellent, ranking 16th of 113 metro areas. Its unemployment rate ranks 2nd, change in unemployment 12th (employment grew by nearly 1 percent while the labor force declined slightly) and its enterprise 80th. Contact: Mayor P. J. Morgan, City of Omaha, 1819 Farnham Street #300, Omaha, NE 68183.

Air Quality: New regulations and standards for waste incinerators have been introduced. In 1988, Omaha exceeded the EPA's standards for lead 3 days, airborne particles 1 day and carbon monoxide 1 day. In 1989 Omaha exceeded EPA standards only for airborne lead (2.13 $\mu g/m^3$) that was caused primarily by an industrial source. Contact: Robert Sink: Environmental Quality Control Manager, City of Omaha, 5600 S. 10th Street, Omaha, NE 68107 (402) 734-6060.

Hazardous Waste: Economy Products, a site of pesticide waste, is on the EPA's Superfund list. Public awareness of the impact of household wastes on ground water via landfills has grown. Contact: Robert Sink, Environmental Quality Control Manager, City of Omaha, 5600 S. 10th Street, Omaha, NE 68107 (402) 734-6060.

Water Quality: Omaha's water supply comes from both surface and ground water sources. The pH of the drinking water is a high 9, but otherwise its quality is superior. Contact: Z. Kerekes, Director of Water Quality, Metropolitan Utilities District, Omaha, NE 68107.

Weather: The average temperature is below average at 49.5. Humidity and precipitation are slightly above average.

Average Daily Temperature (degrees F)	49.5
High	59.5
Low	39.4
Average Humidity	
Morning (percent)	81
Afternoon (percent)	62
Annual Precipitation (inches)	29.9
Average Total Snowfall (inches)	32.3
Ozone, Days over 0.12 ppm (one hour)	0

℞ | Omaha offers all basic public health-education programs and emergency hotlines. Omaha has had media campaigns for drug and alcohol-prevention programs. The city provides all common preventive-health and treatment programs. The city also sponsors campaigns for mental health, elderly health care, long-term care for the elderly, immunizations and child care. Anti-smoking laws include partial restriction in restaurants, public offices and private offices. Smoking is prohibited on public transportation. Contact: Mr. Daniel Worthing, M.P.H., Douglas County Health Department, 1819 Farnham, Room 401, Omaha, NE 68183 (402) 444-7471.

Health Resources per 1,000 Pop.	Number	Rank
Hospital beds, community hospitals, city	10.22	21/92
Nurses, community hospitals, city	8.82	32/90
Doctors, metro	2.73	39/113

Omaha did not respond to the author's recreational-services survey.

Omaha public schools employ 43 nurses, 28 psychologists and 9 health aides to provide for 42,000 students. Full-time nurses are present in junior and senior high schools and part-time nurses are present in all elementary schools. No physicians, dentists or psychiatrists are hired by the school district. The school system offers all common health-education programs to grades K-12, including an AIDS education program. In 1988, Omaha implemented a K-12 Human Growth and Development curriculum. Contact: Betty Rundlett, Supervisor of Health Services, Omaha Public Schools, 3215 Cumming Street, Omaha, NE 68131-2024 (402) 554-6411.

Orlando, FL

RIP	🚭	$	🌲	℞	🚶	👫	?
✔	✓	✓	✓	✗	✓	?	✗

The Orlando (Orange County) age-adjusted death rate is in the top quarter of cities surveyed; its incidence of heart attacks and cancer is within the top third. The state's infant-mortality rate is a middling 166th of 301, with rural areas worse off than cities and towns.

	Number	Rank
Age-Adjusted Death Rate	−1.14	22/100
Heart Attacks	−0.30	29/100
Cancer	−0.13	34/100

Orlando ranks 85th out of 111 in robberies, but 46th in homicides. More of a problem is the 83rd-place suicide ranking.

Incidence per 1,000 Pop.	Number	Rank
Homicides (1989)	0.07	46/111
Robberies (1989)	3.06	85/111
Suicides	0.16	83/100
Accidental Deaths	0.34	56/100

$ Orlando's 1988 metro population was 971,000—47th out of 113 metro areas. Its economic health at the end of 1990 was below average, ranking 60th of 113 metro areas. Its unemployment rate ranks 84th, change in unemployment 81st (the labor force grew 7.9 percent, even faster than employment, which grew 6.6 percent) and its enterprise 3rd. Contact: Mayor W.D. Frederick, Jr., City of Orlando, 400 South Orange Avenue, Orlando, FL 32801.

Air Quality: The city did not return our air-quality questionnaire. Orlando is 1989 was in compliance with all NAAQS limits on pollutants, but ozone was close, with 0.11 ppm (0.1 ppm short of the ceiling).

Water Quality: All of the water supply in Orlando comes from ground water (e.g., wells). For the 33 years that Orlando has used well water all parameters remain virtually unchanged. Contact Richard A. Dunham, Superintendent of Laboratories, Orlando Utilities Commission, P.O. Box 3193, Orlando, FL 32802; (407) 244-8779.

Weather: Orlando has a hot, humid, rainy climate; freezing temperatures are a rarity, but the mercury hits the 90s on at least 100 days annually.

Average Daily Temperature (degrees F)	72.4
High	82.8
Low	62.0
Average Humidity	
Morning (percent)	89
Afternoon (percent)	55
Annual Precipitation (inches)	47.8
Average Total Snowfall (inches)	Trace

℞ Health care in Orlando is affordable, and facilities include a cardiac rehabilitation center and a hospice. The city did not respond to the health-services survey.

Health Resources per 1,000 Pop.	Number	Rank
Doctors, metro	1.73	98/113

 Orlando has 72 criteria sports facilities per 100,000 residents, ranking 45th out of 82 metro areas. Most popular sports are tennis, golf, swimming and boating. The city offers aerobics classes. Orlando also provides a handicapped recreational program. The city's sports facilities include 27 baseball/softball fields, 6 football/soccer fields, 36 basketball courts, 34 tennis courts, 7 swimming pools, 6 racquetball courts, 1 running track and 1 golf course. Contact: Don Wilson, Bureau Chief, City of Orlando, Recreation Bureau, 400 S. Orange Avenue, Orlando, Florida 32801.

Parkland/Total City Area (percent)   6.8

Orlando did not respond to the school-health survey.

Paterson, NJ

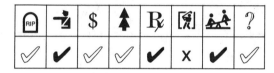

Paterson is located in Passaic County and its metro area includes Bergen County. Although we did not calculate the age-adjusted death rate for the Paterson metro area, the crime data are so different from the Jersey City and Newark metros that we have assigned a middle mortality rating to Paterson. Infant-mortality rates for New Jersey are high among minorities and extremely low among whites (273/301 and 9/301 respectively). Infant-mortality rates are higher in cities than in rural areas of the state.

Although it does not appear in the list of 111 metro areas that we ranked for homicide and robbery, the Paterson metro area (Bergen and Passaic counties) would rate 9th lowest, right after Spokane, on homicides and would rate 46th, with Nashville, on robberies. Assigning more weight to the homicide data, we have given Paterson a top rating on violent crime. Paterson's rankings contrast with those of Newark and Jersey City, which rate 69th and 74th on homicide and 106th and 107th on robberies.

$ Paterson's 1988 metro population (Bergen-Passaic counties) was 1.29 million—37th out of 113 metro areas. Its economic health at the end of 1990 was below average, ranking 67th of 113 metro areas. Its unemployment rate ranks 38th, change in unemployment 91st (employment declined while the labor force grew) and its enterprise 52nd. Contact: Mayor William Pascrell, City of Paterson, 111 Broadway, Municipal Complex, Paterson, NJ 07505.

Air Quality: Paterson did not return the air-quality questionnaire. The Paterson metro is in full compliance with all NAAQS maxima, but it is too close to noncompliance to merit a top rating. In 1989 ozone, for example, was 0.12 ppm, right at the limit. Carbon monoxide was 8 ppm, just 1 ppm below its limit.

Hazardous Waste: Two EPA Superfund sites are located within Passaic County. Passaic County does not have any hazardous-waste disposal sites. Preventive measures are being taken to assure that no hazardous waste is disposed in the county. Hazardous waste generated within the county is disposed of out-of-state. Contact: John J. Ferraioli, County Health Officer, Passaic County Health Department, 317 Pennsylvania Avenue, Paterson, NJ 07503.

Weather: Mild weather with short periods of freezing temperatures and 90-degree days.

Average Daily Temperature (degrees F)	54.5
High	62.2
Low	46.9
Average Humidity	
Morning (percent)	72
Afternoon (percent)	56
Annual Precipitation (inches)	44.1
Average Total Snowfall (inches)	28.6
Ozone, Days over 0.12 ppm (1 hour, 1988)	18

℞ Smoking is prohibited on public transportation and in public offices. Smoking is partially restricted in private offices. The city provides all common health-education programs, emergency hotlines, preventive-health and treatment programs. The city sponsors several programs and services for people with AIDS. The city also sponsors a community education and outreach program for AIDS prevention. Contact: Robin Monkowski, Health Educator, Paterson Division of Health, 176 Broadway, Paterson, NJ 07505.

Health Resources per 1,000 Pop.   **Number**   **Rank**

Doctors, metro   3.12   21/113

Sports leagues sponsored by the Division of Recreation are especially popular in Paterson. The city's sports facilities include 7 softball fields, 8 baseball fields, 6 football/soccer fields, 15 basketball courts, 13 tennis courts, 1 swimming pool and 1 running track. The city offers classes in aerobics and hiking/exploration. Contact: Nick Rocca, Superintendent of Recreation, Division of Recreation, City Hall, 155 Market Street, Paterson, NJ 07505.

Parkland/Total City Area (percent)   3.8

The city school system employs 38 nurses, 15 physicians, 17 psychologists, 1 psychiatrist, 1 dentist and 1 dental health coordinator for its 21,920 students. Nurses are present full-time in all schools. All common health-education programs are offered to students in grades K-12. In addition, AIDS education, mental health, growth and development, dental health, community health and death & dying are also taught. The school system provides all common screens and tests except for immunizations and mental-health exams. Dental treatment is provided for students. Contact: Frank Napier, Superintendent of Schools, Paterson Board of Education, 33 Church Street, Paterson, NJ 07505.

Philadelphia, PA

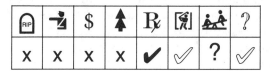

Philadelphia (Philadelphia County) has an age-adjusted death rate that puts it in the bottom quarter of cities surveyed. And while heart attack incidence is below average (41st out of 100), its cancer rate is high, in the bottom quarter. Pennsylvania has extremely high infant-mortality rates among minorities. Contact: Robert G. Sharrar, M.D., M.Sc., Assistant Health Commissioner for Disease Prevention, Philadelphia Department of Public Health, 500 South Broad Street, Philadelphia, PA 19146 (215) 875-5687.

	Number	Rank
Age-Adjusted Death Rate	9.95	77/100
Heart Attacks	−0.16	41/100
Cancer	0.23	79/100

 Philadelphia's crime and accident rates rank in the bottom third of cities surveyed, but its suicide rate is low.

Incidence per 1,000 Pop.	Number	Rank
Homicides (1989)	0.12	85/111
Robberies (1989)	2.81	79/111
Suicides	0.12	31/100
Accidental Deaths	0.36	75/100

$ Philadelphia's 1988 metro population was 4,920,000—4th out of 113 metro areas. Its economic health at the end of 1990 was poor, ranking 87th of 113 metro areas. Its unemployment rate ranks 56th, change in unemployment 96th (employment declined slightly, while the labor force continued to grow by 1.3 percent) and its enterprise 64th. Philadelphia's 1988 metro population of 1,647,000 made it the fifth-largest city surveyed. Contact: Mayor W. Wilson Goode, City of Philadelphia, City Hall #215, Philadelphia, PA 19107.

Air Quality: Major improvements have been made in all air quality levels except ozone, which is a persistent problem on the east coast of the United States. Philadelphia exceeded EPA standards for ozone 21 days in 1988 and carbon monoxide levels for 2 days. The PSI exceeded 100 on 34 days in 1988 and on 18 days in 1989. In 1989 the carbon monoxide level was 12 ppm, well over the maximum NAAQS level of 9 ppm. The city's ozone level was 0.16, well above the 0.12 NAAQS ceiling. Particulates were at 46 $\mu g/m^3$, close to the maximum NAAQS level. Contact: Robert Ostrowski, Acting Director, Air Management Services, Philadelphia Department of Public Health, Air Management Services, 500 South Broad Street, Philadelphia, PA 19146 (215) 875-5623.

Hazardous Waste: The Publicker Industries site is on the EPA Superfund list. The Metal Bank of America, a waste site for PCBs, is also a Superfund site. Philadelphia does not have any disposal sites permitted by the Pennsylvania Department of Environmental Resources. The city has an operating PCB detoxification plant and has two other experimental PCB detoxification/destruction units. Ofra, Inc. is operating a plant that transforms municipal solid waste into recyclable products. Contact: Richard Zipin, Chief of Environmental Engineering, Philadelphia Department of

Public Health, Medical Examiners Building, 321 University Ave., Philadelphia, PA 19104 (215) 875-5658.

Water Quality: Philadelphia's water supply comes entirely from surface water sources. The pH of the drinking water has ranged from 6.4 to a high 9.0 over the 1985–90 period. Three water treatment plants supply the city with drinking water. Of the three, in 1990 one had an average pH of 8.2 (quite high), one was 7.35 and the remaining one was 7.1. The Water Department aggressively monitors the plant intakes, plant effluents and distribution system to comply with the Safe Drinking Water Act. Contact: Theresa M. Iacobucci, Project Engineer, City of Philadelphia, Water Department, 4290 Ford Street, Philadelphia, PA 19131.

Weather: Philadelphia's climate benefits from the moderating influence of its location between the Appalachian Mountains and the Atlantic Ocean. The climate is fairly mild, with few or no zero-degree days, about three months of freezing days (32 degrees or less) and roughly 20 uncomfortably hot days (90 degrees or higher) each year. The city's humidity runs high, however, which can increase the discomfort of warm summer days.

Average Daily Temperature (degrees F)	54.3
High	63.4
Low	45.1
Average Humidity	
Morning (percent)	76
Afternoon (percent)	55
Annual Precipitation (inches)	41.4
Average Total Snowfall (inches)	21.8
Ozone, Days over 0.12 ppm (1 hour, 1988)	21
PSI, Days over 100, 1988	34
PSI, Days over 100, 1989	18

℞ Philadelphia offers all common public health-education programs. The city has increased funding and lengthened hours of city-operated clinics and increased outreach programs for AIDS and prenatal services. All basic emergency hotlines are provided, including domestic violence and mental health services hotlines. The city provides all common preventive-health programs, except blood pressure and cholesterol testing, and treatment programs. It sponsors campaigns for AIDS, prenatal care, fetal alcohol syndrome, fitness and exercise, injury prevention, environmental issues and nutrition. The city's anti-smoking laws include partial restriction on smoking in restaurants, public offices and private offices. Smoking on public transportation is prohibited. Contact: Robert

G. Sharrar, M.D., M.Sc., Asst. Health Commissioner for Disease Prevention, Philadelphia Department of Public Health, 500 South Broad Street, Philadelphia, PA 19146.

Health Resources per 1,000 Pop.	Number	Rank
Hospital beds, community hospitals, city	5.80	58/92
Nurses, community hospitals, city	7.10	51/90
Doctors, metro	3.02	23/113

 Philadelphia has 76 criteria sports facilities per 100,000 people, ranking it 41st out of the 82 cities that provided this information. The city's facilities include 472 baseball fields, 160 football/soccer fields, 399 basketball courts, 228 tennis courts, 86 swimming pools and 5 golf courses. Philadelphia's Recreation and Parks Department sponsors programs for disabled and senior citizens. Several classes (aerobics, hiking and exploration) are offered through the department as are sports and athletics. Contact: Delores Andy, Commissioner, Department of Recreation, City of Philadelphia, 1180 MSB, Philadelphia, PA 19107.

Parkland/Total City Area (percent)   12.8

Philadelphia did not return its school-health questionnaire.

Phoenix, AZ

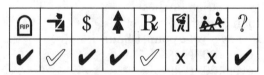

Phoenix and Mesa together make up about 70 percent of the population of Maricopa County, which is the Phoenix metro area. The Phoenix metro area is in the top quarter of major cities in its age-adjusted death rate. Cities and rural areas have the same infant-mortality rates, although statewide, black infants fare worse than white ones. Phoenix ranks in the top half of major cities in its age-adjusted rates of fatal heart attacks and cancer. David Cundiff, M.D., M.P.H., Director for Public Health, Maricopa County Department of Health Services, 1825 East Roosevelt, Phoenix, AZ 85003 (602) 440-6600.

Health Indicators	Number	Rank
Age-Adjusted Death Rate	−1.08	25/100
Heart Attacks	−0.06	47/100
Cancer	−0.16	31/100

 Phoenix's middling crime marks are offset by its high suicide rate, which puts it near the bottom of major cities.

Incidence per 1,000 Pop.	Number	Rank
Homicides (1989)	0.08	59/111
Robberies (1989)	1.72	40/111
Suicides	0.18	95/100
Accidental Deaths	0.41	88/100

$ Phoenix's 1988 metro population was 2,030,000—19th out of 113 metro areas. Its economic health at the end of 1990 was excellent, ranking 26th of 113 metro areas. Its unemployment rate ranks 31st, change in unemployment 22nd (employment rose faster than the labor force) and its enterprise 57th. Contact: Mayor Paul Johnson, City of Phoenix, 251 West Washington Street, Phoenix, AZ 85003; or: Lionel D. Lyons, Assistant to the Mayor (602) 262-7111.

↑ **Air Quality:** Phoenix exceeded the EPA standards on ozone 1 day in 1988. It exceeded standards on carbon monoxide 2 days. Contact: John Power, Director of Environmental Health Services, Maricopa County Health Department, 1825 East Roosevelt, Phoenix, AZ 85003 (602) 258-6381.

Hazardous Waste: Several sites are on the EPA's Superfund list, including Motorola 52nd Street Site, 19th Ave. Landfill, Hassayaga Landfill, Phoenix Goodyear and Motorola Mesa. Within Maricopa County there are no permitted hazardous-waste disposal facilities. Recently, the state hazardous waste facility was established 30 miles southwest of Phoenix. Contact: Norm Weiss, Assistant Director, Hazardous and Solid Waste, Environmental Quality Department, 2005 N. Central, 7th Floor, Phoenix, AZ 85004; 602-257-6829.

Water Quality: The source of Phoenix's drinking water is 95 percent surface water and 5 percent ground water. The pH of the drinking water is 7.8. Mesa's drinking water comes 90 percent from surface water sources; the remainder comes from ground water. Contact: Ron Miller, Assistant Director, Office of Water Quality, 2005 N. Central, Room 302, Phoenix, AZ 85004 (602) 257-2305. Or: John Power, Director of Environmental Health

Services, Maricopa County Health Department, Division of Public Health, 1845 East Roosevelt, PO Box 2111, Phoenix, AZ 85001.

Weather: The weather is generally mild and sunny year-round, with low annual rainfall and low humidity. Winter days are fairly warm, with temperatures in the 60s and 70s, while the temperature only rarely drops below freezing during winter nights. Light snow falls once every six or seven years. Summers are very hot, but residents say it's bearable because of the area's low humidity. Despite the desert surroundings, the landscape is far from desolate. One or more mountain ranges can be seen from almost any point in Phoenix. The famed Superstition Mountains lie to the east.

Average Daily Temperature (degrees F)	71.2
High	85.1
Low	57.3
Average Humidity	
Morning (percent)	52
Afternoon (percent)	23
Annual Precipitation (inches)	7.11
Average Total Snowfall (inches)	Trace
Ozone, Days over 0.12 ppm (1 hour, 1988)	1

℞ The city has good health-care facilities. All common public health-education programs are offered including immunization, injury prevention, cardiovascular screening and prevention, dental health and food handler's training. The city has several basic emergency hotlines and also provides hotlines for battered women, rape, American Red Cross and mental health. The city provides all common preventive-health programs, plus health care for the homeless, community-health nursing and dental care. Phoenix provides treatment programs for drug rehabilitation, alcoholism, mental-health therapy and sexually transmitted diseases. Phoenix has three teaching hospitals—the Good Samaritan Hospital, Maricopa County General Hospital and St. Joseph's Hospital and Medical Center—six cardiac rehabilitation centers and four hospices. Because Phoenix is a competitive health-care environment and is in the forefront of state-of-the-art medical technology, top health-care professionals are easily attracted to the area. Contact: David Cundiff, M.D., M.P.H., Director for Public Health, Maricopa County Department of Health Services, 1825 East Roosevelt, Phoenix, AZ 85003 (602) 440-6600.

Health Resources per 1,000 Pop.	Number	Rank
Hospital beds, community hospitals, city	4.41	80/92
Nurses, community hospitals, city	5.22	70/90
Doctors, metro	2.23	70/113

Phoenix has 46 criteria sports facilities per 100,000 residents, ranking 68th out of the 82 cities for which we have sufficient information. Most recreational facilities are privately owned—swimming pools abound, although it will take a sustained civic effort to keep the water that replenishes the pools flowing. The city's mountain parks, including South Mountain Park, the world's largest municipal park, offer outdoor enthusiasts ample opportunities for hiking, picnicking and enjoying breathtaking views of the Valley of the Sun. Some of this land has been designated mountain preserve, protecting it from the development that has gobbled up land for miles around Phoenix. The Salt River lakes offer water-sports enthusiasts a place for this type of activity. The Valley of the Sun offers year-round play on nearly 100 private golf courses and 1,000 private tennis courts. Public sports facilities include 61 baseball fields, 20 football fields, 43 soccer fields, 100 basketball courts, 196 tennis courts, 5 golf courses and 27 swimming pools. Contact: Director, City of Phoenix, Recreation and Library Department, 2333 N. Central Avenue, Phoenix, AZ 85004; (602) 262-6861.

Phoenix itself did not respond to the school-health survey, but suburban Mesa did. For a total of 61,500 students in the Mesa public-school system, there are 38 nurses and 45 health assistants. A full-time nurse is available in all of the secondary schools and a part-time nurse is available in the elementary schools. The school-health program has a new AIDS policy for students and employees. All common health-education programs are offered to students in grades K-8. The school system provides all common screens and tests except for immunizations, mental-health exams and well-child physical exams. No medical, dental or psychiatric treatment is provided for students.

Pittsburgh, PA

🪦	🛏	$	⬆	℞	🏃	🧑‍🏫	?
X	✔	X	X	✓	✔	?	✓

Pittsburgh (Allegheny County) ranked near the bottom of major cities in age-adjusted death rate, heart attack and cancer, categories. Infant-mortality rates for Pennsylvania are extremely high among minorities. Infant-mortality rates are higher in cities than in rural areas of the state.

	Number	Rank
Age-Adjusted Death Rate	1.75	91/100
Heart Attacks	0.71	91/100
Cancer	0.54	91/100

Pittsburgh's homicide rate is very low, which puts it at the top of the cities surveyed. Robbery, suicide and accident rates are also lower than average.

Incidence per 1,000 Pop.	Number	Rank
Homicides (1989)	0.03	10/111
Robberies (1989)	1.57	34/111
Suicides	0.12	49/100
Accidental Deaths	0.32	36/100

$ Pittsburgh's 1988 metro population was 2,094,000—18th out of 113 metro areas. Its economic health at the end of 1990 was below average, ranking 75th of 113 metro areas. Its unemployment rate ranks 56th, change in unemployment 58th (the labor force grew by 3.5 percent, faster than employment, which grew by 3.0 percent) and its enterprise 75th. Contact: Mayor Sophie Masloff, 512 City-County Building, 414 Grant Street, Pittsburgh, PA 15219.

Air Quality: Pittsburgh did not return our air-quality questionnaire. Our data are from the EPA. The number of days that Pittsburgh's PSI exceeded 100 was 31 in 1988 and 11 in 1989. In 1989 its ozone level was 0.13 ppm, over the NAAQS ceiling of 0.12 ppm. Carbon monoxide was just under the ceiling of 9 ppm. Particulates were 43 $\mu g/m^3$, a bit under the NAAQS ceiling of 50.

Hazardous Waste: Pittsburgh has two hazardous-waste sites: one in Alsco Park, Harrison Township, and the Pico-Hercules Site at Jefferson Borough. Pennsylvania has no active hazardous-waste disposal sites. Therefore, wastes are transported to other states. Contact: Donald Berman, Director, Allegheny County Waste Management, 441 Smithfield Street, Pittsburgh, PA 15219 (412) 355-5594.

Water Quality: The nitrate content of Pittsburgh's water, 1.7 mg/l, is relatively high, 10th highest of 61 cities for which we have this information. But its pH is 7.8, close to the ideal of 7 and Pittsburgh officials say the quality is excellent. Turbidity is average (34th out of 57 cities) at .23 t.u. The quality of the drinking water is excellent. In the past ten years the University of Pittsburgh has done a great deal to ensure that the quality of the city water supply continues to exceed EPA standards. The Pittsburgh

Water & Sewer Authority is currently in the middle of a seven-year, $190 million capital-improvement program to upgrade the Water Department's distribution systems. Contact: Dawn Botsford, Executive Director, Pittsburgh Water & Sewer Authority, Suite 700 Porter building, Pittsburgh, PA 15219 (412) 255-8935.

Weather: The average temperature is slightly low at 50.3.

Average Daily Temperature (degrees F)	50.3
High	59.9
Low	40.7
Average Humidity	
Morning (percent)	78
Afternoon (percent)	57
Annual Precipitation (inches)	36.3
Average Total Snowfall (inches)	44
PSI, Days over 100, 1988	31
PSI, Days over 100, 1989	11

℞ Pittsburgh provides all basic public health-education programs and emergency hotlines. The city provides all common preventive-health and treatment programs. The city sponsors public awareness campaigns dealing with poison prevention, pedestrian and traffic safety, infant mortality, recycling, smoke-free environments and minority health problems. Smoking is prohibited on public transportation and in public offices and is partially restricted in restaurants and private offices. Recently, the city has built Wellness Centers and sponsored a recycling law and smoking ordinance. New health-treatment programs include an adolescent HIV program in the schools, a university training center for AIDS/STD and an injury-prevention effort with Children's Hospital and the Allegheny County Health Department. Contact: Albert Brunwasser, 3333 Fores Avenue, Pittsburgh, PA 15213.

Health Resources per 1,000 Pop.	Number	Rank
Hospital beds, community hospitals, city	17.50	2/92
Nurses, community hospitals, city	22.37	1/90
Doctors, metro	2.88	31/113

Pittsburgh has 146 sports facilities per 100,000 residents, ranking 11th of 82 cities. The Great Race, the nation's sixth-largest 10 km. race, has 13,000 participants. The city has added health and fitness rooms to its recreation center. The city's sports facilities include 128 baseball fields, 64 football fields, 26 soccer fields, 180 basketball courts, 150 tennis courts, 1 golf course, 2 running tracks and 34 swimming pools. Contact:

Louise Brown, Director, City of Pittsburgh Department of Parks and Recreation, 400 City and County Building, Pittsburgh, PA 15219 (412) 255-2632.

Parkland/Total City Area (percent)   7.2

 Pittsburgh did not respond to the school-health survey.

Portland, ME

 RIP	🏃	$	⬆	R	🏃	👫	?
X	✔	X	✔	✔	?	✔	✔

Portland (Cumberland County) scores near the bottom of 100 cities with its age-adjusted death rates. It has the 8th lowest longevity. Infant mortality in Maine cities is significantly higher than in rural areas.

	Number	Rank
Age-Adjusted Death Rate	2.48	93/100
Heart Attacks	0.64	87/100
Cancer	0.82	98/100

 Portland has the 8th lowest rate for robberies of 111 metro areas. Homicides and accidental deaths are also below average.

Incidence per 1,000 Pop.	Number	Rank
Homicides (1989)	0.04	19/111
Robberies (1989)	0.58	8/111
Suicides	0.15	81/100
Accidental Deaths	0.30	23/100

$ Portland's 1988 metro population was 212,000—104th out of 113 metro areas. Its economic health at the end of 1990 was below average, ranking 75th of 113 metro areas. Its unemployment rate ranks 38th, change in unemployment 104th (the labor force grew faster than employment) and its enterprise 47th. Contact: Mayor Esther B. Clenott, City of Portland, City Hall, Portland, ME 04101.

▲ **Air Quality:** The city did not return our air-quality questionnaire. According to EPA data, Portland—surprising to those who think of Maine as the embodiment of environmental purity—violated the NAAQS limit on ozone in 1989. The city's ozone level was 0.13 ppm, above the ozone limit of 0.12 ppm. For a small community like Portland, ringed by ocean and countryside, our first thought was that this exceedance was less forgivable than one by a city ringed by more conurbations beyond its control. We were going to assign Portland our lowest environment rating in protest. But according to the Corporate Environmental Data Clearinghouse, a project of the Council on Economic Priorities in New York City, prevailing air currents carry pollution from the Midwest to southern Maine; so this is an extenuating circumstance. Fortunately, other air-pollution data for Portland were comfortably below the NAAQS levels (particulates and carbon monoxide were about half the ceiling).

Water Quality: The water supply comes entirely from lakes and the pollution program has been effective in maintaining the excellent quality. The tap water has improved due to the corrosion control program aimed at controlling lead, copper and iron found in residences and commercial buildings. Contact: Phillippe Boissonneault, Quality Assurance Supervisor, Portland Water District, 225 Douglass Street, Portland, ME 04104 (207) 774-5961.

Weather: Portland is cool, with an average temperature of 45 degrees. Precipitation is above the national average at 43.5 inches annually, while snowfall is extremely high at 71.5 inches annually.

Average Daily Temperature (degrees F)	45.0
High	55.0
Low	35.0
Average Humidity	
Morning (percent)	79
Afternoon (percent)	59
Annual Precipitation (inches)	43.5
Average Total Snowfall (inches)	71.5

℞ Portland provides public health-education programs for CPR training, AIDS education, nutrition, prenatal and infant care, family planning and sexually transmitted diseases. Emergency hotlines are available for child abuse, suicide and AIDS information. The city provides all common preventive-health programs except prenatal and infant medical care or food provision; it also provides adolescent primary health care. It provides treatment for sexually transmitted diseases, but not for drug abuse, alcoholism or mental illness. A new primary health care service for homeless clients has been established and a walk-in service for nursing-related assessments of treatments has been enlarged. The city addresses AIDS education, sexually transmitted diseases, nutrition and parenting in health-awareness campaigns. An interesting new change is the multiple intervention risk reduction program that will target smoking, nutrition, obesity and lifestyle. There are no smoking ordinances. Contact: Meredith Tipton, Public Health Director, City of Portland, 389 Congress Street, Portland, ME 04101.

Health Resources per 1,000 Pop.	Number	Rank
Doctors, metro	3.40	15/113

Portland did not respond to the recreational-services survey.

For a total of 9,000 students in the public-school system there are five nurses, two psychologists and one physician on call. A part-time nurse is available in only 5 percent of the schools. The school system offers all common health-education programs to students in grades K-12. The school system also has an AIDS education program. The school system provides all common screens and tests except for mental-health exams and well-child physical exams. Medical treatment is provided for students. Contact: Josephine Piampiano, Director, School Health Program, Portland Public Schools, 331 Veranda Street, Portland, ME 04103.

Portland, OR

🪦	🏋	$	🌲	℞	🎿	🧑‍🤝‍🧑	?
X	✔	✔	✔	✓	✓	?	✓

Portland (Multnomah County) ranks a high 85th in the age-adjusted death rate. Cancer and heart attack rates are also high. Infant-mortality rates for Oregon are high among blacks and relatively low among other minorities and whites. Infant-mortality rates are slightly higher in rural areas than in cities.

	Number	Rank
Age-Adjusted Death Rate	1.14	85/100
Heart Attacks	0.36	78/100
Cancer	0.28	84/100

Portland has a very high suicide rate, 9th highest of 100 metro areas, possibly reflecting its exposure to Pacific cultures where suicide is more commonly accepted than in the West. It also has high accident rates. Homicides are below average and robberies are slightly above average.

Incidence per 1,000 Pop.	Number	Rank
Homicides (1989)	0.05	31/111
Robberies (1989)	2.70	74/111
Suicides	0.18	92/100
Accidental Deaths	0.42	89/100

$ Portland's 1988 metro population was 1,188,000—40th out of 113 metro areas. Its economic health at the end of 1990 was good, ranking 31st of 113 metro areas. Its unemployment rate ranks 29th, change in unemployment 43rd (employment grew 5.2 percent, slightly faster than the labor force) and its enterprise 49th. Contact: Mayor J.E. Bud Clark, City of Portland, 1220 Southwest Fifth, Portland, OR 97204.

Air Quality: Despite continuing population growth, Portland has experienced small to moderate improvement in carbon monoxide and ozone levels. Portland did have 1 carbon monoxide exceedance and 2 ozone exceedances in 1988. Contact: Nick Nikkila, Department of Environmental Quality, 811 SW 6th, Portland, OR 97204.

Hazardous Waste: There are 2 EPA Superfund sites in the Portland area: Gould/NL Industries and Allied Planting. There are no commercial hazardous-waste disposal sites in the county. There has been a reduction in the amount of hazardous waste generated within the county apparently due to the state's new toxic use and hazardous waste reduction law. On the solid waste side, the Portland area is building a 185,000 tons-per-year composting facility that is planned to recycle half of the region's solid waste into a useful soil conditioner. Contact: Bob Danko, Senior Analyst, Hazardous & Solid Waste Division, Department of Environmental Quality, 811 SW 6th Avenue, Portland, OR 97204.

Weather: The average daily temperature is about average at 53. Humidity is slightly above average.

Average Daily Temperature (degrees F)	53.0
High	62.0
Low	44.0
Average Humidity	
Morning (percent)	86
Afternoon (percent)	60

Annual Precipitation (inches)	37.4
Average Total Snowfall (inches)	6.8
Ozone, Days over 0.12 ppm (1 hour, 1988)	2

℞ The city has teen clinics and outreach programs located in high schools. All common health-education programs are provided by the county. The county sponsors all basic emergency hotlines, with the exception of a sexually transmitted diseases hotline. The city provides all common preventive-health and treatment programs except that its cholesterol screening program is limited. State smoking laws prohibit smoking on public transportation and in public offices. Smoking is partially restricted in restaurants. Contact: Billie Odegaard, Multnomah County Health Division, 426 SW Stark, Portland, OR 97204.

Health Resources per 1,000 Pop.	Number	Rank
Doctors, metro	2.85	35/113

Portland has 83 sports facilities per 100,000 residents, ranking it 35th of 82 cities. Walking, jogging, running and aerobics are especially popular in Portland. The city's sports facilities include 15 baseball fields, 12 football fields, 100 soccer fields, 110 basketball courts, 112 tennis courts, 4 golf courses, 14 running tracks, 100 softball fields and 14 swimming pools. Contact: Rich Gunderson, Director of Recreation, Bureau of Parks & Public Recreation, 1120 SW 5th Avenue, Portland, OR 97204.

All common health-education programs are offered to students in grades K-8 and one year in high school. Oregon has a state-wide wellness curriculum that emphasizes skills and information for a healthy lifestyle. The city did not respond to the personnel or screens and tests portions of the school-health survey. Contact: Ann Shelton, Health Specialist, Portland Public Schools, 501 North Dixon, Portland, OR 97227.

Providence, RI

🪦	🏊	$	⬆	℞	🏌	👫	?
X	✔	X	X	✔	X	✓	✓

The Providence metro area includes Pawtucket. Providence ranks a high 81st in the age-adjusted mortality rate. Rhode Island has comparatively low infant-mortality rates among minorities. Infant-mortality rates are only slightly higher in cities than in rural areas. Contact: Dr. Barbara De Buono, Director, Rhode Island Department of Health, Disease Control, 3 Capitol Hill, 106 Cannon Bldg., Providence, Rhode Island 02908 (401) 277-2362.

	Number	Rank
Age-Adjusted Death Rate	0.83	81/100
Heart Attacks	0.68	89/100
Cancer	0.24	80/100

 Rates for homicides, robberies, suicides and accidental deaths in Providence are all below average.

Incidence per 1,000 Pop.	Number	Rank
Homicides (1989)	0.06	36/111
Robberies (1989)	1.36	29/111
Suicides	0.12	34/100
Accidental deaths	0.32	43/100

$ Providence's 1988 metro population was 647,000—64th out of 113 metro areas. Its economic health at the end of 1990 was poor. It ranks 108th of 113 metro areas. Its unemployment rate ranks 90th, change in unemployment 111th (employment dropped a hefty 7.7 percent, faster than the labor force, which shrunk 4.1 percent) and its enterprise 85th. Contact: Mayor Joseph R. Paolino, City of Providence, 25 Dorrance Street, Providence, RI 02903.

↑ **Air Quality:** The city did not return our air-quality questionnaire. EPA data indicate that in 1989 Providence's ozone level was 0.13 ppm, exceeding the NAAQS ceiling of 0.12 ppm. Particulates were also high, 39 μg/m³, but were below the NAAQS limit.

Weather: Because of its location on the Atlantic coast, Providence is subject to capricious weather patterns, characterized by sudden storms. The average January temperature is 29.9 degrees, while July averages 72.8 degrees.

Average Daily Temperature (degrees F)	50.3
High	59.3
Low	41.2
Average Humidity	
Morning (percent)	74
Afternoon (percent)	54
Annual Precipitation (inches)	45.9
Average Total Snowfall (inches)	36.3

℞ Seven hospitals are located in Providence. The city is served by the
    Metropolitan Nursing and Health Services Association of Rhode
Island. The city also has 17 nursing homes, with a combined bed capacity
of 1,400. The Rhode Island Group Health Association, one of the first
health-maintenance organizations in the country, is located in Providence.
Contact: Wayne Farrington, Department of Health, Facilities Regulation,
75 Davis Street, Providence, RI 02908 (401) 277-2566.

Health Resources per 1,000 Pop.	Number	Rank
Doctors, metro	3.64	11/113

Providence has 52 sports facilities per 100,000 residents, ranking
63rd out of 82 cities. Basketball, softball and baseball are very
popular with the young people of the city. Playground programs have been
reinstituted for children aged 6 to 12. The city is also home to several yacht
clubs. The Providence Civic Center can house 10,000 for hockey games
and up to 13,000 for other events. The city's sports facilities include 30
baseball fields, 6 football fields, 9 soccer fields, 30 basketball courts, 6
tennis courts, 1 golf course, 1 running track, 1 volleyball court and 7
swimming pools. Contact: Ray Brown, Providence Recreation Department, 1 Reservoir Avenue, Providence, RI 02901.

Parkland/Total City Area (percent)	10

To serve 20,000 students in the public-school system are 21 nurses,
1 physician and 10 psychologists. A part-time nurse is available in
all schools. All basic health-education programs are offered in various
grades. The school system provides all common screens and tests except
for immunizations. Mental-health exams and learning-disabilities screens
are provided only to special-education students. Dental treatment is provided for students. Contact: Dr. Betty Mathieu, Medical Director, Providence School Department, 480 Charles Street, Providence, Rhode Island
02904 (401) 456-9317.

Raleigh, NC

RIP	🔁	$	⬆	℞	🤸	👫	?
✔	✔	✔	✔	✔	✔	✔	✔

The consolidated area of Raleigh includes Durham. Durham is located in Durham County. Raleigh ranks 17th in the age-adjusted
mortality rate. Infant-mortality rates for North Carolina are high among

minorities and low among whites. Infant-mortality rates are higher in cities than in rural areas of the state.

	Number	Rank
Age-Adjusted Death Rate	−1.29	17/100
Heart Attacks	−0.40	25/100
Cancer	−0.28	22/100

 Raleigh has relatively low rates of homicides, robberies, suicides and accidental deaths.

Incidence per 1,000 Pop.	Number	Rank
Homicides (1989)	0.07	45/111
Robberies (1989)	1.25	27/111
Suicides	0.87	11/100
Accidental deaths	0.31	30/100

$ Raleigh-Durham's 1988 metro population was 684,000—60th out of 113 metro areas. Its economic health at the end of 1990 was excellent, ranking 11th of 113 metro areas. Its unemployment rate ranks 6th, change in unemployment 71st (employment fell slightly while the labor force increased slightly) and its enterprise 7th. Contact: Mayor Avery Upchurch, City of Raleigh, PO Box 590, Raleigh, NC 27602.

Air Quality: The number of carbon-monoxide exceedances decreased from 22 in 1984 to 2 in 1988. The number of ozone exceedances, however, increased significantly through 1988. In 1989 carbon monoxide was at 11 ppm, substantially above the NAAQS cailing of 9 ppm. Ozone was at 0.12 ppm, exactly at the NAAQS ceiling. Contact: Lee Daniel, Acting Air Quality Chief, N.C. State Board of Environmental Contact (Air Quality), PO Box 27687, Raleigh, NC 27611-7687 (919) 733-7015.

Hazardous Waste: A hazardous-waste-disposal site has been proposed, to be sited in nearby Granville County. Raleigh has no inactive waste sites. It has two household-hazardous-waste collection days a year. Contact: Lynn Baird, Public Works Director, City of Raleigh, PO Box 590, Raleigh, NC 27602 (919) 890-3415.

Water Quality: Raleigh rates in the middle on turbidity. Its pH is very good at 7.3, very close to the ideal. Its nitrates are also low, ranking 11th out of 61 cities. Overall water quality, while it has always met all EPA standards, has been further improved due to the addition of potassium permanganate

for manganese control as well as for taste and odor. Contact: Carl Sim-
mons, Public Utilities Director, City of Raleigh, PO Box 590, Raleigh, NC
27602 (919) 890-3400.

Weather: Overall, Raleigh and Durham's climate is mild, but the summers
are humid. Even so, while the area averages 80 freezing days (32 degrees
and below) during winter, the summer is characterized by only about three
weeks' worth of 90-degree days.

Average Daily Temperature (degrees F)	59.0
High	70.3
Low	47.7
Average Humidity	
Morning (percent)	85
Afternoon (percent)	54
Annual Precipitation (inches)	41.8
Average Total Snowfall (inches)	7.5
Ozone, Days over 0.12 ppm (1 hour, 1988)	10

℞ The area's excellent, low-cost medical facilities include four teaching hospitals, two medical schools (Duke and Chapel Hill), two
comprehensive cancer treatment centers (Duke and Chapel Hill) and three
hospices. Raleigh has six hospitals, while Durham has five; Durham likes
to call itself the "City of Medicine," which is not unjustified in view of the
reputation and quality of research at the Duke University Medical Center
and because of the multimillion-dollar biomedical research and development industry that has grown up at the nearby Research Park.

Health Resources per 1,000 Pop.	Number	Rank
Doctors, metro	5.18	4/113

Wake County sponsors most of the health-care programs in the city. Wake
County has built a new public health center in Raleigh. The county also
addresses health promotion, disease control, environmental health, family
planning, children's services, prenatal care and dental care in its public
awareness campaigns. Public health-education programs include CPR
training, AIDS education, nutrition, anti-smoking, anti-drug, prenatal and
infant care, family planning and sexually transmitted diseases. All basic
emergency hotlines are provided. The county provides all common
preventive-health and treatment programs. The city as of 1991 had passed
no laws restricting smoking, but workplace limitations were under consideration. Contact: Dr. Leah Devlin, Director, Wake County Health Department, PO Box 949, Raleigh, NC 27602 (919) 755-0761.

Raleigh has 112 sports facilities per 100,000 residents, ranking 21st out of 82 cities. The city offers aerobics and arts and craft classes and hiking and exploration groups. The Greenway System offers 24 miles of paved trails. The award-winning Parks and Recreation Department offers active and passive leisure services for all city residents at over 200 sites. The department also offers classes in aerobics and hiking/exploration as well as special events for the blind, deaf, and physically challenged. A $13.5 million bond was approved for Parks and Recreation facilities. Funds will be used to construct an indoor aquatics facility, softball complex, develop two new community parks and provide improvements to all the parks in the area. The city's sports facilities include 42 baseball fields, 6 football fields, 6 soccer fields, 64 basketball courts, 91 tennis courts, 2 golf courses, 1 running track, 14 volleyball courts and 9 swimming pools. Contact: Jack Duncan, Parks & Recreation Department, PO Box 590, Raleigh, NC 27602.

Parkland/Total City Area (percent)   7

For a total of 62,462 students in the public-school system, there are 26 psychologists, 7 physical therapists, 3 audiologists and 7 occupational therapists. A part-time nurse is present in all schools. A health services plan for the next three to five years has been developed. The major goal is to add 24 to 25 school nurse positions. The school system offers an extensive health-education program including such topics as wellness, consumer health, mental health (self-esteem), dental health, safety, chronic diseases, growth and development, environmental health and communicable diseases. Health education is taught in grades K-12. The school system provides all common screens and tests except for mental-health exams; it also provides dental screening, clinical services, individual health appraisals and referrals. Dental treatment, audiological evaluations, physical therapy and occupational therapy for children with special needs are also provided. Contact: Wake County Public Schools, 3600 Wake Forest Road, Raleigh, NC 27602.

Richmond, VA

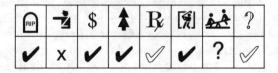

 Cities in Virginia are not part of the surrounding counties; they are independent entities. Richmond ranks a low 13th in the age-adjusted mortality rate. Cancer and heart attack rates are also low. Infant-mortality rates for Virginia are high among minorities and low among whites. Infant-mortality rates are higher in cities than in rural areas of the state. Contact: Ms. Irma C. Reeder, Planning and Evaluation Manager, Richmond City Health Department, 600 East Broad Street, Richmond, VA 23219 (804) 780-4239.

	Number	Rank
Age-Adjusted Death Rate	−1.67	13/100
Heart Attacks	−0.66	12/100
Cancer	−0.30	20/100

Richmond has an extremely high homicide rate. Rates for robberies, suicides and accidental deaths are all below average.

Incidence per 1,000 Pop.	Number	Rank
Homicides (1989)	0.16	100/111
Robberies (1989)	1.85	48/111
Suicides	0.12	33/100
Accidental deaths	0.32	44/100

$ Richmond's 1988 metro population was 844,000—55th out of 113 metro areas. Its economic health at the end of 1990 was good, ranking 23rd of 113 metro areas. Its unemployment rate ranks 25th, change in unemployment 58th (the labor force grew by 4.2 percent, faster than employment, 3.8 percent) and its enterprise 21st. Contact: Mayor Geline Williams, City of Richmond, Room 201 City Hall, Richmond, VA 23219.

Air Quality: In 1988, Richmond had eight days of ozone exceedances of EPA standards. In 1989, however, Richmond had no ozone exceedances. Weather conditions have a significant effect on ozone levels. Contact: Albert E. Spencer, Chief, Division of Environmental Health,

Richmond City Health Department, 600 East Broad Street, Room 618, Richmond, VA 23219 (804) 780-4595.

Water Quality: Richmond's supply of drinking water comes from surface water sources. The pH of the drinking water was 7.12 in 1988. The quality of the drinking water has improved from a turbidity standpoint. Contact; Albert E. Spencer, Chief, Division of Environmental Health, Richmond City Health Department, 600 East Broad Street, Room 618, Richmond, VA 23219 (804) 780-4595.

Weather: Richmond's daily temperature is close to the national average at 57.7. Humidity and precipitation are above average.

Average Daily Temperature (degrees F)	57.7
High	68.8
Low	46.5
Average Humidity	
Morning (percent)	83
Afternoon (percent)	53
Annual Precipitation (inches)	44.1
Average Total Snowfall (inches)	14.6
Ozone, Days over 0.12 ppm (1 hour, 1988)	8

℞ Richmond did not respond to the health-services survey.

Health Resources per 1,000 Pop.	Number	Rank
Hospital beds, community hospitals, city	15.85	3/92
Nurses, community hospitals, city	19.57	2/90
Doctors, metro	2.97	27/113

Richmond has 137 sports facilities per 100,000 residents, ranking it 12th out of 82 metro areas. The department of recreation and parks offers classes in aerobics. Especially popular is the Festival of Arts, a summer-long festival of drama, art, music and dance at the city's outdoor amphitheatre. The city's sports facilities include over 40 football/soccer fields, 40 baseball fields, 145 tennis courts, 6 running courses and 11 swimming pools. Contact: Director, Recreation and Parks Department, Office of the Mayor, Richmond City Hall, Room 201, Richmond, VA 23219.

Parkland/Total City Area (percent)	5

 Richmond did not respond to the school-health survey.

Riverside, CA

🪦	🏃	$	🌲	℞	🏃	👫	?
x	x	x	x	x	?	x	✓

🪦 The Riverside metro area includes San Bernardino, which is located in the County of San Bernardino. Riverside ranks a high 79th in the age-adjusted mortality rate. Heart-attack rates are also high. Infant-mortality rates for California are high among blacks and relatively low among whites. Infant-mortality rates are higher in cities than in rural areas.

	Number	Rank
Age-Adjusted Death Rate	0.79	79/100
Heart Attacks	0.58	84/100
Cancer	0.07	62/100

🏃 Riverside has the 2nd highest rate of accidental deaths and the 10th highest rate of suicides for 100 metro areas. Homicide and robbery rates are in the bottom third of 111 metro areas.

Incidence per 1,000 Pop.	Number	Rank
Homicides (1989; Riverside only)	0.12	83/111
Robberies (1989; Riverside only)	3.95	98/111
Suicides	0.17	91/100
Accidental deaths	0.48	99/100

$ Riverside's 1988 metro population was 2.28 million—16th out of 113 metro areas. Its economic health at the end of 1990 was poor, ranking 96th of 113 metro areas. Its unemployment rate ranks 106th, change in unemployment 104th (the labor force grew even more rapidly than employment) and its enterprise 28th. Contact: Mayor Albert Brown, City of Riverside, 3900 Main Street, Riverside, CA 92522.

🌲 **Air Quality:** The city did not return our air-quality questionnaire. EPA data show that Riverside in 1989 violated NAAQS ceilings for both particulates and ozone. Particulates were 93 μg/m^3, nearly double the standard. Ozone was 0.28 ppm, more than double the standard. Its carbon monoxide was just short of the ceiling, 8 ppm.

Water Quality: 93 percent of Riverside's drinking water comes from ground water sources. The remaining 7 percent comes from surface water. The pH of the drinking water was 7.7 in 1989. The city has a comparatively high nitrate level (22.9 mg/l in 1989) in the drinking water. A drought could result in serious water shortages. Contact: David Garcia, Water Engineering Manager, City of Riverside, 3900 Main Street, Riverside, CA 92522 (714) 782-5285.

Weather: Riverside is centrally located; one hour from Los Angeles, the beach, skiing and Palm Springs. Precipitation is low at around 12 inches annually.

℞ Riverside did not respond to the health-services survey.

Health Resources per 1,000 Pop.	Number	Rank
Hospital beds, community hospitals, city	4.20	81/92
Nurses, community hospitals, city	4.83	74/90
Doctors, metro	1.68	100/113

 Riverside did not respond to the recreational-services survey.

 To serve the 29,000 Riverside public-school students are 10 nurses and 16 psychologists. Nurses are present part-time in all schools. All common health-education programs are offered to students in grades K-12. Of the common screens and tests, the school system provides *only* hearing, vision and scoliosis tests. No medical, dental or psychiatric treatment is provided. Contact: Virginia Brawner, Coordinator, Child Welfare and Attendance, Riverside Unified School District, PO Box 2800, Riverside, CA 92516.

Rochester, NY

🪦 RIP	🚱	$	🌲	℞	🏌	🧑‍🏫	?
✓	✓	✓	✓	✓	✓	✓	✓

🪦 Rochester ranks 65th in the age-adjusted mortality rate. New York has high infant-mortality rates among minorities and in urban areas. Contact: Andrew S. Doniger, Director, Monroe County Health

Department, 111 Westfall Road, Caller 632, Rochester, NY 14692 (716) 274-6077.

	Number	Rank
Age-Adjusted Death Rate	0.42	65/100
Heart Attacks	0.41	81/100
Cancer	0.10	66/100

Rochester has extremely low homicide and accident rates. Robberies and suicides are also below average, making Rochester a fairly safe city to live in.

Incidence per 1,000 Pop.	Number	Rank
Homicides (1989)	0.02	5/111
Robberies (1989)	1.72	38/111
Suicides	0.12	36/100
Accidental deaths	0.28	12/100

Rochester's 1988 metro population was 980,000—44th out of 113 metro areas. Its economic health at the end of 1990 was good, ranking 29th of 113 metro areas. Its unemployment rate ranks 11th, change in unemployment 30th (the labor force shrunk 2.8 percent, slightly faster than employment, which shrunk 2.4 percent) and its enterprise 77th. Contact: Mayor Thomas Ryan, City of Rochester, 30 Church Street, Rochester, NY 14614.

Air Quality: Rochester's air quality is characterized as "good" according to the EPA's Pollution Standards Index (PSI), but the city exceeded the ozone standard in 1988 and in 1989 was on the edge of noncompliance with a ozone level of 0.11 ppm, just below the 0.12 ppm maximum. Compliance depends on the weather. Contact: Richard S. Elliott, P.E., Director of Environmental Health, Monroe County Health Department, 111 Westfall Road, Caller 632, Rochester, NY 14632 (716) 274-6067.

Hazardous Waste: Rochester has one industrial hazardous-waste incinerator and no landfills. Recently there have been investigations of contamination of Kodak properties and local and state Health Departments are in the process of assessing risks to nearby residential areas. Rochester has initiated the collection of household hazardous wastes. Contact: Mark Gregor, Environmental Analyst, City of Rochester, Department of Environmental Services, 30 Church Street, Suite 300-B, Rochester, NY 14614 (716) 428-5978.

Water Quality: Rochester's drinking water supply comes from surface water sources. The pH of the water ranged from 7.0 to 7.5 in 1989. The city will soon complete a new water filtration plant. Contact: Art Wachs, Director, Water Bureau, City of Rochester Department of environmental services, 10 Felix Street, Rochester, NY 14608 (716) 428-7509.

Weather: The average daily temperature is slightly below the national average at 47.9. Humidity and precipitation are slightly above average.

Average Daily Temperature (degrees F)	47.9
High	57.2
Low	38.7
Average Humidity	
Morning (percent)	81
Afternoon (percent)	62
Annual Precipitation (inches)	31.3
Average Total Snowfall (inches)	88.9
Ozone, Days over 0.12 ppm (1 hour, 1988)	1.1

℞ Rochester did not respond to the health-services survey.

Health Resources per 1,000 Pop.	Number	Rank
Hospital beds, community hospitals, city	12.89	10/92
Nurses, community hospitals, city	12.34	15/90
Doctors, metro	2.85	34/113

Rochester has 116 sports facilities per 100,000 residents, ranking it 18th out of 82 cities. In 1987, the city completed construction of a fully enclosed ice arena for ice skating and hockey. In cooperation with the University of Rochester Rowing Club, the city has developed a rowing facility to encourage participation. New sections of hiking trails have been developed along the Genesee River. Softball and volleyball are the most popular organized sports and ice hockey and ice skating are also gaining popularity. Lake Ontario sport fishing has become increasingly popular over the past ten years. Sports facilities include 102 baseball fields, 35 football/soccer fields, 64 basketball courts, 65 tennis courts, 3 golf courses, 11 running tracks, 5 ice rinks and 26 swimming pools. Contact: Thomas August, Commissioner, Department of Parks, Recreation and Human Services, City Hall, 30 Church Street, Room 200-B, Rochester, NY 14614 (716) 428-6750.

Parkland/Total City Area (percent)	13.6

 Rochester employs 39 nurses, 2 physicians, 50 social workers, 93 speech/language teachers, 2 audiologists, 20 occupational and physical therapists and assistants, 7 child-development assistants, 56 psychologists and 34 school-health aides in its public-school system of 32,000 students. The school system's AIDS policy and guidelines have been revised to include district employees as well as students. The school system offers a comprehensive health education program (including AIDS education) to students in grades K-6, 7 and 11. No medical or psychiatric treatment is provided. The school system requires but does not perform immunizations; it obtains 99 percent compliance on school entry. Well-child physical exams are conducted for school children the Monroe County Health Department. The school system provides all common screens and tests except for immunizations. Dental treatment is provided only for students in the district under contract with the Monroe County Health Department. Contact: Joan Willis, Director of Pupil Personnel Services, Rochester City School District, 131 West Broad Street, Rochester, NY 14614 (716) 325-4560.

Sacramento, CA

🪦 RIP	🔻	$	↟	℞	🏃	🏖	?
✔	✓	✓	X	✓	?	X	✓

Sacramento (Sacramento County) has the 10th best age-adjusted mortality rate of 100 metro areas. Heart-attack and cancer rates are also very low, ranking 11/100 and 15/100, respectively. Infant-mortality rates for California are high among blacks and relatively low among whites. Infant-mortality rates are higher in cities than in rural areas.

	Number	Rank
Age-Adjusted Death Rate	−1.95	10/100
Heart Attacks	−0.67	11/100
Cancer	−0.35	15/100

 Sacramento has a high number of suicides and robberies. Homicide and accident rates, however, are relatively low.

Incidence per 1,000 Pop.	Number	Rank
Homicides (1989)	0.06	39/111
Robberies (1989)	3.89	62/111
Suicides	0.14	70/100
Accidental deaths	0.29	20/100

| $ | Sacramento's 1988 metro population was 1.38 million—32nd out of 113 metro areas. Its economic health at the end of 1990 was below |

Sacramento's 1988 metro population was 1.38 million—32nd out of 113 metro areas. Its economic health at the end of 1990 was below average, ranking 74th of 113 metro areas. Its unemployment rate ranks 81st, change in unemployment 71st (the labor force grew by 2.1 percent, substantially faster than employment, which grew by 1.5 percent) and its enterprise 34th. Contact: Mayor Anne Rudin, City of Sacramento, 915 I Street, #205, Sacramento, CA 95814.

Air Quality: Sacramento was out of compliance in 1989 with two pollutants. It exceeded ozone standards 30 days in 1988. The city also exceeded carbon monoxide standards 10 days in 1988. In 1989 its carbon monoxide level was 13 ppm, exceeding by a substantial margin the NAAQS maximum of 9 ppm. Its 1989 ozone level was 0.14, again exceeding the NAAQS ceiling of 0.12 ppm. Particulate levels were also high in 1989. Contact: Norman Covell, County Air Quality Officer, County of Sacramento, 8475 Jackson Road, Room 220, Sacramento, CA 95814.

Hazardous Waste: Sacramento has three sites on the EPA's Superfund list: Southern Pacific Transportation Co. (copper, lead, zinc), Union Pacific Railroad Yard (asbestos, arsenic, cadmium, zinc), and Pacific Gas and Electric (lamp black). In 1991 no facilities in Sacramento County were capable of legally disposing of hazardous waste. Aerojet General Corp. and Pacific Gas and Electric have applied for State Health Department and EPA permits to incinerate hazardous material on the site where they produce waste. Contact: Reginald Young, Deputy Director, Public Works, 915 I Street, Sacramento, CA 95814.

Water Quality: Surface water provides Sacramento with 85 percent of its drinking water. The other 15 percent comes from ground water sources. The pH of the drinking water is 8.6. Contact: Reginald Young, address cited above.

Weather: With low humidity, mild winters and hot but not uncomfortable summers, Sacramento has a very pleasant climate. It almost never snows, and freezing days number about 14 a year; on the other extreme, Sacramento has only about a month and a half of days in the 90s each year.

Average Daily Temperature (degrees F)	60.6
High	73.4
Low	47.8
Average Humidity	
Morning (percent)	82
Afternoon (percent)	46
Annual Precipitation (inches)	17.10

Average Total Snowfall (inches)   0.1
Ozone, Days over 0.12 ppm (1 hour, 1988)   30

℞ Sacramento has increased its AIDS and prenatal services. The county has also increased medical services in jails. The county provides all common preventive-health services and treatment programs. Anti-smoking laws in the city include partial restriction in restaurants, public offices and private offices. Smoking on public transportation is prohibited. The city offers all common health-education programs (except sexually transmitted diseases) to residents. The county provides all common emergency hotlines (except an alcoholism emergency hotline). Contact: Bette Hinton, M.D., Director of Health, County Health Department, 3701 Branch Center Road, Sacramento, CA 95827.

Health Resources per 1,000 Pop.	Number	Rank
Hospital beds, community hospitals, city	6.49	50/91
Nurses, community hospitals, city	8.92	30/90
Doctors, metro	2.32	65/113

Current recreational development is focused on spectator sports. Sacramento did not return the recreational-facilities questionnaire.

Sacramento's public-school system employs 35 nurses for its 47,000 students. Nurses are present full-time in 5 percent of the schools and part-time in 95 percent of the schools. A Tobacco-Free School District Policy was passed. The school system also has a policy for the admission of children with HIV/AIDS. The schools provide all common screens and tests except for immunizations, mental-health exams and speech therapy. They also conduct TB skin tests. No medical, dental or psychiatric treatment is provided for students. Contact: Keith T. Larick, Superintendent, Sacramento City Unified School District, PO Box 2271, Sacramento, CA 95812.

Salt Lake City, UT

🪦	✈	$	🌲	℞	🏃	👫	?
✔	✔	✔	X	✓	?	X	✓

Salt Lake City (Salt Lake County) has the 7th best age-adjusted mortality rate of 100 metro areas. Cancer and heart attack rates are also amazingly low, ranking 2/100 and 8/100, respectively. The overall infant-mortality rate for Utah is lower than normal. Infant-mortality rates among blacks are only slightly higher than among whites. Infant-mortality rates among other minorities are lower than those among whites. Rates are higher in rural areas than in cities.

	Number	Rank
Age-Adjusted Death Rate	−2.46	7/100
Heart Attacks	−0.77	8/100
Cancer	−0.78	2/100

Salt Lake City has the 11th lowest homicide rate and the 11th lowest robbery rate of 111 metro areas. However, the suicide rate for the city is very high.

Incidence per 1,000 Pop.	Number	Rank
Homicides (1989)	0.03	11/111
Robberies (1989)	0.78	11/111
Suicides	0.16	87/100
Accidental deaths	0.32	46/100

Salt Lake City's 1988 metro population was 1,065,000—43rd out of 113 metro areas. Its economic health at the end of 1990 was ranked 25th of 113 metro areas. Its unemployment rate ranked 14th, change in unemployment 34th (employment grew by 3.4 percent, faster than the labor force, 3.1 percent) and its enterprise 61st. Contact: Mayor Palmer DePaulis, Salt Lake City, 300 City-County Building, Salt Lake City, UT 84111.

Air Quality: Salt Lake City in 1989 was out of compliance with two pollutants. It exceeded ozone standards one day in 1988. It was recently discovered that PM10 (total suspended particles) is also a problem in Salt Lake County. Regulations will be in place in 1991 that are expected to reduce emissions from all major PM10 sources substantially. In 1988, the city exceeded PM10 standards for 3 days and carbon monoxide standards for 1 day. Air-pollution strategies have significantly reduced ozone and carbon monoxide air pollution and the city and county expect carbon monoxide attainment by 1993 and ozone attainment by 1995. Contact: Jim Brande, Director of Air Quality, Salt Lake City-County Health Department, 610 South 200 East, Salt Lake City, UT 84111.

Water Quality: Salt Lake City has increased monitoring and surveillance of surface water watershed areas. There is a possible trend toward increased total dissolved solids in wells. Surface water provides 80 percent of the city's drinking water; ground water supplies 15 percent and the remaining

5 percent is supplied by natural springs. The pH of the water was 8.1 in 1989. Contact: Leroy Hooten, Director, Salt Lake City Public Utilities, 1530 South-West Temple, Salt Lake City, UT 84115.

Weather: Salt Lake City's climate has its extremes: hot summers (but with low humidity) and cold winters with lots of snow. Each year there are several zero-degree days, over 100 freezing days and about a month and a half of days in the 90s.

Average Daily Temperature (degrees F)	51.7
High	64
Low	39.3
Average Humidity	
Morning (percent)	67
Afternoon (percent)	43
Annual Precipitation (inches)	15.31
Average Total Snowfall (inches)	58.2
Ozone, Days over 0.12 ppm (one hour in 1988)	1

℞ Health care in the Salt Lake area is of high quality and low cost. Health Department clinics in the city have been reorganized to be multi-dimensional full health clinic facilities (medical services, treatment of sexually transmitted diseases, immunizations). The city sponsors awareness campaigns for cholesterol, Earth Day, Public Health Awareness Week, and physical fitness (bike to work with the mayor). The city provides medical assistance and clinical care to the homeless, co-sponsored with private organizations. At homeless shelters, medical care is provided daily. All common health-education programs and emergency hotlines are provided by the city. Recently, environmental and recycling campaigns have been popular. The county provides all common preventive-health services and treatment programs, *except* treatment for alcoholism (if you maneuver past the Mormon-inspired attempts to make alcohol hard to get to, and then you drink too much, you are on your own). The city's anti-smoking laws include partial restrictions in restaurants and private offices. Smoking on public transportation and in public offices is prohibited. Contact: Dr. Harry Gibbons, Salt Lake City County Health Department, 610 South 200 East, Salt Lake City, UT 84111.

Health Resources per 1,000 Pop.	Number	Rank
Doctors, metro	2.31	66/113

In addition to its strong economy and relatively-low-to-average cost of living, Salt Lake City has great scenic beauty. The city and environs are a sports paradise. Though unparalleled in its proximity to powder-covered ski slopes in the winter, Salt Lake City also is home to hikers who venture into the area's eight canyons during the summer. Salt Lake City does have a long, snowy winter, but the summer is more than long enough for residents to make use of the city's 14 golf courses, 253 football/soccer fields, 134 baseball fields, 58 softball fields, 57 volleyball courts, 23 handball/racquetball courts, 2 ice skating rinks, 28 quarter-mile tracks, 30 swimming pools and 14 recreation centers. The fact that the Mormon majority frowns on drinking alcoholic beverages and the state has laws prohibiting privately owned package stores and liquor by the drink sets a healthy tone for the area—although drinking does go on in members-only clubs that are easily joined.

An elementary health curriculum is currently being written for Salt Lake City's lower schools. Plans are under way to update CPR and First Aid training for staff members. The school system employs 2 nurses and 1 health aide to provide for its 24,266 students. Nurses are on call full-time in all of the schools. All common health-education programs, including AIDS education, are offered to students in grades K-7 and 10. The school system provides all common screens and tests except for mental-health exams and well-child physical exams. It conducts a two-year growth study in elementary schools. Medical treatment is provided for students. Contact: Salt Lake City School District, 440 East 100 South, Salt Lake City, UT 84111.

San Antonio, TX

RIP	🏃	$	🌲	℞	🏃	👥	?
✓	X	X	✔	✓	?	?	XX

San Antonio ranks a middling 43rd in the age-adjusted mortality rate. Infant-mortality rates for Texas are high among minorities and relatively low among whites. Infant-mortality rates are higher in cities than in rural areas of the state.

	Number	Rank
Age-Adjusted Death Rate	−0.28	43/100
Heart Attacks	−0.26	34/100
Cancer	−0.11	39/100

San Antonio has a very high homicide rate (95/111), but the suicide rate is below average. Rates for robberies and accidents are average.

Incidence per 1,000 Pop.	Number	Rank
Homicides	0.14	95/111
Robberies	2.22	64/111
Suicides	0.11	28/100
Accidental deaths	0.33	48/100

$ San Antonio's 1988 metro population was 1,323,000—35th out of 113 metro areas. Its economic health at the end of 1990 was poor. It ranks 103rd of 113 metro areas. Its unemployment rate ranks 105th, change in unemployment 71st (labor force grew slightly, employment shrank slightly) and its enterprise 86th. Contact: Mayor Lila Cockrell, City of San Antonio, City Hall, San Antonio, TX.

Air Quality: San Antonio did not respond to the air-quality survey. EPA data indicate that its air quality is within NAAQS maxima. Its 1989 ozone level was 0.11 ppm, below the 0.12 NAAQS maximum. Carbon monoxide was 7 ppm, below the 9 ppm standard. Particulate pollution was about half of the NAAQS maximum.

Water Quality: San Antonio did not provide up-to-date information, but *The Book of American City Rankings* (Facts on File, 1983) lists its dissolved solids as a relatively high 386 mg/l, among the highest dozen of 63 cities; this contributes to turbidity. The city also had the 8th highest concentration of dissolved minerals, 237 ppm, which makes for very hard water. Water above 180 ppm requires softening before use. The city also had a high pH factor of 8.2. San Antonio also had the 14th highest concentration of nitrates of 66 cities.

Weather: The average temperature in San Antonio is warm at 68.7 degrees. Humidity is also above average.

Average Daily Temperature (degrees F)	68.7
High	79.6
Low	57.8
Average Humidity	
Morning (percent)	83
Afternoon (percent)	55
Annual Precipitation (inches)	29.13
Average Total Snowfall (inches)	0.8

Health Resources per 1,000 Pop.	Number	Rank
Doctors, metro	2.27	68/113

℞ San Antonio did not respond to any of the environmental, health services, recreational services, or school health questionnaires.

San Diego, CA

RIP	⚡	$	♠	℞	🏃	🏖	?
✓	✓	✓	X	✓	?	✔	✓

 San Diego (San Diego County) ranks a relatively low 37th in the age-adjusted mortality rate. Infant-mortality rates for California are high among blacks and relatively low among whites. Infant-mortality rates are higher in cities than in rural areas of the state.

	Number	Rank
Age-Adjusted Death Rate	−0.59	37/100
Heart Attacks	−0.01	54/100
Cancer	−0.04	45/100

⚡ San Diego has about average rates for homicides, suicides and accidents. San Diego's robberies rate is slightly above average.

Incidence per 1,000 Pop.	Number	Rank
Homicides (1989)	0.08	55/111
Robberies (1989)	2.32	67/111
Suicides	0.13	54/100
Accidental deaths	0.33	53/100

$ San Diego's 1988 metro population was 2,370,000—14th out of 113 metro areas. Its economic health at the end of 1990 was below average, ranking 62nd of 113 metro areas. Its unemployment rate ranks 70th, change in unemployment 88th (the labor force grew faster than employment) and its enterprise 11th. Contact: Mayor Maureen O'Conner, City of San Diego, 202 C Street, San Diego, CA 92101.

Air Quality: While downtown San Diego experienced only 2 days of ozone exceedances in 1988, the surrounding areas of Alpine, Del Mar, El Cajon and Oceanside exceedances ranged from 7 to 34 days. Contact: Mahmood I. Hossain, Senior Air Pollution Chemist, Air Pollution Control District, 9150 Chesapeake Drive, San Diego, CA 92123.

Hazardous Waste: San Diego has no active or inactive waste sites. In 1986, 39,359 tons of hazardous waste were generated. 200,000 tons of this came from a single location and consisted of a single pile of automobile shredded waste that is still on-site pending a final decision of disposal. Permanent household hazardous waste collection sites is a current priority for the city. Six planned locations in Orange County (one in San Diego), were scheduled to be opened in April, 1990. Unfortunately, there has been an alarming increase in illegal dumping of hazardous waste on public and private properties. There is a need for economical waste disposal for the small generator businesses. Contact: Rich Hays, Director of Waste Management, City of San Diego, 525 B Street, San Diego, CA 92101.

Water Quality: San Diego's water supply comes from surface water sources, except for 0.1 percent which comes from ground water sources. The city has increased monitoring for trace organic chemicals. Contact: Roger Frauenfelder, Deputy City Manager, City of San Diego, 202 C Street, San Diego, CA 92101.

Weather: San Diego enjoys mild weather with few extreme fluctuations in temperature—no freezing days and only a handful of days in the 90s during the year. It has relatively few rainy days.

Average Daily Temperature (degrees F)	63.8
High	70.5
Low	57.0
Average Humidity	
Morning (percent)	76
Afternoon (percent)	62
Annual Precipitation (inches)	9.3
Average Total Snowfall (inches)	Trace
Ozone, Days over 0.12 ppm (1 hour in 1988)	2

Smoking is prohibited on all public transportation and public offices. It is partially restricted in restaurants and private offices. Public awareness campaigns are in effect against AIDS, sexually transmitted diseases, smoking, seat belts, immunizations, household hazardous materials, child health and child passenger safety seats. The county sponsors a peer-education program for AIDS education. It also established an AIDS Prevention and Follow-up Center to provide HIV-infected persons with preventive medical care and educational programs. San Diego County opened a new psychiatric hospital in 1989. All common health-education programs and emergency hotlines are sponsored by the county, *except* that the county does no cholesterol testing. Telephone-information lines are available for influenza vaccinations. The county provides all common preventive-health services and treatment programs. Contact: Dr. J. William Cox, Director, San Diego County Department of Health Services, 1700 Pacific Highway, San Diego, CA 92101.

Health Resources per 1,000 Pop.	Number	Rank
Hospital beds, community hospitals, city	4.71	71/91
Doctors, metro	2.51	51/113

The city's sports facilities include 50 baseball fields, 43 football/soccer fields, 43 basketball courts, 128 tennis courts, 16 swimming pools and 4 golf courses. San Diego also has 43 miles of beach and bay front areas for fun in the sun. Contact: George Loveland, Director, Parks & Recreation Department, Balboa Park, San Diego, CA 92101.

Parkland/Total City Area (percent)	1.7

The San Diego public-school system employs 125 nurses, 2 physicians, 60 psychologists and 61 health aides for its 121,000 students. Nurses are present full-time in 40 percent of the schools and part-time in the remainder of the schools. All common health-education programs are offered to students in grades K-6, 8 and 10. AIDS education is taught to students in grades 6-12. The school system coordinates treatment programs with private physicians. The school system provides all common screens and tests. Contact: Ed Fletcher, Director, San Diego City Schools, 2716 Marsi Avenue, San Diego, CA 92113.

San Francisco, CA

⚰️ RIP	🛏️	$	↑	℞	🏌️	👥	?
✔	✔	✔	✔	✔	X	X	✔

San Francisco (San Francisco County) metro area ranks 27th in the age-adjusted mortality rate. Heart attack and cancer rates are relatively low, ranking 15th and 29th, respectively. Infant-mortality rates for

California are high among blacks and other minorities and low among whites. Infant-mortality rates are higher in cities than in rural areas of the state. Contact: Jeanne Duggan, Vital Statistics, Department of Public Health, 101 Grove Street, San Francisco, CA 94102.

	Number	Rank
Age-Adjusted Death Rate	−0.98	27/100
Heart Attacks	−0.53	15/100
Cancer	−0.17	29/100

 San Francisco ranks in at a high 95th for robberies and 80th for suicide. Accident rates are also above average.

Incidence per 1,000 Pop.	Number	Rank
Homicides (1989)	0.07	50/111
Robberies (1989)	3.68	95/111
Suicides	0.15	80/100
Accidental deaths	0.35	65/100

$ San Francisco's 1988 metro population was 1,590,000—27th out of 113 metro areas. Its economic health at the end of 1990 was good, ranking 36th of 113 metro areas. Its unemployment rate ranks 17th, change in unemployment 58th (employment fell faster than the labor force) and its enterprise 55th. Contact: Mayor Art Agnos, City of San Francisco, City Hall, Room 200, San Francisco, CA 94102.

Air Quality: Air quality has been good for the past decade, except for one or two isolated carbon monoxide buildups on stagnant fall or winter nights. San Francisco exceeded the carbon-monoxide standard only once in 1988. In 1989 San Francisco's PSI remained below 100 all year (it had been one day above 100 in 1988). Its 1989 ozone level was 0.09 ppm, comfortably below the 0.12 ppm NAAQS maximum. The city's nitrogen dioxide level at 0.026 ppm was half the NAAQS maximum. Carbon mono-dioxide level at 0.026 ppm was half the NAAQS maximum. Carbon monoxide, however, was at 8 ppm, just below the 9 ppm NAAQS standard. g/m^3, well within the NAAQS maximum of 50 $\mu g/m^3$. Contact: Ted McHugh, Director of Public Information, Bay Area Air Quality Management Control Board, 99 Ellis Street, San Francisco, CA 94109.

Hazardous Waste: There are no hazardous waste sites in San Francisco on the EPA's National Priorities List for "Superfund"; however, one site, Hunter's Point Naval Shipyard, is proposed. Contact: Bill Lee, Director of Toxics, Health and Safety Services, City & County of San Francisco, 101 Grove Street, Rm. 207, San Francisco, CA 94102.

Weather: The Bay Area has a pleasant, mild, two-season climate. Compared to Los Angeles, it is free of the uncomfortably hot summer weather. Compared to Seattle, it has fewer days of freezing weather.

Average Daily Temperature (degrees F)	56.6
High	64.9
Low	48.3
Average Humidity	
Morning (percent)	84
Afternoon (percent)	62
Annual Precipitation (inches)	19.7
Average Total Snowfall (inches)	Trace
PSI, Days above 100, 1988	1
PSI, Days above 100, 1989	0

℞ The overall quality of health care in San Francisco is high. With one of the finest medical schools in the country at the University of California at San Francisco (UCSF), the city attracts exceptionally talented and committed physicians and students. Thirteen acute-care hospitals are located in the city. The city has fluoridated water and only minimal air pollution. It also supports nonsmokers rights in restaurants, worksites, and public places. Contact: San Francisco Department of Health, 101 Grove Street, San Francisco, CA 94102.

Health Resources per 1,000 Pop.	Number	Rank
Hospital beds, community hospitals, city	7.29	41/91
Nurses, community hospitals, city	5.84	60/90
Doctors, metro	4.97	5/113

San Francisco has 41 sports facilities per 100,000 residents, ranking the city a poor 73rd out of 82 metro areas. The sports facilities include 151 tennis courts, 68 basketball courts, 66 baseball/softball fields, 18 football/soccer fields, 9 swimming pools, 5 golf courses and 2 running tracks; it has four beaches and a marina that provide a place for boat launches, pier fishing and water sports. Contact: Mary Burns, Director, Recreation & Parks Department, McLaren Lodge, Golden Gate Park, San Francisco, CA 94117.

The San Francisco Unified School System employs 10.4 nurses and 11 health aides to service 63,000 students. All common health-education programs are taught to students in grades K-12. The city provides all common screens and tests. Contact Dr. Beverly Bradley, Health Program Supervisor, SF Unified, 1512 Golden Gate Ave., San Francisco, CA 94115 (415) 749-3400.

San Jose, CA

⚰️ RIP	⚡	$	🌲	℞	🚑	👪	?
✔	✔	✔	✗	✔	✗	✔	✓

 San Jose (Santa Clara County) metro area includes Fremont. It ranks 21st in the age-adjusted mortality rate. Infant-mortality rates for California are high among blacks and relatively low among whites. Infant-mortality rates are higher in cities than in rural areas of the state.

	Number	Rank
Age-Adjusted Death Rate	−1.19	21/100
Heart Attacks	−0.31	28/100
Cancer	−0.19	27/100

San Jose has a relatively low homicide and robbery rates, a middling suicide rate.

Incidence per 1,000 Pop.	Number	Rank
Homicides	.04	17/111
Robberies	1.02	16/111
Suicides	.12	40/100
Accidental deaths	.05	14/100

$ San Jose's 1988 metro population was 1,432,000—30th out of 113 metro areas. Its economic health at the end of 1990 was good, ranking 34th of 113 metro areas. Its unemployment rate ranks 44th, change in unemployment 78th (employment declined even faster than the labor force) and its enterprise 4th. Contact: Mayor Thomas McEnery, City of San Jose, 801 North 1st Street, San Jose, CA 95110.

Air Quality: In 1988, San Jose exceeded the NAAQS carbon monoxide standard twice. In 1989 its carbon monoxide level was 12 ppm, well above the NAAQS maximum of 9 ppm and its ozone level was 0.13 ppm, above the NAAQS ceiling of 0.12 ppm. Particulates are also quite high, 41 $\mu g/m^3$.

Hazardous Waste: San Jose did not respond. Fremont has a household hazardous-waste disposal program. A substantial reduction of quantity and toxicity of hazardous waste in Fremont resulted from corporate and industrial recycling efforts. Contact: Elizabeth Stowe, Hazardous Materials Administrator, City of Fremont, 39572 Stevenson Place, Suite 125, Fremont, CA 94538.

Water Quality: San Jose did not return the water-quality survey, but *The Book of American City Rankings* (1983) lists its nitrate level as the second-worst of 66 cities, 15 mg/l. EPA is paying more attention to nitrates as a pollutant and is upgrading them to a primary pollutant starting in 1992.

Weather: San Jose is on the inland side of the bay, whereas San Francisco is at the mouth, but otherwise their pleasant climate is similar—mild weather for most of the year, with two-month winters.

Average Daily Temperature (degrees F)	56.7
High	62.5
Low	51.0
Average Humidity	
Morning (percent)	85
Afternoon (percent)	66
Annual Precipitation (inches)	19.33
Average Total Snowfall (inches)	Trace
Ozone Days over 0.12 ppm, Fremont (1 hour in 1988)	1

℞ San Jose did not respond to the health-services survey. Fremont prohibits smoking in public offices and partially prohibits smoking in restaurants and on public transportation. Contact: Yvonne Ingram, Fitness and Wellness Officer, City of Fremont, 39700 Civic Center Drive, Fremont, CA 94531.

Health Resources per 1,000 Pop.	Number	Rank
Doctors, metro (San Jose-Fremont)	2.85	33/113

San Jose has only 23 sports facilities per 100,000 residents giving it the 2nd lowest ranking (81/82 cities). The Camden Lifetime Activities Center features a fitness and wellness program and was the first city-owned and operated gymnasium/weight room. The city offers classes and programs in hiking/exploration and aerobics. San Jose Youth Services provides many activities and programs throughout the city. The San Jose Office on Aging offers programs and services for senior citizens. The city's sports facilities include 55 basketball courts, 52 sports fields (softball, football, soccer), 61 tennis courts, 12 swimming pools and 5 golf courses. Fremont's 5-km. walk and 10-km. run are especially popular. Fremont has established a walking club. Contact: Brad Brown, Planner, Recreation, Parks and Community Services, 333 West Santa Clara Street, Suite 800, San Jose, CA 95113. Or: Jack Rogers, Director, City of Fremont Leisure Services, 3375 Country Drive, Fremont, CA 94536.

Parkland/Total City Area (percent)   15.1

San Jose's public-school system employs 12 nurses, 12 psychologists, 13 elementary counselors and 41 health aides for its 28,548 students. Fremont has twice San Francisco's nursing staff for half the number of pupils—6 nurses, 12 psychologists and 7 program specialists for its 26,682 students. Fremont students are provided with some medical services. A full-time nurse is available in 25 percent of Fremont schools; a school nurse, counselor and health aide work together as a team with at-risk students. Fremont offers health-education programs to students in grades K-12. It provides first aid services when trained staff or a nurse is available. The Fremont school system provides all common screens and tests except for mental-health exams. Contact: M. Thomas, Supervisor of Health Services, San Jose Unified School District, 1605 Park Avenue, Building 2, San Jose, CA 95126. Or: Bill Walker, Director of Pupil Services, Fremont Unified School District, 4210 Technology Drive, Fremont, CA 94538.

Savannah, GA

🪦	⚰	$	🌲	℞	🎿	👥	?
?	X	✔	✔	X	✔	✔	✓

Savannah (in Chatham County) was not ranked using the age-adjusted death rate. Infant-mortality rates for Georgia are very high among minorities and moderate among whites. Infant-mortality rates are much higher in cities than in rural areas of the state.

Savannah's homicide and robbery rates are slightly above average.

Incidence per 1,000 Pop.	Number	Rank
Homicides (1989)	0.10	78/111
Robberies (1989)	2.58	69/111

Savannah's 1988 metro population was 244,000—100th out of 113 metro areas. Its economic health at the end of 1990 was excellent, ranking 14th of 113 metro areas. Its unemployment rate ranks 40th, change in unemployment 12th (employment grew faster than the labor force, which barely increased) and its enterprise 39th. Contact: Mayor John P. Rousakis, City of Savannah, City Hall, Savannah, GA 31402.

Weather: The average temperature is a warm 65.9 degrees. Humidity and precipitation are high.

Average Daily Temperature (degrees F)	65.9
High	76.7
Low	55.1
Average Humidity	
Morning	85
Afternoon	53
Annual Precipitation (inches)	49.7
Average Total Snowfall (inches)	0.3

 Savannah did not respond to the health-services survey.

Health Resources per 1,000 Pop.	Number	Rank
Doctors, metro	2.02	81/113

Savannah has 130 sports facilities per 100,000 residents, ranking 15 out of 82 metro areas. Savannah is only 17 miles from the ocean and public beaches, marinas and fishing facilities. The city offers several recreation and arts programs for children. Supervised playgrounds are provided year-round. Recreational programming has been taken into public housing communities to provide physical and cultural alternatives for leisure time with major emphasis on drug awareness programs. Savannah's sports facilities include 66 basketball courts, 44 baseball fields, 41 football/soccer fields, 39 tennis courts, 13 swimming pools and 1 golf course. Half-rubber, a stick ball game originated in Savannah, has become increasingly popular. Contact: Joe Shearouse, Director, City of Savannah Leisure Services Bureau, PO Box 1027, Savannah, GA 31402.

Parkland/Total City Area (percent)	1.0

The school system employs 42 nurses, 12 psychologists, 66 counselors and 8 social workers for its 33,318 students. 79 percent of the schools have a full-time nurse and 21 percent have a part-time nurse. All common health-education programs are offered to students in grades K-12. The school system provides all common screens and tests except for immunizations, mental-health exams and well-child physical exams. Medical and dental treatment is provided for students. The "New Futures Initiative" is a new program addressing students at risk of becoming pregnant, failing or dropping out of school. Contact: Donna Vincent, Savannah-Chatham Board of Education, 208 Bull Street, Room 213, Savannah, GA 31401.

Seattle-Tacoma, WA

RIP	✈	$	🌲	R̶	🏃	👫	?
✔	✔	✔	✔	✔	?	?	X

Seattle (King County) has the 8th lowest age-adjusted mortality rate. Heart attack and cancer rates are also extremely low, 3/100 and 11/100 respectively. Tacoma (Pierce County) ranks 31st in the age-adjusted mortality rate. Infant-mortality rates for Washington are high among minorities and relatively low among whites. Infant-mortality rates are higher in cities than in rural areas of the state.

	Number	Rank
Age-Adjusted Death Rate		
Seattle	−2.22	8/100
Tacoma	−0.84	31/100
Heart Attacks		
Seattle	−0.94	3/100
Tacoma	−0.51	16/100
Cancer		
Seattle	−0.45	11/100
Tacoma	−0.13	35/100

Seattle has the 17th lowest homicide rate of 111 metro areas. Accident rates for Seattle city are relatively low; suicide rates are slightly above average. Tacoma has the 5th highest suicide rate among cities. Rates for robberies in Tacoma are also high.

Incidence per 1,000 Pop.	Number	Rank
Homicides (1989)—Seattle	0.04	17/111
Tacoma	0.08	58/111
Robberies (1989)—Seattle	1.84	49/111
Tacoma	2.94	84/111

Suicides—Seattle	0.14	68/100
Tacoma	0.19	96/100
Accidental deaths—Seattle	0.32	33/100
Tacoma	0.31	25/100

$ Seattle's 1988 metro population was 1.86 million—23rd out of 113 metro areas. Its economic health at the end of 1990 was excellent, ranking 4th of 113 metro areas. Its unemployment rate ranks 14th, change in unemployment 19th (employment grew by a healthy 6.3 percent while the labor force fell behind at 5.5 percent) and its enterprise 26th. Nearby Tacoma's 1988 metro population was 559,000—73rd out of 113 metro areas. Its economic health at the end of 1990, in contrast to that of Seattle, was below average, ranking 78th of 113 metro areas. Its unemployment rate ranks 56th, change in unemployment 22nd (employment grew 3.6 percent, the labor force 2.9 percent) and its enterprise 113th. Contact: Mayor Norman Rice, City of Seattle, City Hall, Seattle, WA 98104. Or: Mayor Doug Sutherland, City of Tacoma, 747 Market Street, Suite 1220, Tacoma, WA 98402.

▲ **Air Quality:** Air pollution associated with the fast population growth of the area has offset improvements made in restricting emissions from point sources. In 1989 Seattle's Pollutant Standards Index (PSI) exceeded the 100 ceiling on 4 days, down from 8 in 1988. The city's ozone level in 1989 was acceptable at 0.09 ppm, below the 0.12 ppm ceiling, but its carbon monoxide was unacceptable at 13 ppm, well above the NAAQS ceiling of 9 ppm. Contact: Lou Dooley, Director, Environmental Health Division, Tacoma-Pierce County Health Department, 3629 South D Street, Mail Stop EH-3118, Tacoma, WA 98408.

Hazardous Waste: Pierce County has 7 EPA Superfund sites. But no regulated hazardous waste has been disposed of in the county since 1987. Contact: Lou Dooley, Director, Environmental Health Division, Tacoma-Pierce County Health Department, 3629 South D Street, Mail Stop EH-3118, Tacoma, WA 98408.

Weather: People in Seattle have less to talk about weather-wise than elsewhere because the weather tends to be cloudy and mild, year-round. Because of its proximity to the ocean and to an inland lake, Seattle proper doesn't get much snow. The city has an average of 160 rainy days per year and annual rainfall of 39 inches.

Average Daily Temperature (degrees F)	52.7
High	59.7
Low	45.6

Average Humidity	
Morning (percent)	82
Afternoon (percent)	62
Annual Precipitation (inches)	38.8
Average Total Snowfall (inches)	7.4
PSI, Days over 100, 1988	8
PSI, Days over 100, 1989	4

℞ Health care in Seattle is of high quality and low cost. Area facilities include five teaching hospitals, a medical school and specialized treatment centers for cardiac ailments and cancer. Tacoma and Pierce County established 3 medical centers for the homeless and dental clinics for low income adults and families. They sponsor awareness campaigns for smoking and AIDS, lifestyles and health, and the health professions. They provide all common health-education programs. They sponsor emergency hotlines for child abuse, suicide and alcoholism as well as a general emergency hotline. Tacoma and Pierce County provide all common preventive-health and treatment programs except food for the needy. Smoking is prohibited on public transportation and partially restricted in restaurants, public offices and private offices. Contact: Nancy Cherry, Assistant Director, Community Policy Development, Tacoma-Pierce County Health Department, 3701 Pacific Avenue, Mail Stop Ad-3111, Tacoma, WA 98408.

Health Resources per 1,000 Pop.

(Seattle, 1988)	**Number**	**Rank**
Hospital beds, community hospitals, city	6.84	46/91
Nurses, community hospitals, city	8.89	31/90
Doctors, metro	3.00	24/113

Seattle did not respond to the recreational-services survey or the school-health survey.

 Tacoma employs 29 nurses, 1 physician and 2 audiologists for its 29,500 students. Nurses are present full-time in all high schools and part-time in all other schools. All common health-education programs are offered to students. The school system provides all screens and tests except for immunization and well-child physical exams. Contact: Donna L. Gamble, M.N., Coordinator of Health Services, Tacoma Public Schools, PO Box 1357, Tacoma, WA 98401.

Shreveport, LA

🪦	⚰	$	↟	℞	🏚	👥	?
X	X	X	✔	✓	X	✓	✔

🪦 Shreveport (Caddo Parish) ranks an unhealthy 92nd in the age-adjusted mortality rate. Heart attack and cancer rates for Shreveport are also extremely high. Infant-mortality rates for Louisiana are high among minorities and relatively low among whites. Infant-mortality rates are higher in cities than in rural areas of the state.

	Number	Rank
Age-Adjusted Death Rate	2.14	92/100
Heart Attacks	0.80	93/100
Cancer	0.58	93/100

⚰ Shreveport has the 4th highest homicide rate of 111 metro areas and the 6th highest accident rate of 100 metro areas. Robbery and suicide rates are closer to the median of the communities we surveyed.

Incidence per 1,000 Pop.	Number	Rank
Homicides (1989)	0.20	108/111
Robberies (1989)	2.64	72/111
Suicides	0.12	47/100
Accidental deaths	0.46	95/100

$ Shreveport's 1988 metro population was 359,000—92nd out of 113 metro areas. Its economic health at the end of 1990 was below average but has shown recent improvement. It ranks 85th of 113 metro areas. Its unemployment rate ranks 96th, change in unemployment 3rd (employment barely increased, but the labor force dropped over 2 percent) and its enterprise an unpromising 112th. Contact: Mayor Hazel Beard, City of Shreveport, PO Box 31109, Shreveport, LA 71130.

↟ **Air Quality:** Shreveport was in compliance with NAAQS limits, although its ozone level was 0.12 ppm, very close to noncompliance.

Hazardous Waste: No hazardous-waste-disposal sites have been named in northwest Louisiana. Citizens of Shreveport are becoming more aware of how to dispose of their hazardous waste. Contact: Monroe Penrod, Environmental Coordinator, Department of Environmental Quality, 1525 Fairfield Avenue, Room 11, Shreveport, LA 71101.

Water Quality: All of the water supply in Shreveport is surface water (e.g., reservoirs). The city has added an ozonation plant to improve the quality of the water. Contact: Glen Shelton, Water Programs Supervisor, Health Department Northwest Regional Office, 1525 Fairfield Avenue, Shreveport, LA 71130.

Weather: The average temperature is warm at 65.4. Humidity and precipitation are high.

Average Daily Temperature (degrees F)	65.4
High	76.2
Low	54.6
Average Humidity	
Morning (percent)	87
Afternoon (percent)	58
Annual Precipitation (inches)	43.8
Average Total Snowfall (inches)	1.9

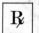 Shreveport did not respond to the health-services survey.

Health Resources per 1,000 Pop. (1988)	**Number**	**Rank**
Hospital beds, community hospitals, city	8.82	25/91
Nurses, community hospitals, city	8.56	36/90
Doctors, metro	2.80	37/113

Shreveport has 46 sports facilities per 100,000 residents, ranking 68th out of 82 metro areas. The city completely renovated 15 neighborhood and community parks, added 7 miles of exercise trails, and constructed a 50-meter pool and center. The center combines horseshoes, volleyball, etc. within the outdoor space of the pool. The city also constructed a waterslide and kiddie water playground. The city's sports facilities include 54 tennis courts, 34 basketball courts, 12 swimming pools, 9 baseball fields, 3 football/soccer fields and 3 golf courses. Contact: Director of Parks & Recreation, 800 Snow Street, Shreveport, LA 71101.

Parkland/Total City Area (percent)	4.7

 The Shreveport public-school system employs 18 nurses and 16 psychologists for the 52,000 students in the school system. All common health-education programs are offered to students in various grades. The school system provides all common screens and tests except that mental-health exams, well-child physical exams, and speech-therapy and learning-disability tests are given only to students for whom a need is suspected. Medical, dental and psychiatric treatment is not routinely provided. Contact: Dr. E. J. Holt, Asst. Superintendent of Support Schools, Caddo Parish School System, PO Box 32000, Shreveport, LA 71130-2000.

Sioux Falls, SD

🪦	🏃	$	🔺	℞	🚶	👪	?
?	✔	✔	✔	✔	✔	✓	✔

 Sioux Falls is located in Minnehaha County. We did not calculate age-adjusted death rates for this city. Infant-mortality rates for South Dakota are low among blacks, but extremely high among other minorities. Infant-mortality rates among whites are slightly higher than blacks. Rates are higher in rural areas than in cities.

Average Daily Temperature (degrees F)	52.7
High	59.7
Low	45.6
Average Humidity	
Morning (percent)	82
Afternoon (percent)	62
Annual Precipitation (inches)	38.8
Average Total Snowfall (inches)	7.4

Sioux Falls ranks among the four safest metro areas in the nation based on homicide and robbery rates.

Incidence per 1,000 Pop.	Number	Rank
Homicides	0.02	3/111
Robberies	0.27	4/111

$ Sioux Falls' 1988 metro population was 126,000—110th out of 113 metro areas. Its economic health at the end of 1990 was extremely strong, ranking 2nd of 113 metro areas. Its unemployment rate ranks 3rd, change in unemployment 22nd (employment grew slightly while the labor force shrunk by 1.1 percent) and its enterprise 13th. Contact: Mayor Jack White, City of Sioux Falls, City Hall, Sioux Falls, SD 57102.

Air Quality: Prior to 1987 sulfur dioxide, nitrogen dioxide and lead were monitored, but levels were so low monitoring was discontinued. Particulates were less than half the NAAQS maximum in 1989. Contact: Thomas M. Olson, M.P.H., Public Health Director, Sioux Falls Health Department, 1320 South Minnesota Avenue, Sioux Falls, SD 57105.

Hazardous Waste: Minnehaha County has no hazardous-waste sites. Work is being done in the areas of additional storage for recycling and transport of toxic materials to a hazardous waste site. The city has programs for waste reduction and recycling. Contact: Thomas M. Olson, M.P.H., Public Health Director, Sioux Falls Health Department, Sioux Falls, SD 57105.

Water Quality: Seven percent of the water supply in Sioux Falls comes from surface water and 93 percent comes from ground water. The pH of the drinking water was 8.82 in 1988. Contact: Thomas M. Olson, M.P.H., Public Health Director, Sioux Falls Health Department, 1320 South Minnesota Avenue, Sioux Falls, SD 57105.

Weather: The average temperature is cool at 45.3. Normal annual precipitation is about average.

Average Daily Temperature (degrees F)	45.3
High	56.7
Low	33.9
Average Humidity	
Morning (percent)	81
Afternoon (percent)	60
Annual Precipitation (inches)	24.1
Average Total Snowfall (inches)	39.7

R⃥ The city did not respond to the health-services questionnaire.

Health Resources per 1,000 Pop. (1988)	Number	Rank
Doctors, metro	2.86	32/113

 The city is working on a family-aquatics center and a new golf course. There are over 14 miles of bike trails and parks along the Big Sioux River Greenway that encircles the city. The city's sports facilities include 79 softball fields, 41 tennis courts, 29 football/soccer fields, 21 basketball courts, 7 swimming pools, 7 ice rinks and 3 public golf courses. Recreational facilities include several indoor recreation centers. The city provides supervised summer playgrounds and swimming, tennis and golf lessons. Contact: Lowen Schuett, Director, Sioux Falls Parks & Recreation Department, 224 West 9th Street, Sioux Falls, SD 57102.

Parkland/Total City Area (percent)	5.5
Aerobics classes	yes
Hiking or exploration groups	yes

The Sioux Falls public-school system employs 12 nurses, 6 psychologists, 32 counselors, 5 health clerks, 6 occupational therapists, 4.5 physical therapists and part-time physicians for athletic physicals. Nurses are present part-time in all of the schools. The school system has a K-12 health curriculum and an employee wellness program. The school system provides all common screens and tests except for immunizations; it also provides a dental screen. Medical treatment is provided for students. Contact: Mary Lerssen, Supervisor of Health Services, Sioux Falls Public Schools, 201 East 38th Street, Sioux Falls, SD 57117.

Spokane, WA

Spokane (Spokane County) ranks an average 56th in the age-adjusted mortality rate. Infant-mortality rates for Washington are high among minorities and relatively low among whites. Infant-mortality rates are higher in cities than in rural areas of Washington.

	Number	Rank
Age-Adjusted Death Rate	0.08	56/100
Heart Attacks	0.07	60/100
Cancer	1.88	38/100

 Spokane has the 8th lowest homicide rate of the surveyed cities. The city's suicide rate, however, is very high.

Incidence per 1,000 Pop.	Number	Rank
Homicides (1989)	0.03	8/111
Robberies (1989)	1.22	24/111
Suicides	0.15	82/100
Accidental deaths	0.36	68/100

$ Spokane's 1988 metro population was 356,000—94th out of 113 metro areas. Its economic health at the end of 1990 was below average, ranking 80th of 113 metro areas. Its unemployment rate ranks 64th, change in unemployment 34th (employment grew 3.1 percent compared to the labor force, 2.8 percent) and its enterprise 103rd. Contact: Mayor Vicki McNeill, City of Spokane, 808 West Spokane Falls Blvd., Spokane, WA 99201.

↑ **Air Quality:** Air quality is improving. In 1987, there were over 60 days of non-attainment of carbon monoxide standards, and in 1988 it was down to 34. Non-attainment was only by two or three points. Contact: Dale Arnold, Acting Environmental Programs Director, 808 West Spokane Falls Blvd., Spokane, WA 99201.

Hazardous Waste: There are no hazardous waste sites in the county, but six sites where activities have placed them on the National Priorities List. Four landfills inadvertently accepted wastes, mainly organic solvents, which created environmental concerns. The remainder are industries whose activities created environmental pollution. Contact: Dale Arnold, Acting Environmental Programs Director, 808 West Spokane Falls Blvd., Spokane, WA 99201.

Water Quality: 100 percent of the water supply in Spokane is from ground water. Measures to protest the sole source aquifer are ongoing. Aquifer quality remains steady and of high quality. Contact: Dale Arnold, Acting Environmental Programs Director, 808 West Spokane Falls Blvd., Spokane, WA 99201.

Weather: The average temperature is cool at 47.2 degrees. Precipitation is low at 16.71 inches annually.

Average Daily Temperature (degrees F)	47.2
High	57.1
Low	37.2
Average Humidity	
Morning (percent)	77
Afternoon (percent)	52
Annual Precipitation (inches)	16.71
Average Total Snowfall (inches)	51.2

℞ Anti-smoking legislation in Spokane prohibits smoking in restaurants and public offices and on public transportation. All common health-education programs and emergency hotlines are provided by the city. The county provides all common preventive health and treatment programs. Contact: Lee Mellish, Administrator, Spokane County Health District, West 1101 College Avenue, Spokane, WA 99201.

Health Resources per 1,000 Pop. (1988)	Number	Rank
Hospital beds, community hospitals, city	8.15	31/91
Nurses, community hospitals, city	9.15	27/90
Doctors, metro	2.49	52/113

 Spokane did not respond to the recreational-services survey.

The Spokane school system employs 8.8 nurses, 17 psychologists, 8 occupational therapists and 6 physical therapists for its 27,615 students. In addition, physicians are employed on a consulting basis. The nurses are present on a full-time basis in 3 percent of the schools and on a part-time basis in the remainder. The school system contracts with Public Health for screening programs in order to free the nurses to work more closely with the children with specific health needs. They also have a school program with a full-time nurse for medically fragile elementary students. All common health-education programs are offered to students in grades K-7 and 9-12. The school system provides all common screens and tests except for well-child physical exams. Impedence screens are provided in grades K-3. No medical, dental or psychiatric treatment is provided for students. Contact: Carol Kerkering, Health Department, School District #81, North 200 Bernard, Spokane, WA 99201.

Springfield, MA

🪦 RIP	🏊	$	🌲	℞	🥾	🧑‍🏫	?
X	✔	X	✓	✓	✔	✔	✔

Springfield (Hampden County) ranks an unhealthy 94th in the age-adjusted mortality rate. Heart attack and cancer rates are also high. Infant-mortality rates for Massachusetts are high among minorities and very low among whites. Infant-mortality rates are somewhat higher in cities than in rural areas of Massachusetts.

	Number	Rank
Age-Adjusted Death Rate	2.50	94/100
Heart Attacks	0.63	86/100
Cancer	0.53	91/100

Springfield ranks 6th of the cities surveyed for homicides, but has an average suicide rate.

Incidence per 1,000 Pop.	Number	Rank
Homicides	0.02	6/111
Robberies	2.14	59/111
Suicides	0.13	51/100

$ Springfield's 1988 metro population was 522,000—76th out of 113 metro areas. Its economic health at the end of 1990 was the poorest of 113 metro areas. Its unemployment rate ranks 93rd (11th worst), change in unemployment 108th (5th worst—employment dropped by 5.2 percent while the labor force shrunk by 2.2 percent) and its enterprise 108th (5th worst). Contact: Mayor Mary E. Hurley, City of Springfield, 36 Court Street, Springfield, MA 01103.

Air Quality: Springfield did not return the air-quality survey. EPA data for 1989 indicate that the city was in violation of the NAAQS 0.12 ppp ozone limit, with an ozone level of 0.13 ppm. Carbon monoxide was also just below the NAAQS ceiling.

Hazardous Waste: Hampden County's hazardous waste site on the EPA's National Priorities List for "Superfund" is PSC/Palmer, which is contaminated with solvents and PCBs. The county has no legal hazardous-waste-disposal facilities. Efforts are being made through legislation, education and state/industry cooperation to implement hazardous-waste source reduction. Contact: Alan Weinberg, Division of Environmental Protection, State House West, 436 Dwight Street, Springfield, MA 01103.

Weather: Springfield is a cool city with an average temperature of 49.8 degrees. Average annual precipitation is high at 44.4 inches.

Average Daily Temperature (degrees F)	49.8
High	60.1
Low	39.5
Average Humidity	
Morning (percent)	77
Afternoon (percent)	52
Annual Precipitation (inches)	44.4
Average Total Snowfall (inches)	48.8

℞ The city has a private transportation system, Peter Pan, which provides wheel-chair buses free of charge for agencies needing transportation for the elderly to day care centers. A private hospital also provides day care to the elderly and has a van that travels to senior centers to give ophthalmological services. Eyes are tested without charge. The city sponsors public health messages addressing substance abuse, adolescent pregnancies, pre/post natal care, infant mortality, low-birth weight babies, anti-smoking, over-medication of the elderly, AIDS, food-borne diseases, recycling, anti-pollution, and water contamination by solid and liquid waste. The city conducts public forums on TV. Topics include AIDS, adolescent pregnancies, substance abuse, homeless housing, infant mortality, family planning, elderly care, protection from violence and illiteracy. All common health-education programs and emergency hotlines are provided by the city. The city provides all common preventive-health and treatment services; it also provides fluoride mouth rinses in grades 1-6 and provides dental care to the homebound and disabled. Current anti-smoking legislation prohibits smoking on public transportation and partially restricts it in restaurants and public offices. The public health council is reviewing an ordinance that will restrict smoking in the workplace as well. Contact: John Cipolla, Springfield Public Health Department, 1414 State Street, Springfield, MA 01109.

Health Resources per 1,000 Pop. (1988)	**Number**	**Rank**
Doctors, metro	2.48	54/113

Springfield has 106 sports facilities per 100,000 residents, ranking 26th out of 82 metro areas. Activities offered by the city of Springfield include a Halloween haunted house, park reservation program, and an environmental center. The city's sports facilities include 53 baseball fields, 53 tennis courts, 26 basketball courts, 27 football/soccer fields, 11 swimming pools, 2 golf courses and 1 running track. Contact: Edward Moariarty, Deputy Superintendent of Recreation, Parks Department, Administration Bldg., Forest Park, Springfield, MA 01108.

Parkland/Total City Area (percent)	9.9

The Springfield public-school system employs 27 nurses, 6 physicians, and 14 licensed practical nurses for its 28,144 students. A nurse is present on a full-time basis in 10 percent of the schools and part-time in the remainder. All common health-education programs are offered to students in grades K-12. The school system provides all common screens and tests except for speech therapy; it also provudes dental screening. Medical, dental and psychiatric treatment is provided for students. Contact: John Cipolla, Commissioner, Public Health Department, 1414 State Street, Springfield, MA 01109.

Springfield, MO

[RIP]	⬇	$	🌲	℞	🚶	👫	?
?	✔	✔	✔	✔	✔	✔	✔

[RIP] Springfield is located in Greene County. Age-adjusted death rates were not calculated. Infant-mortality rates for Missouri are high among minorities and relatively low among whites. Infant-mortality rates are higher in cities than in rural areas of the state.

⬇ Springfield is probably one of the safest cities around. It has the 11th lowest homicide rate, 12th lowest robbery rate and 3rd lowest accident rate. Suicide rates were unavailable.

Incidence per 1,000 Pop.	Number	Rank
Homicides (1989)	0.034	11/111
Robberies (1989)	0.859	12/111
Accidental deaths	0.159	3/100

$ Springfield's 1988 metro population was 234,000—101st out of 113 metro areas. Its economic health at the end of 1990 was below average, ranking 66th of 113 metro areas. Its unemployment rate ranks 44th, change in unemployment 58th (labor force growth outpaced employment growth) and its enterprise 78th.

🌲 **Air Quality:** Springfield is experiencing increased winter carbon monoxide levels due to residential wood-burning. Sulfur emissions from a coal-fired power plant have caused sulfur dioxide levels that threaten the EPA standard. But so far the city has complied with the NAAQS standards. Ronald Boyer, Chief, Air Pollution Control, Springfield/Greene County Health Department, 227 East Chestnut Expressway, Room 104, Springfield, MO 65802.

Water Quality: Springfield has a proactive watershed protection program. 73 percent of its water is surface water, 6 percent ground water, and 21 percent natural springs. Contact: John Witherspoon, Director of Water Laboratories, Springfield City Utilities, 301 East Central, Springfield, MO 65802.

Weather: The mean temperature in Springfield is about average for the nation. Humidity and precipitation are both high.

Average Daily Temperature (degrees F)	55.9
High	67.4
Low	44.3
Average Humidity	
Morning (percent)	82
Afternoon (percent)	58
Annual Precipitation (inches)	39.47
Average Total Snowfall (inches)	17.1
Ozone, Days over 0.12 ppm (one hour in 1988)	0

℞ Springfield sponsors health awareness campaigns addressing AIDS, environmental health effects, prenatal care and anti-drug use. Smoking legislation prohibits smoking in public offices. The city has expanded its indigent outpatient primary care and prenatal care for indigent pregnant females. All common health-education programs and emergency hotlines are provided by the city/county health authority. The authority also provides all common preventive-health programs, and treatment for sexually transmitted diseases but not for drug abuse, alcoholism or mental illness. Contact: Harold Bengsch, Director of Public Health, Springfield/Green County Health Department, 227 East Chestnut Expressway, Springfield, MO 65802.

Health Resources per 1,000 Pop. (1988)	**Number**	**Rank**
Doctors, metro	2.00	82/113

Springfield has 67 sports facilities per 100,000 residents, ranking 52nd out of 82 metro areas. Softball and tennis are especially popular in Springfield. The city's sports facilities include 56 tennis courts, 18 baseball fields, 9 soccer fields, 13 basketball courts, 6 swimming pools, 3 golf courses and 2 running tracks. Contact: Dan Kinney, Director of Parks, Springfield Parks & Recreation, 1923 North Weller, Springfield, MO 65803.

Springfield public schools employ 17 nurses, 3 psychologists, 1 physical therapist, and 1.5 occupational therapists. Nurses are present in all of the schools on a part-time basis. All common health-education programs are offered to students in grades K-9. The school system provides all common screens and tests except for well-child physical exams. Medicaland dental treatment is provided for students. Contact: Ginny Staley,

RN, Supervisor of Health Services, Springfield Public Schools, 940 North Jefferson, Springfield, MO 65802.

St. Louis, MO

🪦	🔪	$	🌲	℞	🚗	🏃	?
✓	X	X	X	✓	X	✔	✔

The St. Louis metro area includes East St. Louis, IL. St. Louis ranks a moderate 54th in the age-adjusted mortality rate. Infant-mortality rates for Missouri are high among minorities and relatively low among whites. Infant-mortality rates are higher in cities than in rural areas of the state.

	Number	Rank
Age-Adjusted Death Rate	0.00	54/100
Heart Attacks	0.33	76/100
Cancer	0.03	52/100

St. Louis ranks a high 81st out of 111 for homicides and 73 out of 100 for accidents. Rates for suicide and robberies are also above average.

Incidence per 1,000 Pop.	Number	Rank
Homicides (1989)	0.11	81/111
Robberies (1989)	2.52	68/111
Suicides	0.13	58/100
Accidental deaths	0.36	73/100

St. Louis' 1988 metro population was 2,467,000—12th out of 113 metro areas. Its economic health at the end of 1990 was poor, ranking 98th of 113 metro areas. Its unemployment rate ranks 90th, change in unemployment 58th (employment declined slightly while the labor force grew slightly) and its enterprise 93rd. Contact: Mayor Vincent Schoemehl, City of St. Louis, 200 City Hall, St. Louis, MO 63103.

Air Quality: The years 1985–90 have seen a gradual decline in the number of days when ozone is above the NAAQS. Contact: Arnold Montgomery, Air Pollution Control, 1200 Carr Lane, St. Louis, MO 63104.

Hazardous Waste: St. Louis is facing a rapid decrease in available landfill capacity for disposing of wastes, with three alternatives being worked on: composting of yard waste, recycling of residential waste and a waste-to-energy facility. St. Louis has six confirmed waste "Superfund" sites. The Thompson Chemical/Superior Solvents site has polynuclear aromatic hydrocarbons, volatile organic compounds and dioxin. The Todd site contains Stoddard solvent which after remedial actions to the site remains in the soil and ground water. Ground water in the area is not used for drinking. The Hamill Transfer location is contaminated with dioxin from waste oil sprayed on-site. There is moderate potential for ground water contamination. Dioxin also contaminates the Acetylene Gas Co. location; at present there are no known environmental problems due to paving of the site. Solvent residue has been spilled at the ACF site, and following remediation, residual contamination remained in the soil subsurface and shallow ground water. Contact: George Jenkerson, Hazardous Materials Program Manager, Room 402, City Hall, St. Louis, MO 63103.

Water Quality: 100 percent of the water supply in St. Louis is from surface water, e.g., the Mississippi and Missouri rivers. Contact: David Visintainer, Water Division, Department of Public Utilities, 10450 Riverview Blvd., St. Louis, MO 63137.

Weather: The weather changes rather frequently. Summers are hot and humid and winters are long and bring about 20 inches of snow. Rainy days are plentiful.

Average Daily Temperature (degrees F)	55.4
High	65.5
Low	45.3
Average Humidity	
Morning (percent)	84
Afternoon (percent)	60
Annual Precipitation (inches)	33.91
Average Total Snowfall (inches)	19.7
Ozone, Days over 0.12 ppm (one hour in 1988)	2

℞ Health-awareness programs address infant mortality, AIDS, sexually transmitted diseases, lead poisoning, teen-age pregnancy, homelessness, environmental health and health issues relating to the elderly. All common health-education programs and emergency hotlines are provided by the city, including: TeenAge Health Consultants, a peer education program for adolescents; Growing Younger, a wellness program for seniors; HealthStreet, outreach community centers for health promotion; ChildSave, infant-mortality prevention and Community Outreach for Risk Reduction, AIDS education in the at-risk drug community. The city provides all common preventive-health services except provision of food to the needy. It provides treatment for sexually transmitted diseases, but not for drug abuse, alcoholism or mental illness. Smoking legislation was being debated as this book went to press. Contact: Dian Sharma, Ph.D., Health Commissioner, PO Box 14702, St. Louis, MO 63178-4702.

Health Resources per 1,000 Pop. (1988)	**Number**	**Rank**
Hospital beds, community hospitals, city	18.16	1/91
Nurses, community hospitals, city	18.88	3/90
Doctors, metro	2.49	53/113

St. Louis has 55 sports facilities per 100,000 residents, ranking 60th out of 82 metro areas. It offers extensive recreational facilities and services. Many participate in the city's softball, basketball and volleyball leagues. The city has recently contracted management of its public golf courses, resulting in considerable capital improvements and upgrading of the courses. St. Louis' sports facilities include 144 baseball fields, 57 soccer fields, 25 basketball courts, 8 running tracks, 8 swimming pools and 4 golf courses. The city also offers classes and programs in aerobics, arts and crafts, hiking, boxing, archery, croquet and fishing. Contact: Evelyn Rice, Director of Parks, Recreation and Forestry, 5600 Clayton Road, Forest Park, St. Louis, MO 63110.

Parkland/Total City Area (percent)	7.7

The St. Louis public-school system employs 96 nurses, 3 physicians, 48 psychologists, 48 social workers and 118 counselors for its 60,000 students. A nurse is present on a full-time basis in 95 percent of the schools and part-time in 5 percent. The school system has an extensive health education program. All common programs are offered to students in preschool and grades K-12 including programs in AIDS education, family life, CPR/First aid, dental health, menstrual health, teen pregnancy, and weight control and eating disorders. The school system provides all common screens and tests. Medical, dental and psychiatric treatment is provided for students. Contact: Jerome Jones, Superintendent, St. Louis Public Schools, 911 Locust Street, 6th Floor, St. Louis, MO 63101.

Stockton, CA

🪦	✈	$	⬆	℞	📷	👥	?
?	x	x	x	x	x	✓	✔

 Stockton is located in San Joaquin County. We did not calculate age-adjusted death rates for this community. Infant-mortality rates for California are high among blacks and relatively low among whites. Infant-mortality rates are higher in cities than in rural areas of the state.

Homicide and robbery rates are high, among the highest 17 of the 111 metro areas we compare.

Incidence per 1,000 Pop.	Number	Rank
Homicides	0.13	91/111
Robberies	3.10	86/111

$ Stockton's 1988 metro population was 456,000—82nd out of 113 metro areas. Its economic health at the end of 1990 was poor, ranking 95th of 113 metro areas. Its unemployment rate ranks 113th, change in unemployment 109th (employment declined 2.7 percent while the labor force grew slightly) and its enterprise 14th. Contact: Mayor Barbara Fass, City of Stockton, Stockton City Hall, Stockton, CA 95201.

Air Quality: Stockton did not return our air-quality survey. EPA data indicate that in 1989 the city was in violation of both the carbon monoxide NAAQS limit of 9 ppm (Stockton's level was 10 ppm) and the 50 $\mu g/m^3$ maximum for particulates (Stockton's level was 51 $\mu g/m^3$).

Water Quality: 94 percent of Stockton's water supply comes from ground water, e.g., wells. The remainder is from surface water. The pH of the drinking water was 7.6 in 1989. Contact: Duane Cox, Superintendent of Water/Sewers, Stockton Municipal Utilities District, 2500 Navy Drive, Stockton, CA 95203.

Weather: The mean temperature in Stockton is slightly above average at 61.6. Precipitation is very low at 13.77 inches annually.

Average Daily Temperature (degrees F)	61.6
High	74.5
Low	48.6
Average Humidity	
Morning (percent)	78
Afternoon (percent)	44
Annual Precipitation (inches)	13.77
Average Total Snowfall (inches)	Trace
Carbon monoxide level, 1989	10
	ppm
Particulates level (PM10), 1989	51

℞   The city did not respond to the health-services questionnaire.

Health Resources per 1,000 Pop.	Number	Rank
Doctors, metro	1.52	106/113

Stockton has 44 sports facilities per 100,000 residents, ranking it 70th out of 82 cities. Organized youth and adult sports, especially softball and baseball, are very popular. Stockton has recently reinstituted an Afterschool Playground Program, aiding many "latch-key" children. The city's sports facilities include 54 tennis courts, 19 basketball courts, 10 baseball fields, 4 swimming pools, 2 golf courses and 3 soccer fields. There are also 6 community centers. Contact: Emil Seifert, Director, Parks & Recreation Department, 425 North El Dorado Street, Stockton, CA 95202.

Parkland/Total City Area (percent)	2.5

The Stockton Unified School District employs 5 nurses, 17 psychologists and 6.5 health clerks for its 33,000 students. Nurses are present part-time in all of the schools. All common health-education programs are offered to students in grades K-12. The school system provides all common screens and tests, and also provides dental-hygiene screening. No medical, dental or psychiatric treatment is provided for students. Contact: Gayle Martins, Administrator of Health Services, Stockton Unified School District, 701 North Madison, Stockton, CA 95202.

Syracuse, NY

⚰️ RIP	🏃	$	🌲	℞	🏭	🧑‍🤝‍🧑	?
X	✔	✓	✓	✓	✔	?	✓

 Syracuse (Onondaga County) ranks a high 72nd in the age-adjusted death rate. Cancer and heart attack rates are above average. Infant-mortality rates for New York are high among minorities and relatively low among whites. Infant-mortality rates are significantly higher in cities than in rural areas of the state.

	Number	Rank
Age-Adjusted Death Rate	0.59	72/100
Heart Attacks	0.24	72/100
Cancer	0.22	78/100

Syracuse has extremely low rates of homicide, suicide and robberies. Accident rates are about average for cities.

Incidence per 1,000 Pop.	Number	Rank
Homicides (1989)	0.03	7/111
Robberies (1989)	0.88	13/111
Suicides	0.08	7/100
Accidental deaths	0.32	45/100

$ Syracuse's 1988 metro population was 650,000—63rd out of 113 metro areas. Its economic health at the end of 1990 was good, ranking 53rd of 113 metro areas. Its unemployment rate ranks 36th, change in unemployment 47th (employment and the labor force both shrunk by 1 percent) and its enterprise 76th. Contact: Mayor Thomas Young, City of Syracuse, City Hall, Syracuse, NY 13202.

Air Quality: Syracuse had one day of carbon monoxide exceedance in 1988. Ozone continues to approach the standard on hot, sunny, summer days; the level was at 0.10 ppm for 1989, close to the maximum. Syracuse exceeded the carbon monoxide limit of 9 ppm in 1989; the level was 10 ppm. Contact: Norman Boyce, Superintendent, Air Quality Department, New York State Department of Environmental Conservation, 615 Erie Blvd. West, Syracuse, NY 13204.

Weather: Syracuse's average temperature is cool at 47.7. Precipitation is slightly above average at 39.11 inches annually, but snowfall is extremely high at 109.4 inches annually.

Average Daily Temperature (degrees F)	47.7
High	56.9
Low	38.4
Average Humidity	
Morning (percent)	81
Afternoon (percent)	61
Annual Precipitation (inches)	39.11
Average Total Snowfall (inches)	109.4

℞ Syracuse has instituted new outreach programs to assist in making prenatal care more accessible to high-risk pregnant women. The county addresses the following health issues: flu immunization for senior citizens, prenatal care, well-child care, injury control, traffic safety/bicycle awareness, poison prevention, lead poison prevention, and fire prevention. The county offers all common public health-education programs. The county provides emergency hotlines for child abuse, suicide and AIDS information. The county provides all common preventive-health programs except food to the needy. It provides treatment for sexually transmitted diseases but not for drug abuse, alcoholism or mental illness. Anti-smoking legislation prohibits smoking on public transportation and in public offices. It is also partially restricted in restaurants, private offices and public areas. The county established a campaign to educate school children in prevention of disease transmission by encouraging handwashing. Contact: Dr. James R. Miller, Commissioner, Onondaga County Health Department, 421 Montgomery Street, Syracuse, NY 13202.

Health Resources per 1,000 Pop. (1988)	**Number**	**Rank**
Doctors, metro	2.60	47/113

Syracuse has 137 sports facilities per 100,000 residents, ranking it 12th out of 82 cities. Broomball, a form of ice hockey with a rubber ball, cut-off brooms and no skates is very popular in Syracuse. The city's sports facilities include 92 basketball courts, 63 tennis courts, 39 baseball fields, 16 football/soccer fields, 10 swimming pools, 3 running tracks, 3 ice rinks and 2 golf courses. There are popular sports leagues for softball, basketball, volleyball and broomball. Contact: Gerald Wilcox, Department of Parks & Recreation, 412 Spencer Street, Syracuse, NY 13204.

Parkland/Total City Area (percent)	5.6
Aerobics classes	yes
Hiking or exploration groups	no

Syracuse did not respond to the school-health survey.

Tampa-St. Petersburg, FL

⚰️RIP	🔪	$	↟	℞	🏃	👥	?
✓	✓	✓	✔	✓	✓	✓	✔

Tampa (Hillsborough County) and St. Petersburg (Pinellas County) have above-average mortality rates even after adjusting for age, rating 61 out of 100 metro areas. Infant-mortality rates in the state are high, especially for non-whites. Infant-mortality rates are higher in rural areas than in cities.

	Number	Rank
Age-Adjusted Death Rate	0.33	61/100
Heart Attacks	3.08	66/100
Cancer	2.77	56/100

 The city has very high rates of robberies, suicides and accidents. Homicide rates are slightly above average.

Incidence per 1,000 Pop.	Number	Rank
Homicides (1989)	0.09	64/111
Robberies (1989)	3.81	96/111
Suicides	0.18	93/100
Accidental deaths	0.36	74/100

$ Tampa's 1988 metro population was 1,995,000—21st out of 113 metro areas. Its economic health at the end of 1990 was good, ranking 49th of 113 metro areas. Its unemployment rate ranks 70th, change in unemployment 58th (the labor force grew faster than employment) and its enterprise 23rd. Contact: Mayor Sandra Freedman, City of Tampa, 306 East Jackson, Tampa, FL 33602.

Air Quality: While ozone problems are ever-present in a warm climate like Tampa's, the city and Hillsborough County and in 1987, Hillsborough County recorded six days with ozone exceedances, in the difficult year of 1988 the county came through with a clean record. In 1989 no NAAQS limits were exceeded and ozone was 0.2 ppm below the limit. Contact: Roger Stewart, Director, Environmental Protection Commission, Hillsborough County, 1900 9th Avenue, Tampa, FL 33604.

Weather: Freezing temperatures are a rarity in the Tampa Bay area, but 90 degree days abound. The average summer temperature is 82 degrees, and the average winter temperature is 60.4 degrees; the summer months are punctuated with frequent thunderstorms.

Average Daily Temperature (degrees F)	72.0
High	81.4
Low	62.5
Average Humidity	
Morning (percent)	88
Afternoon (percent)	58
Annual Precipitation (inches)	46.73
Average Total Snowfall (inches)	Trace
Ozone, Days over 0.12 ppm (one hour in 1988)	0

℞ Most of the local awareness campaigns are joint ventures of the city, county and state health agencies. Local newspapers, radio and TV stations assist the health team in addressing such issues as immunization, AIDS, indigent health care, elderly care, substance abuse, sexually transmitted diseases and mental health issues. Emergency hotlines are available for all the common subjects and several others, including sexual abuse, hazardous materials, poison information, victims assistance programs, and disabled and elderly abuse. Smoking is prohibited on public transportation and in public offices and is partially restricted in restaurants and private offices. Conscious of poor infant-mortality rates, the city has increased its attention toward the reduction of substance abuse during pregnancy through intervention and assistance, promoting safer pregnancies and reducing the number of low-birthweight and substance-addicted babies. Hillsborough County provides all common preventive-health and treatment programs. Contact: Joyner Sims, Ph.D, Senior Public Health Administrator, Hillsborough County Public Health Unit, Tampa, FL 33675-5135.

Health Resources per 1,000 Pop. (1988)	Number	Rank
Hospital beds, community hospitals, city		
Tampa	12.67	12/91
St. Petersburg	8.64	27/91
Nurses, community hospitals, city		
Tampa	13.08	13/90
St. Petersburg	7.56	44/90
Doctors, metro, Tampa-St. Petersburg	2.11	73/113

Tampa has 102 baseball-softball fields, 13 football-soccer fields, 146 tennis-racquetball-multipurpose courts, 13 swimming pools, 2 beaches, 3 golf courses, 2 gymnasiums, 60 playgrounds, 24 community centers, and 2 marine boat docks. Its criteria sports facilities rank in the top of the second third of cities in our survey.

The Tampa school district employs 8 registered nurses, 16 licensed practical nurses and 42 psychologists for its 124,000 students. In addition, the public health unit employs 14 registered nurses. The 16 schools with exceptional students have nurses present on a full-time basis. The other 89 percent of the schools have a nurse present on a part-time basis. All common health-education programs are offered through 6th grade and then again in 9th and 10th. The school system offers all screens and tests except mental-health exams; also, the well-child physical exams are provided only on entrance into the school. While medical treatment is available, students are not provided with any dental or psychiatric treatment. Contact: Mary Ellen Gilleyye, Hillsborough County Schools, Health Division, 900 East Kennedy Blvd., Tampa, FL 33602.

Toledo, OH

🪦 RIP	🕊	$	🌲	℞	🏃	👥	?
X	✓	X	✔	✓	?	✓	✓

Toledo (Lucas County) ranks 99th of 100 major cities in age-adjusted death rate. Toledo also has the second highest heart attack rate and the fourth highest cancer rate of 100 metro areas. Ohio's infant-mortality rate in rural areas is very low (16/301) compared to the urban rate (153/301). Infant-mortality rates are high among minorities and relatively low among whites. Contact: Carole Lanier, Registrar, Toledo Health Department, 635 North Erie Street, Toledo, OH 43604.

	Number	Rank
Age-Adjusted Death Rate	3.70	99/100
Heart Attacks	1.27	99/100
Cancer	0.74	97/100

Toledo has the highest accident rate of 100 metro areas. Robberies and suicides in the city are also above average.

Incidence per 1,000 Pop.	Number	Rank
Homicides (1989)	0.74	53/111
Robberies (1989)	1.79	77/111
Suicides	0.16	84/100
Accidental deaths	0.48	100/100

$ Toledo's 1988 metro population was 616,000—68th out of 113 metro areas. Its economic health at the end of 1990 was poor, ranking 90th of 113 metro areas. Its unemployment rate ranks 93rd, change in unemployment 81st (labor force grew 1.3 percent, versus employment growth of 0.1 percent) and its enterprise 46th. Contact: Mayor John McHugh, City of Toledo, 1 Government Center, Suite 2200, Toledo, OH 43604.

Air Quality: Toledo remained within NAAQS limits in 1989, although ozone was 0.11, just 0.1 ppm from the maximum. Carbon monoxide and particulates were comfortably within their limits.

Hazardous Waste: Lucas County has no hazardous-waste sites on the EPA's National Priorities List for Superfund. Contact: Michael White, Director, City of Toledo Utilities Department, 1 Government Center, Suite 1500, Toledo, OH 43604.

Water Quality: The water supply in Toledo comes from surface water sources. Contact: Michael White, Director, City of Toledo Utilities Department, 1 Government Center, Suite 1500, Toledo, OH 43604.

Weather: The average temperature is cool at 48.6. The humidity is above average.

Average Daily Temperature (degrees F)	48.6
High	58.8
Low	38.3
Average Humidity	
Morning (percent)	84
Afternoon (percent)	61
Annual Precipitation (inches)	31.78
Average Total Snowfall (inches)	38.3
Ozone, Days over 0.12 ppm (one hour in 1988)	6

℞ Health-awareness campaigns include immunization for influenza, preschool surveillance, Rocky Mountain spotted fever and lyme disease, hypertension, heart disease, women's health, infant car seats, accidental poisoning, AIDS, sexually transmitted diseases, head lice and encephalitis. Recent additions consist of teen pregnancy, HIV counseling and testing, cocaine babies, cholesterol triglyceride testing and education, proper diet, animal bites and rabies, smoking, polluted water and drug counseling. The city provides all common health-education programs and emergency hotlines, and all common preventive-health programs. However, the city only treats the general public for sexually transmitted diseases; it also treats city employees for alcohol or drug abuse or for mental illness. Anti-smoking laws prohibit smoking on public transportation and elevators. Smoking is partially restricted in restaurants and public and private offices. In an attempt to make health care more available, Toledo has a variety of mobile health services, support groups, health resource guides, Lifeline system (a home-to-hospital communication system that assists the elderly and handicapped), housing for homeless families with children, respite care services to adult care-givers, and immunizations at malls and dental sealant program in area schools. All common emergency hotlines are available. Sixty of 180 buses have lift equipment; all buses running on Saturday and Sunday have lift equipment. Contact: Joyce Chapel, Acting Director, City of Toledo Board of Health, 635 North Erie Street, Toledo, OH 43604.

Health Resources per 1,000 Pop. (1988)	Number	Rank
Hospital beds, community hospitals, city	6.82	47/91
Nurses, community hospitals, city	9.31	26/90
Doctors, metro	2.52	50/113

 Toledo did not respond to the recreational-services survey.

The Toledo public-school system employees 25 nurses and 18 psychologists (plus 2 interns) for its 41,978 students. Nursing services are provided by the school system for all high schools, all junior high schools, and one elementary school. The Toledo Health Department provides services to the other 42 elementary schools. In addition, the school system employs nine nurses who give service exclusively to parochial/private schools (auxiliary services programs) as provided for in Ohio law. All common health-education programs are provided to students in grades 1-10. The school system provides all common screens and tests except for immunizations (which are provided by the Health Department on request) and well-child physical exams; the schools also provide occupational and physical therapy. No medical, dental or psychiatric treatment is provided for students. Contact: Dave Jensen, Director of Pupil Placement & Adjustment Services, Toledo Public Schools, Manhattan and Elm Streets, Toledo, OH 43608.

Tucson, AZ

RIP	⛟	$	🌲	℞	🏃	🤼	?
✓	✓	✔	✓	✔	✓	✓	✔

 Tucson (Pima County) ranks a moderate 60th in the age adjusted mortality rate. Infant-mortality rates for Arizona are high among minorities and relatively low among whites. Infant-mortality rates are the same in cities as in rural communities. Contact: Mike Checkton, Director of Vital Statistics, Pima County Health Department, 150 West Congress, Tucson, AZ 85726.

	Number	Rank
Age-Adjusted Death Rate	0.32	60/100
Heart Attacks	−0.02	53/100
Cancer	0.05	58/100

Tucson has the 2nd highest rate of suicides and the 7th highest rate of accidents.

Incidence per 1,000 Pop.	Number	Rank
Homicides (1989)	0.08	59/111
Robberies (1989)	1.72	41/111
Suicides	0.23	99/100
Accidental deaths	0.44	94/100

$ Tucson's 1988 metro population was 636,000—65th out of 113 metro areas. Its economic health at the end of 1990 was excellent, ranking 21st of 113 metro areas. Its unemployment rate ranks 21st, change in unemployment 15th (the labor force declined faster than employment) and its enterprise 67th. Contact: Mayor Tom Volgy, City of Tucson, PO Box 27210, Tucson, AZ 85726-7210.

Air Quality: Tucson met the NAAQS challenge in 1989 for ozone and carbon monoxide but exceeded the standard for particulates, with 52 μg/m^3, just above the standard.

Hazardous Waste: There are no approved hazardous waste disposal facilities in Pima County. Hazardous wastes would be those found in wildcat dumps and landfills from the estimated 265,000 households in Pima County. The county has conducted two successful household-oriented hazardous-waste-collection programs. The collected waste was recycled or disposed of outside the state of Arizona. There is a permanent collection site open year-round. Contact: Janet Marcus, Chair, Council Environmental Committee, PO Box 27210, Tucson, AZ 85726 (602) 791-4687.

Water Quality: 100 percent of the water supply in Tucson is from ground water. It has a high level of nitrates, 2.15 mg/l, 6th highest of 61 cities for which we have this information. The pH is good, 7.5, quite close to the target of 7. Contact: Tom Jefferson, Water Quality Administrator, Tucson Water, PO Box 27210, Tucson, AZ 85726.

Weather: Tucson is warm and sunny throughout most of the year. Although there are an average of 139 days with temperatures in the 90s each year, the area's low humidity makes them more comfortable. In addition, temperatures fall after sunset, making summer evenings cool. There are roughly 20 days a year when the temperature drops to freezing.

Average Daily Temperature (degrees F)	68.0
High	81.7
Low	54.2
Average Humidity	
Morning (percent)	52
Afternoon (percent)	25
Annual Precipitation (inches)	11.14
Average Total Snowfall (inches)	1.3
Ozone, Days over 0.12 ppm (one hour in 1988)	0

℞ Tucson did not respond to the health-services survey.

Health Resources per 1,000 Pop. (1988)	Number	Rank
Hospital beds, community hospitals, city	5.49	63/91
Nurses, community hospitals, city	6.92	53/90
Doctors, metro	3.03	22/113

 Tucson has 46 sports facilities per 100,000 residents, ranking 35th out of 82 metro areas. Tucson is one of the few cities in the nation that offers a unique blend of social service and recreation programs. Five new neighborhood centers have allowed the Parks and Recreation Department to expand services to include social, educational, health and welfare and recreational services. The City offers an extremely popular leisure education program. A variety of health and fitness programs and arts programs are offered by the city. Other offerings include sports leagues, community theatre, swimming programs and senior citizen programs. The city's sports facilities include 137 tennis courts, 75 football/soccer fields, 38 multiple-use courts, 19 baseball fields, 51 softball fields, 23 swimming pools, 5 jogging paths, 5 bike paths and 5 golf courses. Contact: Jim Rondstadt, Director, City Parks & Recreation Department, 900 South Randolph Way, Tucson, AZ 85716.

Parkland/Total City Area (percent)   3.7

The *Amphitheatre* school district employs 8.5 nurses and additional health clerks. Seven are present full-time in 50 percent of the schools, one present part-time in 7 percent of the schools. 43 percent of the schools do not have a nurse present during school hours. This is part of a plan to reduce the number of RNs in school and increase parental involvement as a cost containment tactic. The school provides all common screens and tests except for immunization, mental-health exams, well-child physical exams and speech therapy. Contact: Virginia Davis, Director of Health Services, Amphitheatre School District, 701 West Wetmore Road, Tucson, AZ 85705.

The *Sunnyside* school district employs 17 nurses and 11 psychologists for its 13,000 students. A nurse is present on a full-time basis in all the schools. It provides all common screens and tests. Contact: Dr. Alan Storm, Sunnyside School District, PO Box 11280, Tucson, AZ 85734.

The *Flowing Wells* school district employs 7 nurses, three psychologists, two speech therapists and four speech technicians for its 6,500 students. An occupational and physical therapist is on contract as needed. It provides all common screens and tests. Contact: Eileen Smith, Head Nurse, Flowing Wells School District, 1556 West Prince Road, Tucson, AZ 85705.

The *Tucson Unified* school district employs 43 nurses, 1 part-time physician, and 30 psychologists. Nurses are present full-time in 14 percent of the schools and part-time in 86 percent. It provides all common screens and tests except for immunization and well-child physical exams; it does limited mental-health testing. Contact: Barbara McClure, Assistant Director of Health Services, Tucson Unified School District, PO Box 40400, 1010 East 10th St., Tucson, AZ 85719 (602) 882-2401.

All common health-education programs are offered through grade 12 in the Amphitheatre, Sunnyside and Flowing Wells school districts, with the exception of Illnesses in the Amphitheatre district. The Flowing Wells, Amphitheatre and Sunnyside school districts also offer an AIDS education program. Medical treatment is provided to students in Flowing Wells and Sunnyside school districts.

Tulsa, OK

🪦 RIP	☠	$	🌲	℞	🏃	🏖	?
✓	✓	✓	✓	X	✓	✓	✓

 Tulsa (Tulsa County) ranks an average 52nd in the age-adjusted mortality rate. Infant-mortality rates for Oklahoma are high among blacks and relatively low among whites and other minorities. Infant-mortality rates are higher in cities than in rural communities.

	Number	Rank
Age-Adjusted Death Rate	−0.06	52/100
Heart Attacks	0.31	75/100
Cancer	−0.06	44/100

Tulsa has average rates for homicides and robberies. Rates for suicides and accidents are above average.

Incidence per 1,000 Pop.	Number	Rank
Homicides (1989)	6.90	48/111
Robberies (1989)	2.15	60/111
Suicides	0.15	76/100
Accidental deaths	0.36	71/100

$ Tulsa's 1988 metro population was 728,000—59th out of 113 metro areas. Its economic health at the end of 1990 was good, ranking 43rd of 113 metro areas. Its unemployment rate ranks 44th, change in unemployment 10th (employment grew 4.7 percent, labor force 3.4 percent) and its enterprise 94th. Tulsa has benefited from the establishment of an American Airlines maintenance facility and some aerospace (McDonnell Douglas, Rockwell) plants. Contact: Mayor Roger A. Randle, City of Tulsa, 200 Civic Center, Tulsa, OK 74103.

Air Quality: There was great satisfaction in February 1990 when Tulsa achieved Federal attainment status for ozone and total suspended particulates. Its 1989 record showed compliance with all standards, but it was a close call (ozone was at 0.12). The problem was with petrochemical processing in the area as well as the usual motor-vehicle traffic. Tulsa area oil fields are pretty depleted and all are in secondary recovery, which reduces oil-related pollution. The drop in oil and farm prices and the recession have also contributed to a cleaner environment. Contact: Jim Van Sandt, Tulsa City-County Health, 4616 East 15th Street, Tulsa, OK 74116.

Hazardous Waste: Tulsa has two sites on the EPA's National Priorities List for "Superfund", Compass Industries Landfill and Sand Springs Petrochemical Complex. Compass Industries Landfill is believed to have received jet fuels, solvents, caustics, benzene and PCB's. Sand Springs Petrochemical Complex is an abandoned oil refinery with contaminated soils, sludge and liquids. The household waste of current interest in Tulsa includes used motor oil, paints, and abandoned "orphan waste" left on public property. Contact: Bob Pool, Grants Administrator, Water & Sewer Department, 200 Civic Center, Tulsa, OK 74103.

Water Quality: 100 percent of the water supply in Tulsa is supplied by surface water. Contact: Bob Pool, Grants Administrator, Water & Sewer Department, City of Tulsa, 200 Civic Center, Tulsa, OK 74103.

Weather: Hot summers and mild winters. Humidity and precipitation are slightly above average.

Average Daily Temperature (degrees F)	60.3
High	71.3
Low	49.2
Average Humidity	
Morning (percent)	81
Afternoon (percent)	56
Annual Precipitation (inches)	38.77
Average Total Snowfall (inches)	9.3

℞ The Tulsa City-County Health Department recently opened a clinic to serve the homeless. Health awareness messages include prenatal care, AIDS, childhood immunizations, dental education and sexually transmitted diseases. Tulsa offers health-education summer programs in low-rent subsidized-housing projects which cover all the common topics. The city-county authority provides all common preventive-health and treatment programs. Tulsa prohibits smoking on public transportation, and the state partially restricts smoking in restaurants, educational facilities and health care facilities. The handicapped are serviced by special handicapped lift buses which are dispatched to individual calls. Those that the city does not support are provided by civic and social service organizations. Emergency Hotlines are available for all common topics and a "Helpline" is also provided for personal emergencies. Contact: Dr. Jerry Cleveland, Acting Director, Tulsa City-County Health Department, 4616 East 15th Street, Tulsa, OK 74112.

Health Resources per 1,000 Pop. (1988)	Number	Rank
Hospital beds, community hospitals, city	6.52	48/91
Nurses, community hospitals, city	5.83	61/90
Doctors, metro	1.84	93/113

Tulsa has 116 sports facilities per 100,000 residents, ranking 18th out of 82 metro areas. Running and biking are especially popular in Tulsa. The city plans to create an additional 50 miles of trails. Tulsa's abundance of sports facilities include 138 Baseball fields, 16 football fields, 78 soccer fields, 46 basketball courts, 148 tennis courts, 28 swimming pools and 6 golf courses. Contact: Hugh McKnight, Director, Parks and Recreation, 707 South Houston Street, Tulsa, OK 74121.

Parkland/Total City Area (percent)	5.8

Tulsa public-school system employs 17 nurses, 1 physician, 18 psychologists, and 42 health clerks/assistants for its 43,977 students. All common health education topics as well as Safety, minor first aid, dental, and growth and development are offered through 12th grade. The school system provides all common screens and tests. A referral system is used to provide medical, dental or psychiatric treatment for students. Contact: Emily Latimer, Director, Health Services, Tulsa Public Schools, 3027 South New Haven, Tulsa, OK 74147.

Washington, DC

RIP	🏃	$	🌲	℞	🏃	👥	?
✔	X	✔	✓	✔	?	✓	X

The District of Colombia's age-adjusted mortality rate ranks a great 6th out of 100 metro areas. The city has the lowest rate of heart attacks. Cancer rates are also very low. The district's infant-mortality rate for whites is about average at 166/301. Infant-mortality rates for minorities, which are the majority of the city's population, are some of the worst in the nation (300/301 for blacks and 297/301 for other minorities).

	Number	Rank
Age-Adjusted Death Rate	−2.48	6/100
Heart Attacks	0.92	1/100
Cancer	1.55	8/100

Washington, D.C. is among the 10 cities with the highest robbery rates, in part because of the large number of visitors, who are easy marks. It also has a high homicide rate. Its accidental-death rate is, however the 9th lowest. Suicide rates are also below average.

Incidence per 1,000 Pop.	Number	Rank
Homicides (1989)	0.17	102/111
Robberies (1989)	3.35	92/111
Suicides	0.11	21/100
Accidental deaths	0.26	9/100

$ Washington, D.C.'s 1988 metro population was 3,734,000—6th out of 113 metro areas. Its economic health at the end of 1990 was excellent, ranking 20th of 113 metro areas. Its unemployment rate ranks 19th, change in unemployment 80th (employment declined while the labor force grew) and its enterprise 2nd. Contact: Mayor Sharon Dixon, City of Washington, DC, District Building, Washington, DC 20004.

Air Quality: Air quality in Washington does not meet NAAQS requirements. Ozone was 0.12 ppm in 1989 and carbon monoxide was 9 ppm. Ozone exceedances usually occur in the summer and carbon-monoxide exceedances in the late fall and winter. Contact: Joseph Nwude, Chief, Air Quality Control and Monitoring Branch, D.C. Department of Consumer & Regulatory Affairs, 2100 Martin Luther King Jr., Ave., SE, Washington, DC 20020.

Hazardous Waste: Washington has no hazardous-waste sites. Most of the waste is generated by small-quantity generators who are largely exempt from compliance with hazardous-waste laws. Accordingly, Washington has planned a waste-minimization effort. Contact: Angelo Tompros, Chief, Pesticide & Hazardous Waste Management Branch, D.C. Department of Consumer & Regulatory Affairs, 2100 Martin Luther King Jr., Ave., SE, Washington D.C. 20020.

Water Quality: Washington, D.C. did not return its water-quality questionnaire. But according to *The Book of American City Rankings* (Facts on File, 1983), it ranked 18th highest out of 66 cities on the amount of nitrates in the water—0.87 mg/l. Its water was also fairly hard, 18th highest in dissolved minerals out of 69 cities with 150 ppm.

Weather: Summers are hot and muggy. Winters are mild. Precipitation is above average at 39 inches annually.

Average Daily Temperature (degrees F)	53.9
High	65.2
Low	42.5
Average Humidity	
Morning (percent)	74
Afternoon (percent)	53
Annual Precipitation (inches)	39.0
Average Total Snowfall (inches)	17.4
Ozone, Days over 0.12 ppm (one hour in 1988)	15

℞ Washington did not respond to the health-services survey.

Health Resources per 1,000 Pop. (1988)	Number	Rank
Hospital beds, community hospitals, city	7.53	37/91
Nurses, community hospitals, city	9.02	29/90
Doctors, metro	3.39	16/113

Washington did not respond to the recreational-services survey.

 There is a full-time nurse in 10 percent of the schools, and a part-time nurse in 88 percent. The total number of students in all grades is 81,301. The school system appointed a cabinet-level Health Services officer in January 1990, who is responsible for the development and implementation of a Comprehensive Health Plan. The first school-based Senior High School Adolescent Health Center opened during the 1989–90 school year. The school system offers all common health-education programs and HIV/AIDS, physical fitness, anatomy, adolescent growth and development and hypertension through 12th grade. The school system provides all common screens and tests except for mental-health exams and well-child physical exams; it checks on immunizations only if an epidemic of the disease breaks out. It also provides physical appraisals, referrals, follow-ups, parent-staff conferences and statistical reports. Dental treatment is provided for students. Contact: Andrew Jenkings, Superintendent, D.C. Public Schools, 415 12th Street N.W., Washington, DC 20004.

Wichita, KS

🪦	🏃	$	🌲	℞	🖼	🧑‍🤝‍🧑	?
✔	✔	✔	✔	x	?	?	x

🪦 Wichita (Sedgwick County) ranks 30th in the age-adjusted death rate. Infant-mortality rates for Kansas are extremely high among blacks and other minorities. Rates among whites are relatively low. Infant-mortality rates are higher in cities than in rural areas of the state.

	Number	Rank
Age-Adjusted Death Rate	−0.89	30/100
Heart Attacks	−0.10	44/100
Cancer	−0.34	16/100

 Wichita has a relatively high accident rate (78/100). Homicide and suicide rates are below average.

Incidence per 1,000 Pop.	Number	Rank
Homicides (1989)	0.06	41/111
Robberies (1989)	2.00	55/111
Suicides	0.10	23/100
Accidental deaths	0.37	78/100

$ Wichita's 1988 metro population was 483,000—81st out of 113 metro areas. Its economic health at the end of 1990 was good, ranking 46th of 113 metro areas. Its unemployment rate ranks 25th, change in unemployment 30th (employment grew faster than the labor force) and its enterprise 95th. Contact: Mayor Robert Knight, City of Wichita, 455 North Main Street, Wichita, KS 67202.

🌲 **Air Quality:** Wichita met all standards in 1989 and the EPA has reclassified Wichita as in-attainment for carbon monoxide and all other criteria pollutants. Contact: Jack Brown, Acting Director of Environmental Health Services, Department of Community Health, 1900 East 9th Street, Wichita, KS 67214.

Hazardous Waste: Wichita has two hazardous waste sites on the EPA's National Priorities List for "Superfund," John's Sludge Pond and Big River

Sand. Both sites are inactive. Sludges from a re-refined oil factory containing lead and ΓCBs are deposited at John's Sludge Pond. This site has been remediated and is in the process of delisting from the National Priorities List. Paint barrels had been dumped on the Big River Sand property. The barrels have been removed, and the site, remediated with "no further action" required, will be delisted. In 1987, Sedgwick County disposed of 1,804,1511 tons of acid from chemical plant waste streams into an injection well. Contact: Jack Brown, Acting Director of Environmental Health Services, Department of Community Health, 1900 East 9th Street, Wichita, KS 67214.

Water Quality: Wichita water is supplied 40 percent by surface water and 60 percent by ground water. The pH of the drinking water was 8.4 in 1989. Contact: Jack Brown, Acting Director of Environmental Health Services, Department of Community Health, 1900 East 9th Street, Wichita, KS 67214.

Weather: The average temperature in Wichita is 56.4. Precipitation is about average at 28.61 inches annually.

Average Daily Temperature (degrees F)	56.4
High	67.6
Low	45.1
Average Humidity	
Morning (percent)	80
Afternoon (percent)	56
Annual Precipitation (inches)	28.61
Average Total Snowfall (inches)	17
Air Pollution Index (percent of mean)	140
Ozone, Days over 0.12 ppm (one hour in 1988)	0

℞ Smoking is prohibited in Wichita on public transportation and in public offices. It is partially restricted in restaurants and private offices. Wichita sponsors health awareness campaigns addressing cholesterol, high blood pressure, AIDS, back-to-school immunizations, poison prevention, diabetes, children's dental health, birth defects prevention, Great American Smokeout, nutrition, cancer, accident prevention, suicide prevention, rabies, fitness, alcohol awareness, toy safety, fire prevention, elderly, and family sexuality education. The city has some of the common health-education programs and emergency hotlines, but did not advise us on nutrition, family planning, or sexually transmitted disease programs or child abuse, alcoholism, drug abuse, or sexually transmitted diseases hotlines. The city offers all common preventive-health programs except food for the needy, and all common treatment programs except for mental illness, which is provided by the county. Contact: Fred E. Tosh, M.D.,

M.P.H., Director, Department of Community Health, 1900 East 9th Street, Wichita, KS 67214.

Health Resources per 1,000 Pop. (1988)	Number	Rank
Hospital beds, community hospitals, city	6.17	52/91
Nurses, community hospitals, city	7.68	43/90
Doctors, metro	2.07	77/113

 Wichita did not respond to the recreational-services survey or to the school-health survey.

Wilmington, DE

🪦	🏃	$	🌲	℞	🚻	👥	?
✓	✔	x	✓	x	✔	?	x

Wilmington ranks an average 53rd in the age-adjusted mortality rate. Infant-mortality rates for Delaware are extremely high among blacks and other minorities and relatively low among whites. Infant-mortality rates in cities more than double the rates in rural communities.

	Number	Rank
Age-Adjusted Death Rate	−0.04	53/100
Heart Attacks	−0.25	35/100
Cancer	0.12	71/100

 Wilmington has a high suicide rate, ranking 85th of 100 metro areas. Homicide, robbery and accident rates are all below average.

Incidence per 1,000 Pop.	Number	Rank
Homicides (1989)	0.06	34/111
Robberies (1989)	1.39	31/111
Suicides	0.16	85/100
Accidental deaths	0.32	38/100

$ Wilmington's 1988 metro population was 574,000—72nd out of 113 metro areas. Its economic health at the end of 1990 was poor, ranking 93rd of 113 metro areas. Its unemployment rate ranks 92nd, change in unemployment 110th (employment declined slightly while the labor force grew substantially) and its enterprise 30th. Contact: Mayor Daniel Frawley, City of Wilmington, Municipal Building, 1000 North King Street, Wilmington, DE 19801.

 Air Quality: Wilmington exceeded ozone limits with a 0.13 ppm ozone level in 1989, which gives it a middle rating.

Water Quality: All drinking water in Wilmington is supplied by surface water (e.g., reservoirs). Additional mandated testing has shown that the water meets or is purer than EPA water-quality standards. Contact: William G. Turner, Commissioner, Department of Public Works, City of Wilmington, 800 French Street, Wilmington, Del. 19801.

Weather: The average temperature in Wilmington is 54. Precipitation is above average at 41.4 inches annually.

Average Daily Temperature (degrees F)	54.0
High	63.5
Low	44.5
Average Humidity	
Morning (percent)	78
Afternoon (percent)	55
Annual Precipitation (inches)	41.4
Average Total Snowfall (inches)	21.3

 Wilmington did not respond to the health-services survey.

Health Resources per 1,000 Pop.	Number	Rank
Doctors, metro	1.99	83/113

 Wilmington has been developing a cycling series. It has also been acquiring and preserving waterfront land for leisure purposes. The city provides several day and summer camps for children. The city's sports facilities include 23 baseball/softball fields, 18 football/soccer fields, 38 basketball courts, 23 tennis courts, 7 swimming pools, 3 running tracks, and 2 golf courses. Contact: Donald Bowman, Director of Parks and Recreation, City of Wilmington, 800 French Street, Wilmington, DE 19801.

Parkland/Total City Area (percent)	4.4

Wilmington did not respond to the school-health survey.

Worcester, MA

🪦	🏃	$	🌲	℞	🖼️	👥	?
X	✔	X	✔	✔	✓	✔	✔

Worcester (Worcester County) has a very poor age-adjusted death rate, ranked 98 out of 100 cities. The cancer and heart attack rates are also very high (99/100 and 94/100 respectively). Infant-mortality rates for Massachusetts are high among blacks and extremely low among whites. Infant-mortality rates are higher in cities than in rural communities.

	Number	Rank
Age-Adjusted Death Rate	3.43	98/100
Heart Attacks	3.02	94/100
Cancer	0.87	99/100

 Worcester has high suicide and robbery rates. Accident rates for the city are average and homicide rates are relatively low.

Incidence per 1,000 Pop.	Number	Rank
Homicides (1989)	0.05	21/111
Robberies (1989)	2.91	83/111
Suicides	0.15	78/100
Accidental deaths	0.33	50/100

Worcester's 1988 metro population was 416,000—87th out of 113 metro areas. Its economic health at the end of 1990 was very poor, ranking 109th of 113 metro areas. Its unemployment rate ranks 100th, change in unemployment 111th (employment fell nearly 4 percent while the labor force increased slightly) and its enterprise 87th. Contact: Mayor Jordan Levy, City of Worcester, 455 Main Street, Worcester, MA 01608.

Air Quality: Worcester was in compliance with NAAQS ceilings in 1989, but was only slightly below the carbon monoxide with 8 ppm (vs. 9 ppm being the standard) and just below the ozone standard with 0.10 ppm, vs. the 0.12 ppm standard.

Hazardous Waste: Worcester County has no EPA Superfund sites and the

City of Worcester has no hazardous-waste-disposal sites. Contact: John F. Grady, Chief Inspector, Worcester Department of Public Health, 37 Lee Street, Worcester, MA 01602-2120. Or: Massachusetts Department of Environmental Protection, Central Region, 75 Grove Street, Worcester, MA 01605.

Water Quality: Worcester's drinking water comes from surface water sources. The pH of the drinking water is 6.2, slightly acidic. Contact: Robert J. Paterson, Chief Inspector, Worcester Department of Public Health, 25 Meade Street, Worcester, MA; Or: Massachusetts Department of Environmental Protection, 37 Shattuck Street, Lawrence, MA 01843.

Weather: The average temperature in Worcester is cool at 46.8. Precipitation and snowfall are above average at 47.6 and 69.7 inches respectively.

Average Daily Temperature (degrees F)	46.8
High	55.5
Low	38.1
Average Humidity	
Morning (percent)	74
Afternoon (percent)	57
Annual Precipitation (inches)	47.6
Average Total Snowfall (inches)	69.7

℞ Worcester offers all common public health-education programs including programs on heart and lung cancer, cholesterol, and geriatrics. The city provides all common prevent-health and treatment programs, except that it is only indirectly involved in the prenatal and infant medical care programs. Major emergency hotlines are provided by the city. The city has an executive office of elderly affairs, a Mayor's Task Force on drugs and school-based health clinics. New health programs include Health Care for the Homeless, Emergency Trauma Triad, and community involvement groups. Contact: Joseph G. McCarthy, Director of Public Health, Worcester Department of Public Health, 37 Lee Street, Worcester, MA 01602-2120 (508) 799-8531.

Health Resources per 1,000 Pop.	Number	Rank
Doctors, metro	4.46	8/113

Worcester has 70 sports facilities per 100,000 residents, ranking 45th out of 79 metro areas. The city spent $1.2 million on Elm Park, an historic park which includes a walking program. The city's sports facilities include 44 baseball fields, 15 football/soccer fields, 23 basketball courts, 25 tennis courts, 9 swimming pools, 1 running track, 2 volleyball courts, 4 beaches, and 1 golf course. Contact: Thomas W. Taylor, Commissioner, Parks & Recreation, City Hall, 455 Main Street, Worcester, MA 01608 (508) 799-1190.

| Parkland/Total City Area (percent) | 5.1 |

Almost all of the schools (90 percent) have a full-time nurse in attendance; the others (10 percent) are served by a part-time nurse. A school-based health center is situated in one high school. The school system provides all common screens and tests except for mental-health exams, speech therapy and learning disabilities. Medical treatment is provided for students. Contact: Joseph G. McCarthy, Director, Public Health c/o Manager Mulford's Office, City Hall, 455 Main Street, Worcester, MA 01609.

CHAPTER TEN

The Real Truth

So, how healthy is it where you live and work? If you have been reading carefully, you will hear *two different kinds of answers.*

THE FACTS

On one level, this book is about facts. The biggest fact of all is that some places are healthier than others. A little ingenuity can give anyone access to this truth.

For example, Honolulu, Anchorage, Denver, Charlotte and Bridgeport are the five healthiest metropolitan areas, if we adjust mortality rates to take into account the median age of residents, as we demonstrated in Chapter 1. Buffalo, Toledo, Worcester, Newark and Flint are the five least healthy.

Another fact that this book has attempted to establish is that all the air pollution in the worst American city isn't nearly as important to some-one's health as whether or not they smoke cigarettes.

In Chapters 2-4 we showed how to reduce hazards in the home and workplace. Becoming aware of how your health is affected by your imme-diate surroundings is important in the quest for a longer, healthier life.

The Japanese, who in 1955 had a male life expectancy three years shorter than the U.S., by 1986 had a life expectancy four years longer. Chapter 5 identified the five states with the lowest death rates from chronic/preventable diseases: Hawaii, North Dakota, Utah, New Mexico and Texas. The five states with the highest death rates were Michigan, West Virginia, New York, Ohio and Kentucky.

The metropolitan areas with the lowest age-adjusted heart-attack rates are Washington, D.C., Honolulu, Seattle, Denver and Albuquerque; the ones with the highest rates are Buffalo, Toledo, New York, Flint and

Newark. Age-adjusted cancer death rates are lowest in Denver, Salt Lake City, Honolulu, Miami and Charlotte; they are highest in Buffalo, Worcester, Portland, ME, Toledo and Charleston, WV. Homicide rates are lowest in Boise, Lincoln, Rochester, Syracuse and Spokane; they are highest in New Orleans, New York, Miami, Shreveport and Jacksonville.

In Chapters 6-8 we looked at factors that might affect age-adjusted mortality rates—environmental measures, health services availability and accident rates—and how to improve them. Such factors can be changed for the better by community involvement and action and legislation.

In Chapter 9 we examined each major U.S. metropolitan area, highlighting the facts and figures that affect your health and happiness.

INTEGRATING THE FACTS

Another truth is that the facts in this book are passive until you use them. If you have a choice of cities to live or work in, this book will help you make your decision. If your purpose is to find out how healthy someplace is, you can weigh your options by putting together the information for the cities or neighborhoods among which you must choose. You could compare a city with the two that have the highest and lowest age-adjusted death rates, Honolulu and Buffalo.

Honolulu has significantly lower death rates, even though Buffalo has more doctors, nurses and hospital beds. Doctors are like economic-development officials—when they are around, you know something is wrong. However, the hospital occupancy rate for the two cities is almost the same, suggesting that Honolulu's needs are met by fewer physicians, nurses and hospital stays. Honolulu has lower infant mortality rates and fewer deaths from accidents. You are less likely to lose your job in Honolulu, but are more likely to be under stress. Buffalo has a lower urban stress rate based on rates of alcoholism, suicide, divorce and crime. Buffalo's homicide rate is slightly lower. So while Honolulu comes out on top, Buffalo still ranks higher in a few areas.

Table 10-1 compares these two metro areas with those of Indianapolis and Raleigh. You could have put this table together from the material in the book. Make your own.

A DEEPER TRUTH: HOW ATTITUDES AFFECT YOUR HEALTH

But collecting facts is for me a means to an end. I like writing fact books because they are useful to the kind of people I respect—people who are doing something about their lives and their planet. The fact that you have

TABLE 10-1
COMPARING FOUR CITIES

Factor (No. Ranked)	Honolulu	Raleigh	Indianap.	Buffalo
Age-Adj. Death Rate (100)	1	17	62	100
Heart Attacks (100)	2	25	63	100
Robberies (100)	14	27	53	61
Economic Health (113)	6	11	6	41
Air Quality (110)	9	68	47	35
Doctors/Pop. (113)	62	4	43	29

been reading this book is a sign that you are taking charge of your life and how healthy it will be.

The deeper truth is that you are reducing the stress in your life and lowering your risk of a heart attack. No kidding. We have seen that it does make a difference where you live and work. The environment and the availability of health and recreational services do bear a relationship to life and death, and to injury, health and sickness rates, although the relationship needs to be constantly reexamined.

But even more important, where you live and work is a function of individual behavior as well as surrounding conditions. The most important things we can do to improve our health—stop smoking, drink moderate amounts of alcohol, don't overeat, eat nutritious food and get regular exercise—don't depend on our environment. They depend on us.

When a life-threatening illness such as cancer strikes, a positive mental attitude can help us get well. In a recent survey of cancer specialists, 96 percent of the doctors agreed that seeking medical help at an early stage was important; 85 percent said that patient determination to comply with medical recommendations was important, and 80 percent said "a positive approach to the challenge of illness" was important. Patients with a negative attitude (depressed, bitter, frustrated, despairing, recently retired, or recently failed in a life endeavor) were described by some physician respondents as generally experiencing a "rapid progression of their disease."[1] You *can* help yourself get better and stay better; you *should*.

People are more productive, happier and healthier when they feel in control. That's the lure of small business, which in so many other ways is entrepreneurial self-exploitation. Poll after poll shows that people feel better about what they believe they can control or help control. The most stressful jobs are those in which the employee doesn't have control over the pace or organization of work.

If a community is in trouble, the way back from despair is initiative, entrepreneurship, civic leadership. If you started this book to find a place to relocate, stop and ask yourself if you are going to leave your problems behind, or will the problems be a part of your luggage, wherever you go. Ask why you want to leave and what you will give up. The people and companies that most successfully move are the ones *without* special problems. Most companies that fled New York first in the 1960s were weak sisters that had a dismal record after they moved.

The real challenge may be to energize enough individuals in a community to take heart and turn it around. Houston showed how to do it in the face of oil-price declines and its disastrous real-estate market slide.

WHERE *YOU* LIVE

Three out of four Americans live or work in metro areas. So cities are important to us. But our neighborhoods and homes are even more important. Healthy cities can have unhealthy neighborhoods; unhealthy cities can have healthy neighborhoods. Even if you can't move, you can make your home and office much healthier and achieve the same objective as you would by moving.

In Table 10-1 we compared data for four metro areas. If you decide to collect the same information for your city or neighborhood to see how you stack up, send us your report. Some models for doing this are provided in Chapter 9, in the summary for New York City and Yonkers.

In the next edition of this book we may use your contribution, with full credit. Please send it to JTM Reports, 30 Irving Place, New York, NY 10003. We will add it to our computerized data base and improve our understanding of the health of cities.

DARING TO CARE

In the end, how healthy we are depends on where we live and work, not only in the wider sense—our country, our metropolitan area, our neighborhood, home and workplace—but also in the personal sense, how much we care about our own health and that of others. How healthy we are depends on our personal lifestyle and attitudes, and the surroundings we have built for ourselves.

A guru of the macrobiotic school (which places great emphasis on a rigorous dietary regime) has gone so far as to place attitude ahead of diet— saying that a calm, cheerful person is following the essence of the macrobiotic regimen regardless of his or her diet. In other words:

> *Rather eat franks and beer*
> *with thanks and cheer,*
> *than grain and sprouts*
> *with pain and doubts.*[2]

Because you are taking the trouble to examine your environmental and community conditions, you are someone who has a positive attitude toward your health. Keep up this attitude! You are already on your way to good health at home and work!

Notes

Chapter 1. Where You Live and Work

1. Source: U.S. Department of Health and Human Services, *Vital Statistics of the U.S., 1987*, Volume II, Part B, Mortality, Section 8, Table 8-8. Age-Adjusted Rates: The age-adjusted rates were calculated as follows: First, we estimated the coefficients on the following regression model: Death Rate for Metro Area = Intercept + b (Median Age). (The coefficient for age was significant at the .05 level, but the R-squared was low—to be expected given the simple, bivariate character of the regression.) From the model we calculated predicted values and then the difference between actual and predicted values; this residual rate is used as an age-adjusted death rate. Median Age: The median age data were obtained from *Sales and Marketing Magazine*, Survey of Buying Power, 1983 and 1989, for the years 1982 and 1987. The sample of metropolitan areas included in the two issues differed from each other. When a metropolitan area was in both issues, the mean was calculated to approximate the year 1986. In cases where only one year was available (either 1982 or 1987), the data were adjusted up or down in line with the overall trend of the metropolitan areas for which both years were available, which in virtually all cases showed aging of the population. The author thanks Hans Bos for assistance with the age adjustments and related regressions.
2. The statistical computation is from an unpublished paper by Hans Bos, May 8, 1990, which was based on his work as a research consultant for this book.
3. Susan Saegert, "The Meaning of Home in Low-Income Cooperative Housing in New York City," pamphlet put out by the Housing Environments Research Group, Graduate Center, City University of New York.
4. The Gallup Poll in 1988 and 1990 found that respondents rate local officeholders more highly in honesty and ethical standards than state officeholders (14 to 11 in 1988, 21 to 17 in 1990); Senators and Members of Congress fared better than state officeholders. *New York Times*/CBS polls in 1990–91 show that while 69 percent disapprove of the job Congress is doing, 51 percent approve of their own representative in Congress; and while 84 percent believe pollution is a serious problem that's getting worse, only 42 percent think pollution is a serious problem in the area where they live. "Home Sweet (or at Least Sweeter) Home," The New York Times, April 21, 1991, Section 4, p. 6.
5. Neighborhood: A single group of apartment buildings in New York City may have thousands of residents and constitute a neighborhood. A block is usually the first level of U.S. community allegiance, with the block being part of a neighborhood. Statistically, a

neighborhood can be thought of as a ZIP code area or a Census tract, although neither one is necessarily drawn with respect for how residents identify themselves. In many cities, like Houston, people identify themselves as living in a particular neighborhood rather than the city. School system: Sometimes school districts are under an independent board or other jurisdiction, for example in Texas.

6. "American Ways: Transportation and Relocation," *TRW Credentials*, 4:2 (1990). Jack Moskowitz, *What Lies Ahead: Countdown to the 21st Century*, (Alexandria, VA: United Way of America, 1989) p. 73.

7. Felicity Barringer, "Population Tops 29 Million As California Widens Gap," *The New York Times*, August 28, 1990, p. A16.

8. Title IV of the Superfund Amendments of 1986 provides for "Radon Gas and Indoor Air Quality Research." See *Environmental Statutes* (Rockville, MD: Government Institutes, Inc., 1990), pp. 1034 et seq. Also, Title III of the Toxic Substances Control Act, "Indoor Radon Abatement," requires EPA to publish a citizen's guide to radon and to take other steps to control radon; see *ibid.*, pp. 1145 et seq.

9. The bill was originally introduced in 1989 and late that year was reported to the Senate Floor but was not passed by the Senate. Nora Goldstein, "Rx for the Home and Office," *In Business*, March/April 1990, p. 35, updated by an interview in April 1991 with Senate Environment and Public Works Committee, which has oversight over the bill. The bill is concurrently being introduced in the House by Rep. Joseph Kennedy (D-MA).

10. Goldstein, *op. cit.*, p. 34.

11. See John Tepper Marlin, *Cities of Opportunity: A Comprehensive Guide to Finding the Best Place to Work, Live and Prosper in the 1990s and Beyond* (MasterMedia, 1988), pp. 58–59.

12. Moskowitz, *op. cit.*, p. 74.

13. For more discussion of the rationale for linking entrepreneurship (as measured by small-business formation and growth) and community economic health, see Chapter 3 of Marlin, *op. cit.*, pp. 24–36.

14. Unemployment and jobs data provided through the courtesy of Associate Commissioner Tom Plewes, Bureau of Labor Statistics, #2919, 441 G Street, NW, Washington, DC 20212 (202) 523–1180, and Patrick Carey, Local Area Unemployment Service, Bureau of Labor Statistics, #2083, same address (202) 523–1002.

15. Enterprise rankings derived from John Case, "The Most Entrepreneurial Cities in America: Why Some Cities Boom While Others Languish," *Inc.*, March 1990, pp. 42–43. The original list included 192 cities. Rankings that are tied are for cities within metro areas for which only the metro area was ranked by *Inc.* Three cities in our ranking—Billings, Bismarck and Casper—were not in the *Inc.* survey; for them we used the rating assigned to Fargo, ND.

Chapter 2: The Healthy Home

1. This subject is discussed at some length in John Tepper Marlin, *The Catalogue of Healthy Food* (New York: Bantam, 1990), pp. 54–55. See also Patricia Moore, "Clinical Ecology: Medicine for the Chemical-Sensitive?", *Garbage*, March/April 1990, p. 30. A dozen highly chemical-sensitive families have settled in Winbirley, TX., because it is free of chemicals in the air or ground and is near a Dallas clinic that specializes in their problems. Lisa Belkin, "Sufferers Find a Haven in a Chemical World," *The New York Times*, December 2, 1990, p. 1.

2. The NRC's Board on Environmental Studies and Toxicology is the source of the report. Cited in "Controlling Your Own Longevity," *Longevity*, May 1990, p. 28.

3. Moore, *op. cit.*, pp. 34–35.

4. Ana Radelat, "Are Power Lines and Household Appliances Hazardous to Your Health?" *Public Citizen*, May/June, pp. 16–20.

5. Jane E. Brody, "Guidelines for Electrical Safety in the Modern Maze of Home Appliances," *The New York Times*, May 17, 1990, p. B12.

6. One of three major causes: National Safety Council, as reported in *The World Almanac 1990*, p. 837. More than 6,000 people die: Iver Peterson, "Sprinklers in the Home Gain Support," *The New York Times*, June 24, 1990, section 10, p. 1. Sixteen percent: Cited by David Goldbeck, *The Smart Kitchen* (Woodstock, NY: Ceres Press, 1989), p. 39.

7. Burning wood a hazard: Jay Shelton and Andrew B. Shapiro, *The Woodburners Encyclopedia* (Waitsfield, VT: Vermont Crossroads Press, 1977), Chapter 9 ("Safety"), pp. 69–74. Creosote: *Ibid.*, Chapter 12 ("Creosote and Chimney Fires"), pp. 86–87. Foam plastic a problem: William Rose, "Fire Codes and Foam Plastic," *The Journal of Light Construction*, June 1987, p. 22.

8. Goldbeck, *op. cit.*, p. 39.

9. Peterson, *ibid.*, p. 1. Sprinklers installed in homes are usually unobtrusive, being fairly well hidden in walls or ceilings. They do not emit the kind of shower found in most sprinkler systems in commercial locations. Residential sprinkler systems throw a heavy mist of water so as to limit the amount of water damage, and they are generally inexpensive to install during construction of new houses; using plastic pipes instead of iron ones for the sprinkler would further reduce the costs.

10. Source: The Home Ventilating Institute, as cited in *ibid.*, p. 79.

11. Goldbeck, *op. cit.*, p. 61. See also Chapter 6.

12. According to Brobeck and Avery's "Product Safety Book," cited in *ibid.*, p. 63.

13. Deaths from ingesting toxic liquids or solids: National Safety Council, as reported in *The World Almanac 1990*, p. 837. Oregon: Reported by Debra Lynn Dadd, *Nontoxic & Natural* (Los Angeles: Tarcher, 1984), p. 64.

14. Linda Mason Hunter, *The Healthy Home* (New York: Pocket Books, 1989), pp. 105–108.

15. Five sources of natural "recipes" for homemade cleaning products: (1) Debra Lynn Dadd, *Nontoxic, Natural & Earthwise* (Los Angeles: Tarcher, 1990), along with her 1984 and 1986 books previously cited; (2) Hunter, *op. cit.*, pp. 111–114 and elsewhere; (3) Annie Berthold-Bond, *Clean and Green* (Woodstock, NY: 1990, Ceres Press, P.O. Box 87, Woodstock, NY 12498; $8.95, (914) 679–8561); (4) Environmental Health Coalition, 1844 Third Ave., San Diego, CA 92101, excellent series of fact sheets on pest control, paint products and household cleaners; (5) Greenpeace Action, "Stepping Lightly on the Earth," poster, 1436 U Street, N.W., #201A, Washington, DC 20009 (202) 462–8817. Buy green/nontoxic: "Cleaner, Faster, Greener?", *Consumer Reports*, February 1991, pp. 105–106.

16. Renata Kroesa and Judy Christup, "Dioxin: A Primer," in Peter von Stackelberg, "Whitewash: The Dioxin," *Greenpeace*, March/April 1989, p. 9. A link between dioxin and human cancer was based on a NIOSH study that showed workers exposed to dioxin had 46 percent more cancer deaths than the general population; but the causation was not conclusive. Ken Sternberg, "Dioxin Cancer Risk Study Does Little to Quell Safety Concerns," *Chemicalweek*, February 6, 1991, p. 13. The EPA began a National Dioxin Strategy Program in 1983 to study and control the effects of dioxin contamination, the year after it purchased an entire town (Times Beach, Mo.) because of dioxin fears. The statement minimizing dioxin risks is from Dr. Vernon N. Houk, Director of the Center for Environmental Health and Injury Control at the Centers for Disease Control, speaking at the 25th annual conference on Trace Substances in Environmental Health. His comments were supported by Karen Webb, Director of the Division of Environmental and Occupational Health at St. Louis University. See Associated Press, "U.S. Health Aide Says He Erred on Times Beach," *The New York Times*, May 26, 1991, p. A20.

17. G. Tyler Miller, Jr., *Living in the Environment: An Introduction to Environmental Science*, 4th Edition (Belmont), Calif.: Wadsworth Publishing Co., 1985), pp. E80–E82.

18. "Non-Toxic Shoe Polish," *Garbage*, July/August 1990, p. 68.

19. Dadd describes the aluminum as magnetizing the tarnish away. Dadd, *The Nontoxic Home* (Los Angeles: Tarcher, 1986), pp. 26–28. For the full details of making and using nontoxic cleaners consult her books or Hunter, *op. cit.*, pp. 111–114.

20. Environmental Health Watch, "How To Dispose of Toxic Household Materials," *Healthy House Catalog*, 1990, pp. 75, 77, 79.

21. Dadd, *op. cit.* (1990), p. 150, recommends airing dry-cleaned clothing for a full week.

22. Dadd, *op. cit.* (1984), p. 28.

23. The fumes are "polynuclear aromatics" on the EPA list of priority pollutants.

24. Robert Buderi, "Is Your Hair Dryer Out to Get You?" *Business Week*, April 15, 1991, pp. 72B–72C.

25. Philip Shabecoff, "U.S. Sees Possible Cancer Tie to Electromagnetism," *The New York Times*, May 23, 1990, p. A22. Laboratory tests have revealed that children exposed to such radiation seemed to face a higher-than-normal risk of developing leukemia. A U.S. Government (EPA) report concludes that exposure to low-level electromagnetic fields can cause biochemical changes by interfering with gene functioning and may pose a small, but statistically significant, risk of cancer; the report did not eliminate other possible causes and indicated only a statistical, not a causal, link. This paragraph is also based on an interview by the author with an early researcher on the subject who insisted on anonymity because of the volume of mail he receives and cannot answer.

26. Robert O. Becker, M.D., "Electromagnetic Fields: What You Can Do," *East/West*, May 1990, p. 52.

27. Densie Webb, "Eating Well—At Issue: Cookware's Safety," *The New York Times*, December 12, 1990, p. C3.

28. Becker, *op. cit.*, p. 6.

29. David Goldbeck, "Microwave Ovens," *True Food, Wholefoods for Modern Times*, 2:1, Spring 1989, p. 1.

30. Lisa Y. Lefferts and Stephen Schmidt, "Microwaves: The Heat is On," *Nutrition Action Health Letter*, January/February 1990, p. 5.

31. Marian Burros, "Eating Well," *The New York Times*, March 21, 1990, p. C4.

32. Robert Kourik, "Combatting Household Pests Without Chemical Warfare," *Garbage*, March/April 1990, p. 23.

33. Hunter, *op. cit.*, p. 122.

34. *Ibid.*, p. 123 and Group for the South Fork, "Handbook for Toxic-Free Living" (Bridgehampton, NY: self-published pamphlet, 1989).

35. Dr. Jeffrey Sachs, Centers for Disease Control, Atlanta, cited in "Living with Man's Best Friend," *University of California, Berkeley Wellness Letter*, 6:9 (June 1990), p. 7.

36. For examples, see John Tepper Marlin, *The Catalogue of Healthy Food* (New York: Bantam, 1990), p. 13.

37. Warren Schultz, "Natural Lawn Care," *Garbage*, July/August 1990, p. 29.

38. William K. Burke, "Termite War Alternatives," *Garbage*, March/April 1990, p. 28. Dadd (1990), p. 172.

39. Burke, *op. cit.*, p. 29.

40. David Beach, "The Unhealthy House: Pollution Comes Indoors," *1990 Healthy House Catalogue*, 1990, p. 13.

41. John W. Spears, "Builder's Guide To Healthy Houses," *1990 Healthy House Catalog*, 1990, p. 22.

42. *Loc. cit.*

43. "Device Advice," *Inside the Healthy Home*, pp. 31–32.

44. Barry Meier, "The Search for a Safer Humidifier," *The New York Times*, January 12, 1991, p. 48.

45. Barbara Rosewicz, "EPA Issues Rules to Reduce Lead Levels In Drinking Water of American Homes," *The Wall Street Journal*, May 8, 1991, p. B4.

46. Rosewicz, *loc. cit.*

47. National Research Council, Board on Agriculture, *Alternative Agriculture* (Washington,

DC: National Academy Press, 1989), pp. 110–111; Rosewicz, *loc. cit.*, and the EPA Safe Drinking Water Hotline (800) 426–4791.

48. William Mueller, "Testing Your Tapwater," *East/West*, June 1990, p. 68.

49. *Ibid.*, pp. 20, 42. The EPA has required schools to test for lead in their water, but recently found that schools have not been doing so (see Chapter 6). Also, some 600,000 households, mostly in rural areas, drink from wellwater that exceeds the EPA's nitrate standard of 10 parts per million.

50. Renew America, "Drinking Water," *The State of the States 1989*, p. 18. The report notes that over 400 outbreaks of diseases, such as dysentery and gastroenteric problems, affecting over 100,000 persons in the 1970s and early 1980s, could be directly attributed to microorganisms in the water source; in 1983 alone, 21,000 people had illnesses caused by bacteria and viruses in the water supply.

51. *Ibid.*, pp. 43, 83.

52. EPI's argument is in its book *Bottled Water: Sparkling Hype at a Premium Price* (Washington, DC: EPI, 1989). See *ibid.*, pp. 49, 53.

53. Barry Meier, "Lawyers Work to Publicize Risks in Household Products," *The New York Times*, October 14, 1989, p. 31.

Chapter 3: The Healthy Workplace

1. B. Reeve, "The Death Roll of Industry," *Charities and the Commons* 17 (1907), p. 791. Cited in David Rosner and Gerald Markowitz, editors, *Dying for Work: Workers' Safety and Health in Twentieth-Century America* (Bloomington: Indiana University Press, 1989), pp. xi–xii.

2. *Ibid.*, pp. xvi–xvii.

3. OSHA is in the Department of Labor; NIOSH was originally placed in the Department of Health, Education and Welfare, which was later renamed the Department of Health and Human Services.

4. Ruth Ruttenberg and Randall Hudgins, *Occupational Safety and Health in the Chemical Industry* (New York: Council on Economic Priorities, 1981), pp. 122–129.

5. "Workplace Issues: Sensitive Areas," *Inc.*, March 1990, p. 91.

6. Walter A. Kleinschrod, "Piecing Together Comfort, Safety and Utility," *Today's Office*, September 1989, p. 42.

7. The number originally offered by the EPA was 3,800 lung-cancer deaths, as reported by Lawrence K. Altman, "The Evidence Mounts on Passive Smoking," *The New York Times*, May 29, 1990, p. C1. The lung-cancer figure was later reduced slightly, to 3,700. Associated Press, "Criticized Panel Backs E.P.A. Smoking Study," *The New York Times*, December 6, 1990, p. A24.

8. Associated Press, "Secondhand Smoke Assailed in Report," *The New York Times*, May 30, 1991, p. A22.

9. Sheila Machado and Scott Ridley, "Eliminating Indoor Pollution," *The State of the States 1988*, The Renew America Project, May 1988, p. 6.

10. The Gillette Company agreed in early 1990 to reformulate the Liquid Paper products and remove the hazardous elements. Environmental Defense Fund, "Proposition 65 Cleans Up Toxic Office Products," *EDF Letter*, January 1990, p. 1.

11. See, for example, Linda Mason Hunter, *The Healthy Home* (New York: Pocket Books, 1990), pp. 175–176. See also Patricia McCormac, "Role of Light in Health," *Los Angeles Times*, February 17, 1980, part VIII, p. 10. These ideas are becoming more accepted but not universally so.

12. 20 or more times stronger: Robert O. Becker, M.D., "Electromagnetic Fields—What You Can Do," *East West*, May 1990, p. 56. For a fairly balanced presentation of the issues that eventually comes down on the side of saving the planet with some possible low-level

risks to users, see Maria Valenti, "Making the Switch," *New Age Journal*, January/
February 1991, pp. 29–31.

13. The research on lighting was conducted in the Soviet Union; McCormac, *loc. cit.* Scep-
    tics include *The University of California at Berkeley Wellness Letter* as of mid–1991.
14. Kleinschrod, *loc. cit.*
15. Becker, *op. cit.*, p. 109.
16. Andrew Pollack, "San Francisco's Computer Bill Becomes Law," *The New York Times*,
    December 28, 1990, p. B6.
17. "Do Your Eyeglasses Need a Coat?" *University of California at Berkley Wellness Letter*,
    Volume 7, Issue 9, pp. 2–3.
18. Peter T. Kilborn, "Automation: Pain Replaces the Old Drudgery," *The New York Times*,
    June 24, 1990, p. 1. Of 645 Associated Press employees recently surveyed, 61 percent said
    they suffered from neck and back pains. Of 118 clerks at the tax collection office in New
    Jersey, 81 percent complained of hand or wrist pains and 82 percent expressed pains in the
    arms and shoulders.
19. *Ibid.*, p. 22. For example, in February 1990, OSHA cited a 2,000-worker General Motors
    plant in Trenton, N.J., for 40 violations affecting the working conditions of employees
    who needed surgery to correct injuries or disorders they contracted as a result of such
    conditions.
20. "Preventing CTS," *University of California at Berkley Wellness Letter*, April 1991,
    Volume 7, Issue 7, p. 7 and Kilborn, *op. cit.*, p. 22.
21. Marian Sandmaier, "Terminal Pain," *Working Woman*, November 1990, p. 148.
22. "Healthy Lives: A New View of Stress," *University of California, Berkeley Wellness
    Letter*, 6:9 (June 1990), pp. 4–5.
23. Three times greater: Study published in the *Journal of the American Medical Associa-
    tion* and reported on in "Enlarged Hearts Tied to Job Stress," *The New York Times*, April
    11, 1990, p. A19. The survey, involving 215 white- and blue-collar working men between
    the ages of 30 and 60 further found that those who did suffer from job strain (about 21
    percent of the subjects) were generally found to have a significant thickening of the
    heart's left chamber, which is often closely related to and can lead to coronary disease and
    heart attacks. The results of the study suggest that psychological conditions brought
    about by stress and stressful work do have an impact on the physical condition and health
    of the workers, although much work remains to be done in this area.
24. "Labor Month in Review: Job Safety in 1988," *Monthly Labor Review*, December 1989,
    p. 2. All of the facts in this paragraph are from the same source.
25. "Work-Related Illnesses and Injuries," *The Congressional Digest—Occupational Health
    Legislation*, April 1989, p. 101. The study was done by the Council in 1981.
26. *Ibid.*, p. 102.
27. Ruttenberg and Hudgins, *ibid.*, p. 19. Citations: Of the citations referred to as general
    violations, 3 percent were not directly applicable to specific OSHA regulations but
    violated OSHA by not providing a safe and healthy workplace. *Ibid.*, pp. 36, 38, 39, 107,
    119. 84 percent/13 percent: *Ibid.*, p. 109. Of OSHA inspections, about 46 percent resulted
    in citations. Of the violations cited, fewer than 18 percent of the safety violations were
    considered "serious violations" by OSHA standards, while over 50 percent of the health
    violations and 100 percent of the general duty violations were deemed "serious." The
    average number of safety violations cited has decreased, while the average number of
    health and general-duty citations increased.
28. Steven Waldman et al., "Danger on the Job," *Newsweek*, December 11, 1989, pp. 44–46.
29. The information in this paragraph was taken from two fact sheets distributed by the
    Government Accountability Project entitled "Story Issue: Needed Legislation to Protect
    All Employees Who Report Health and Safety Violations" and "Fact Sheet on the Em-
    ployee Health and Safety Whistle-Blower Protection Act, April 1990." Contact: Govern-
    ment Accountability Project, 25 E Street, N.W., Suite 700, Washington, D.C. 20001 (202)
    347–0460.

30. A 1987 suit brought by the Brooklyn District Attorney raised the issue of state rights to protect injury cases. Pymm Thermometer Co. executives were brought up on criminal charges for exposing their workers to mercury poisoning that apparently caused one employee to sustain serious brain damage. The jury convicted the executives, but the judge overruled, saying that such prosecution was properly brought by OSHA, not the states. In February 1989, on the other hand, the Illinois Supreme Court ruled that since OSHA does not prohibit the prosecution of corporate officials on criminal charges by the states for work-related injuries and deaths, the states have the right to do so. Susan Garland, "Safety Ruling Could be Hazardous to Employers' Health," *Business Week*, February 20, 1989, p. 34.

31. "Occupational Health Controversy," *The Congressional Digest*, April 1989, pp. 98 and 103. OSHA issued "Hazard Communication Standards" in 1986 to require employers to inform their workers of hazards and dangers in the workplace; employers must specifically note if the hazards are high in risk.

Chapter 4: The Healthy Building

1. John Bower, "Building Healthy Houses", *The Journal of Light Construction*, August 1989, p. 34. A recent two-year study conducted by the State of Massachusetts determined that half of all illnesses are caused by indoor air pollution.

2. Council on the Environment of New York City et al., "Asbestos in New York City Homes," pamphlet printed by NYU Medical Center, c. 1990. G. Tyler Miller, *Living in the Environment: An Introduction to Environmental Science*, 4th Edition (Belmont, CA: Wadsworth Publishing Co., 1985), p. 407. Linda Mason Hunter, *The Healthy Home* (New York: Pocket Books, 1990), pp. 80–83.

3. William K. Stevens, "Scientists Say Risk From Asbestos Is Higher Than They Had Thought," *The New York Times*, June 8, 1990, p. B7.

4. Joseph Hooper, "The Asbestos Mess," *The New York Times Magazine*, November 25, 1990, p. 38. Michael Fumento, "The Great Asbestos Rip-Out: Dollars for Death," *American Economic Foundation Newsletter*, 5:2, (1989), p. 2, and Sheila Machado and Scott Ridley, "Eliminating Indoor Pollution," *The State of the States 1988*, The Renew America Project, May 1988, pp. 7–8.

5. Chrysotile is the form of fine asbestos insulation derived from the mineral serpentine and found in most homes with asbestos. The other class of asbestos, called amphiboles, is derived from tremolte and other minerals. Only workers: William K. Stevens, "Asbestos Debate Re-emerges in Dispute Over Building Hazard," *The New York Times*, June 26, 1990, p. C4.

6. Asbestos definitions: Stevens, "Scientists Say," *loc. cit.* Pessimists: This point of view was aired at an international asbestos conference in New York in June, 1990. Stevens, "Scientists Say . . . ," *loc. cit.* Animal studies: Dr. Philip Landrigan, co-chairman of the June 1990 New York conference, contends that the methods used by some of the other studies are insufficient in measuring the true risks involved with asbestos, and that there is no way to make a meaningful distinction between occupational and nonoccupational exposure to asbestos as building occupants can also come into contact with chrysotile by disturbing it. Stevens, "Asbestos Debate . . . ," *loc. cit.*

7. "Asbestos in New York City Homes," Pamphlet published by the Council and the Environment of NYC, New York OSHA, NYEPA, and the U.S. Department of Labor. Consensus: The governmental and scientific bodies in this camp include the United Kingdom Advisory Committee on Asbestos, the Ontario Royal Commission on Asbestos, and a recent Harvard University Energy and Environmental Policy Center report.

8. Stevens, "Asbestos Debate . . . ," *loc. cit.*

9. Bower, *op. cit.*, pp. 34–36.

10. Ruth Caplan and the staff of Environmental Action, *Our Earth, Ourselves* (New York: Bantam Books, 1990), p. 69.

11. Toxic gas: Caplan, *op. cit.*, pp. 100–101. EPA: Machado and Ridley, *op. cit.*, p. 10. Laboratory animals: Clint Good and Debra Lynn Dadd, *Healthful Houses* (Bethesda: Guaranty Press, 1988), p. 2.

12. Debra Lynn Dadd, *Nontoxic & Natural* (Los Angeles: Jeremy P. Tarcher, Inc., 1984), p. 128.

13. 300 toxic chemicals: So says a Johns Hopkins University study; see *ibid.*, p. 148. Symptoms: *Edell Health Letter*, 9:6 (June/July 1990), p. 3.

14. Jerry E. Bishop, "Data Cite Perils of Mercury in Latex Paint," *The Wall Street Journal*, October 18, 1990, p. B4.

15. Types of paints: Linda Mason Hunter and editors of Prevention Magazine, *Hints for a Healthy Home*, 1990, p. 28. Milk paint: Dadd, *op. cit.*, p. 148.

16. Good and Dadd, *op. cit.*, p. 52.

17. *Ibid.*, p. 46.

18. New "superwindows" will be available within a few years. They may be quite expensive, but the extra costs necessary to install them will be more than made up in saved energy costs. In the process of development is a glass door that can insulate up to 5 times better than double-paned glass, about the equivalent of an insulated wall. Marnie Stetson, "Windows as Good as Walls," *World Watch*, May/June 1990, p. 38.

19. Iver Peterson, "A Plywood Used in Many Homes is Found to Decay in a Few Years," *The New York Times*, April 11, 1990, p. A1.

20. Dadd, *op. cit.*, p. 165. Hunter, *op. cit.*, p. 173.

21. Chemicals: Bower, *op. cit.*, p. 35. Complaints: "Can Carpets Make You Ill?" *The New York Times*, June 26, 1990, p. 12.

22. Gases: *Ibid.*, p. 2. Sources: Joan Lippert, "Clearing the Air," *Homeowner*, October 1989, p. 28.

23. *Ibid.*, p. 30.

24. *Ibid.*, p. 32.

25. Machado and Ridley, *op. cit.*, p. 9. Of young adults who had been exposed to lead as children, half of them were seven times as likely to drop out of high school and six times as likely to have learning disabilities: University of Pittsburgh study, cited in "Your A-Z Guide to Health: Lead," *U.S. News & World Report*, June 18, 1990, p. 88. Philip Shenon, "Despite Laws, Water in Schools May Contain Lead, Study Finds," *The New York Times*, November 1, 1990, p. A1.

26. Dennis Hevesi, "Bronx Home Offers Refuge From Danger of Lead Paint," *The New York Times*," May 6, 1991, p. B3.

27. Philip J. Hilts, "U.S. Lag Found in Lead Poisoning Tests," *The New York Times*, December 22, 1990, p. L11; "Childhood Lead Poisoning, New York City, 1988," *Morbidity and Mortality Weekly Report*, Volume 39, Number SS-4, p. 1; and Hevesi, *loc. cit.*

28. "Fatal Pediatric Poisoning from Leaded Paint—Wisconsin, 1990," *Morbidity and Mortality Weekly Report*, March 29, 1991, 40:12, p. 194; and Hilts, *loc. cit.*

29. Test children: "Your A-Z Guide to Health," *op. cit.*, p. 88. Stripping paint: *The Journal of Light Construction*, September 1989, p. 48.

30. Machado and Ridley, *op. cit.*, p. 6; Nathaniel Mead, "The Riddle of Radon," *East/West*, July 1990, p. 66; Lippert, *op. cit.*, p. 30.

31. Mead, *op. cit.*, p. 64. "Radon Testing, Remediation," *In Business*, July/August 1990, p. 23.

32. *Ibid.*, p. 66–68. Jane E. Brody, "Some Scientists Say Concerns Over Radon is Overblown by E.P.A.," *The New York Times*, January 8, 1991, p. C4. William K. Stevens, "E.P.A. Moves to Change Environment Priorities," *The New York Times*, January 26, 1991, p. 11. Warren E. Leary, "U.S. Study Finds a Reduced Cancer Danger from Radon in Homes," *The New York Times*, February 2, 1991.

33. "Radon: The Problem No One Wants to Face," *Consumer Reports*, October 1989, pp. 623–624.

34. Machado and Ridley, *loc. cit.*

35. Helmut Ziehe, "Bau-Biologie and Survival," *Introducing Bau-Biologie*, (Clearwater, FL: The International Institute for Bau-Biology and Ecology, Inc., 1990), pp. 5, 8.

36. *Ibid.*, pp. 12–13.

37. "Social architecture" is the American term used that is similar to the idea of "community architecture." Nick Wates and Charles Knevitt, *Community Architecture* (London: Penguin Books, 1987), p. 69.

38. *Ibid.*, pp. 15–19, 164–166.

39. *Ibid.*, pp. 18, 20–21, 25. Also, Robert Haney and David Ballantine (Jonathan Elliott, photographer), *Woodstock Handmade Houses* (New York: Random House, 1974), p. 3.

Chapter 5: Mortality Rates

1. U.S. Department of Health and Human Services, "Advance Report of Final Mortality Statistics, 1987," *Monthly Vital Statistics Report*, September 26, 1989, p. 1.

2. U.S. Bureau of the Census, *World Population Profile*, as reported in *Statistical Abstract of the United States 1990*, 110th Edition, Table 103, p. 72 and Table 1440, pp. 835–36. The preliminary data for 1988 in Table 103 show a slight dip in the life expectancy; we have relied on Table 1440's figure for 1989.

3. Life expectancy: *Statistical Abstract of the U.S. 1990*, Table 1440, p. 835. Life expectancy is predicted to be 76.3 years in 1995 and 77.9 years in 2010.

4. Compare Table 5-1 with the figure for Japan in *Statistical Abstract of the U.S., 1989*, 109th ed., Table 1405, pp. 817–818.

5. Japanese data from M. G. Marmor and George Davey Smith, "Why Are the Japanese Living Longer?" *British Medical Journal*, 299 (December 23–30, 1989), p. 1551. U.S. data from the National Center for Health Statistics, U.S. Department of Health and Human Services, as cited in *World Almanac 1990*, p. 852; 1988 figures are preliminary. The Japanese girl baby did even better, gaining over seven years in relative life expectancy. It should be noted that this trend may not continue, because Japanese urban people are eating more fatty food, twice the fat content of the rural diet. See Marmot and Smith, *op. cit.*, pp. 1549 and 1551. For fuller discussion of the role of diet in determining longevity, see John Tepper Marlin, *The Catalogue of Healthy Food* (New York: Bantam, 1990), pp. 3–9.

6. Daniel Goleman, "A Modern Tradeoff: Longevity for Health," *The New York Times*, May 16, 1991, p. B10.

7. National Center for Health Statistics, Public Health Service, *Vital Statistics of the United States*, Vol. II, *Mortality*, Part B, 1986 and 1987 (Washington, D.C.: U.S. Government Printing Office, 1988 and 1989). Derived from Section 8, Geographic Detail, Table 8-9 "Deaths from Selected Causes."

8. Cause of death data are in all cases from U.S. Government sources as reprinted in: For 1900–04, 1958, and sample intermediate years, *Information Please Almanac, 1960* (New York: McGraw-Hill, 1959), p. 346; for 1970 and 1983, *Reader's Digest Almanac, 1987* (Pleasantville, NY: Reader's Digest Association, Inc., 1986), p. 454; for 1988 (preliminary, and based on a 10 percent sample) *The World Almanac and Book of Facts, 1990* (New York: World Almanac, imprint of Pharos Books, Scripps Howard, 1989), p. 836. The 1900 figure is actually an average of 1900–1904 data. The peak in deaths from heart diseases was not necessarily 1970.

9. Cancer deaths: *Loc. cit.* New cases: U.S. Government data reprinted in *World Almanac 1990*, Table 188, p. 117. The five-year survival rate is based on the period 1979–84. The average five-year survival rate was the same in 1979–84 as it was in 1974–76.

10. Associated Press, "Alzheimer's Disease Rate Up," *The New York Times*, November 2, 1990, p. A17.

11. Figures are deaths from the "chronic but largely preventable" disease areas per 100,000

population. States add up to 51 because the District of Columbia is included. CDC is located in Atlanta, GA. The date are cited in Michael deCourcy Hinds, "Delaware Tries to Erase Image of Its Poor Health," *The New York Times*, January 21, 1990, p. 22. The full citation of the source information is Robert Hahn, Ph.D., "Chronic Disease Reports: Deaths from Nine Chronic Diseases—United States, 1986, *Morbidity and Mortality Weekly Report*, 39:2 (January 19, 1990), pp. 17–20. The *MMWR* is available from the U.S. Government Printing Office in Washington, D.C. for $70 per year; phone (202) 783–3238. Identical information is available from MMS Publications (at *The New England Journal of Medicine*) for $48 per year; phone (617) 893–3800, 8 A.M. to 4 P.M. EST.

12. See Marlin, *op. cit.*, Chapter 5.
13. Editors of the University of California, Berkeley Wellness Letter, *The Wellness Encyclopedia* (Boston: Houghton Mifflin Company, 1991), p. 103.
14. Jane Brody, "Personal Health," *The New York Times*, October 11, 1990, p. B12.
15. "Coronary Heart Disease Attributable to Sedentary Lifestyle—Selected States, 1988," *Morbidity and Mortality Weekly Report*, August 17, 1990, p. 541.
16. Reduces incidence: *Ibid.*, p. 543. Many states: Two handbooks promote physical activity in the community: A. C. King, W. L. Haskell, and S. Blair, *Promotion of Physical Activity in the Community* (Stanford, CA: Stanford Center for Research in Disease Prevention, 1988) and Public Health Service, "Healthy People 2000: National Health Promotion and Disease Prevention Objectives" (Washington, DC: U.S. Department of Health and Human Services, Public Health Service, 1989).
17. Natalie Angier, "Cancer Rates Are Rising Steeply For Those 55 or Older, Study Says," *The New York Times*, August 24, 1990, p. A18.
18. National Cancer Institute, "Farming and Cancer," *Backgrounder*, September 4, 1986, p. 1.
19. National Cancer Institute, "Sun Exposure Causes Many Types of Skin Damage," *Cancer Facts*, November 1988, p. 1.
20. "Family and Other Intimate Assaults—Atlanta, 1984," *Morbidity and Mortality Weekly Report*, 39:31 (August 10, 1990), p. 1.
21. FBI, *Crime in the United States, 1989* (Washington, DC: 1990), pp. 330–358.
22. John McCormick and Bill Turque, "Big Crimes, Small Cities," *Newsweek*, June 10, 1991, pp. 16–19.
23. FBI, *loc. cit.*
24. *Vital Statistics of the U.S., 1987*, Volume II—Mortality, Part B, Section 8, Table 8-8.
25. Possible explanations: I am indebted to Prof. Mitchell L. Moss, Director of the Urban Research Center at New York University, for these two reasonable hypotheses. Support groups: While many groups like the Samaritans help people avoid suicide, some provide information to assist those who want to attempt suicide. See George Howe Colt, "Suicide," *Harvard Magazine*, September–October 1983, pp. 47–66. For community factors that make for a healthy community, see John Tepper Marlin, *Cities of Opportunity* (New York: MasterMedia, 1988), p. 44.
26. Jack Moskowitz, *What Lies Ahead: Countdown to the 21st Century*, (Alexandria, VA: United Way of America, 1989), p. 102.
27. *Statistical Abstract of the United States, 1990*, Table 119, p. 83.
28. *Ibid.*, Table 187, p. 117.
29. Bonnie Burman and Gayla Margolin, "Marriage and Health," *Advances* (New York: Institute for the Advancement of Health), 6:4 (1989), pp. 51–58.
30. *Statistical Abstract of the United States 1990*, Table 103, p. 72 and Table 1440, pp. 835–36. The peak year for marriages was 10.9 marriages per 1,000 people, in 1972, when baby boomers were in their mid–20s. The marriage rate has dropped to 9.7 per 1,000 people in 1988. But divorces have dropped as well, from a peak of 5.3 per 1,000 people in 1979 and 1981, to 4.8 per 1,000 in 1988. *Statistical Abstract, 1990*, Table 80, p. 62.
31. National Center for Health Statistics as reported in Associated Press, "U.S. Health Gap is Getting Wider," *The New York Times*, March 23, 1990, p. A8.

32. Barbara Kantrowitz et. al., "Can the Boys Be Saved?" *Newsweek*, October 15, 1990, p. 67.
33. Nearly entirely because of increased use of guns: Dr. Robert Froehlke, the main author of a report by the Centers for Disease Control, attributes 95 percent of the increase to gun usage. Seth Mydans, "Homicide Rate Up for Young Blacks," *The New York Times*, December 7, 1990, p. A26. Factors: "Homicide Among Young Black Males—United States, 1978–1987," *Morbidity and Mortality Weekly Report*, December 7, 1990, Volume 39, Number 48, pp. 869–873.
34. "Asthma Deaths Are Found to Rise Steadily in U.S.," *The New York Times*, October 3, 1990, p. A24.

Chapter 6: The Environment

1. Adam Clymer, "Polls Show Contrasts in How Public and EPA View Environment," *The New York Times*, May 22, 1989.
2. Toxic accidents and hazardous materials teams: Denise Kalette, "Team Tackles Toxic Trouble," *USA Today*, August 2, 1989.
3. "Witch's Brew at Hanford," *The Economist*, June 2, 1990, p. 25.
4. Phillip Shabecoff, "Military is Accused of Ignoring Rules On Hazardous Waste," *The New York Times*, June 14, 1988, p. C4.
5. EPA, *Toxics in the Community 1988: National and Local Perspectives* (September 1990), pp. 47, 48.
6. EPA, in Keith Schneider, "Toxic Pollution Shows Drop in 1989," *The New York Times*, May 17, 1991, p. A32.
7. *Colorado Air Quality Data Report 1988*, Air Pollution Control Division of the Colorado Department of Health, p. 99.
8. EPA, *op. cit.*, p. 32.
9. Solid Waste: The Council on Environmental Quality, *Environmental Quality*, 1987–1988, pp. 5–6. Waste Production: *Ibid.*, p. 2.
10. Ruth Caplan and the Staff of Environmental Action, *Our Earth, Ourselves* (New York: Bantam Books, 1990), p. 171–172.
11. Benjamin A. Goldman, James A. Hulme and Cameron Johnson, *Hazardous Waste Management* (Washington, DC: Island Press, 1986), pp. 91–92.
12. Jon R. Luoma, "Cities Turn to a New Generation of Incinerators for Garbage," *The New York Times*, August 2, 1988, p. C4.
13. Sulfur Dioxide: Caplan, *op. cit.*, p. 175. Airborne Emissions: Luoma, *op. cit.*, p. C4. In many cases, preventing initial airborne emissions during incineration increases the concentration of toxic pollutants in the ash.
14. Caplan, *op. cit.*, p. 186.
15. Paper: Allan Davis and Susan Kinsella, "Recycled Paper," *Garbage*, May/June 1990, p. 49.
16. Eric N. Berg, "McDonald's Planning to Cut its Garbage," *The New York Times*, April 17, 1991, p. A12.
17. Degradable Plastics: William K. Stevens, "Degradable Plastics Show Promise in Fight Against Trash," *The New York Times*, April 11, 1989, p. C1. Biodegradable Products: *Ibid.*, p. C12. Normally, plastics are made up of tightly bound polymers, which makes them impenetrable by microscopic orjanisms like fungi and bacteria.
18. Increasing Dangers: Nathaniel Mead, "Oh Those Hazy Days of Summer," *East/West*, June 1991, p. 54. ALA: Hilary French, "You Are What You Breathe," *World Watch*, May/June 1990, p. 27. Currently, about 150 million people live in areas where the EPA considers the air quality unhealthy.
19. NAAQS: *Colorado Air Quality . . .*, *op. cit.*, p. 1. Reduction Deadlines: Phillip Shabecoff, "Senators Achieve Accord With Bush on Clean Air Bill," *The New York Times*, March 2,

1990, p. A18. Under the law, states focus on such pollution sources as factories, commercial buildings and dumps, while the Federal Government has authority over the pollution from mobile sources, or cars and trucks.

20. Automobile Pollution: Caplan, *op. cit.*, p. 77. Violation Days: *Ibid.*, p. 79.

21. Keith Schneider, "Lawmakers Reach an Accord On Reduction of Air Pollution," *The New York Times*, October 23, 1990, pp. A1, A18.

22. Allan R. Gold, "Critics Say Cars Got Break on Clean Air," *The New York Times*, October 30, 1990.

23. US EPA, "Ozone," *Environmental Progress and Challenge: An EPA Perspective*, June 1984, p. 19. Following the setting of EPA standards under the Clean Air Act, ozone levels did decrease between 1975 and 1982, even during the high-ozone summer months, but the levels in many cities were increasing between 1986 and 1988 and many argue that the EPA standards need to be more stringent. See the Council on Environmental Quality, *op. cit.*, pp. 57–79. Major cities: "Big Cities Lag in Clean Air, U.S. Says," *The New York Times*, August 17, 1990, p. A6. Tightened restrictions: *Ibid.*, p. 51.

24. The Council on Environmental Quality, *op. cit.*, p. 360.

25. Furnaces: EPA, *op. cit.*, p. 26. Sulfur Dioxide: *Colorado Air Quality . . . , op. cit.*, p. 43. Health effects: Caplan, *op. cit.*, p. 78.

26. Power plants: Shabecoff, "Senators Achieve Accord . . . ," *op. cit.*, p. A18. Sulfuric Acid: EPA, *op. cit.*, p. 26.

27. Caplan, *op. cit.*, p. 78.

28. Particulate pollution: Caplan, *loc. cit.* Diesel cars: EPA, *op. cit.*, pp. 22–23. Particulates decreased: French, *op. cit.*, p. 29.

29. Irritation: EPA, *op. cit.*, p. 28. Particulate matter in the air: *Colorado Air Quality . . . , op. cit.*, p. 49.

30. Body exposure: *Ibid.*, p. 76. Lead is retained: EPA, *op. cit.*, p. 28. Children and fetuses: Caplan, *op. cit.*, p. 78.

31. EPA, *op. cit.*, p. 29.

32. Federal environmental agencies have experimented with different ways of combining pollutants to come up with a single measure of air quality for a city. The Pollutant Standards Index (PSI) was generated by the Council on Environmental Quality for its annual report, based on measures of five pollutants in the EPA's SAROAD data base. The critical cutoff point for the PSI is 100; above 100 is "unhealthful," and people with heart conditions are warned to reduce physical exertion and outdoor activity. See *The Book of American City Rankings* (Facts on File, 1983), pp. 17–19. The EPA publishes a PSI only for very large cities. The author therefore developed a simple way of ranking overall air quality by ranking the cities first by the pollutant with the most number of violations, i.e. ozone, with 35 cities out of compliance. Then the ties were broken within rankings by ranking the pollutant with the next highest frequency of noncompliance, i.e. carbon monoxide (CO), with 24 cities out of compliance. Finally, the third step was to break any remaining ties with the third pollutant, which had 12 violations, particulates (PM10).

33. Population grew 84 percent over the 1947–87 period and the number of automobiles increased 49 percent between 1970 and 1987. Council on Environmental Quality, *Twentieth Annual Report, 1990*, Tables 1 and 42, cited in *Barron's*, April 22, 1991, p. 34.

34. EPA, "National Water Quality Inventory: 1986 Report to Congress," p. 2.

35. Metals and PCBs: *Ibid.*, p. 14. Other pollutants: EPA, "National Water . . ." *op. cit.*, p. 14.

36. *Ibid.*, pp. 3, 20.

37. Stephen S. Hall "The Dirty 13," *Hippocrates*, July/August 1989, p. 55.

38. *Ibid.*, p. 59.

39. Storage tank: John Rather, "Storage Tank Rules Aim to Retain Water Purity," *The New York Times*, June 24, 1990, p. 1. Petroleum products: Stephen L. Kass and Michael B. Gerrard, "Storage Tanks: Multiple Regulations Govern Underground, Aboveground Facilities," *Environmental Law in New York*, July 1990, p. 12.

40. Mississippi: Conger Beasley Jr., "Of Pollution and Poverty Part 2: Keeping Watch in

Cancer Alley," *Buzzworm: The Environmental Journal*, vol. 2, no. 4, July/August 1990, p. 41. High death rates: Greenpeace Report prepared by Public Data Access, *Mortality and Toxics Along the Mississippi* (Washington, DC: Greenpeace, September 1988), p. 4.

41. Jerry Adler, "Troubled Waters," *Newsweek*, April 16, 1990, pp. 72–73.

42. Keith Schneider, "E.P.A. Says It's Ready to Battle Farm and City Water Pollution," *The New York Times*, May 22, 1991, p. A22.

43. Keith Schneider, "U.S. Mandates Tests for Lead in Tap Water," *The New York Times*, May 8, 1991, pp. A1, A24.

44. Jay M. Gould, *Quality of Life in American Neighborhoods: Levels of Affluence, Toxic Waste, and Cancer Mortality in Residential ZIP Code Areas* (Boulder: Westview Press, 1986), shows that cancer-mortality rates in a dozen New Orleans area ZIP codes were in the aggregate 68 percent higher than the national average, and that the Hahnville ZIP code area (70057) had a cancer-mortality rate about 18 times higher than normal. The previously mentioned Greenpeace Report, *Mortality and Toxics Along the Mississippi River*, p. 8, shows that the highest excess-death rates along the Mississippi are in Orleans County (LA), St. Louis County (MO), and Shelby County (TN)—i.e., in New Orleans, St. Louis and Memphis. The EPA in September 1990 continues to list four Louisiana cities as among the top ten generators of toxic waste in the U.S.—Westwego (Jefferson county, right next door to the City of New Orleans, upstream on the Mississippi River, and part of its metro area), Norco (St. Charles county, upstream next to Jefferson county), Donaldsville (St. James and Ascension counties, upstream ten miles on the Mississippi) and Geismar (Ascension county). See EPA, *Toxics in the Community 1988: National and Local Perspectives* (Washington, DC: EPA, September 1990; document #560/4-90-017, for sale by the GPO), p. 113.

45. The table is based on an analysis of the following characteristics of a city's drinking water: presence of microbial contaminants (bacteria); turbidity; presence of inorganic chemicals: arsenic, barium, cadmium, chlorine (residual), chromium, lead, mercury, nitrate, selenium and silver; presence of nonvolatile organic chemicals: endrin, lindane, methoxychlor, 2,4-D, 2,4,5-TP, toxaphene and trihalomethanes; presence of volatile organic chemicals: trichloroethylene, vinyl chloride, benzene, 1,1-dichloroethylene, carbon tetrachloride, 1,2-dichloroethane, para-dichlorobenzene and 1,1,1-trichloroethane; prejsence of radionuclides: alpha particle activity, beta particle and photon activity and radium-226/228; and finally pH. The procedure for construction of a final score was as follows: Firskt, we ranked the cities by each test criterion separately. We normalized each result by expressing it in terms of standard deviations from the mean. We summed and averaged the individual scores, multiplying them by the standard deviation of their ranking to give the more discriminating comparisons additional weight. Although this method reduces the effects of missing data to a minimum, the table might have been slightly different if all the cities had provided us with data on all the pollutants that were compared.

46. "Acid Rain," *An EPA Journal Special Supplement*, United States Environmental Protection Agency, September 1986, p. 5.

47. pH of 5.0: Caplan, *op. cit.*, p. 92. Precipitation: Volker A. Mohnen, "The Challenge of Acid Rain," *Scientific American*, August 1988, p. 30. Chemical changes: Some alkaline soils can help to neutralize the acid, and in already highly acidic soils the acids can also be "buffered." The initial absorption of the chemicals into water droplets in the atmosphere is actually a self-cleaning process, as the atmosphere seeks to cleanse itself of the particles and gases. The chemicals can also combine with dust and other airborne particles to form what is classified as "dry" acid deposition. Mohnen, *op. cit.*, p. 32.

48. Caplan, *op. cit.*, p. 92; and "Acid Rain Migrates Across U.S. Borders—Both Ways," *EDF Letter*, May 1986, p. 1.

49. NAPAP: The National Surface Water Survey is the part of the program that researches the impact of acid rain on lakes and streams in various parts of the country. The Forest Response Project of the EPA is seeking to monitor the effects of acid rain on trees and

other vegetation. Forest Response Project: *Ibid.*, pp. 7–8. Acid Deposition: EPA, *op. cit.*, p. 35.

50. "Acid Rain," *op. cit.*, p. 10.
51. Could increase by 3 to 9 degrees: Phillip Shabecoff, "The Heat Is On: Calculating the Consequences of a Warmer Planet Earth," *The New York Times*, June 26, 1988, sec. 4, p. 1.
52. Bill McKibben, "Reflections: The End of Nature," *The New Yorker*, September 11, 1989, p. 52.
53. Emily Smith, "Scientists Are Leaving the 'Greenhouse' Door Open," *Business Week*, April 22, 1991, p. 90.
54. I owe this far-sighted idea to Shalheveth Freier of the Weizmann Institute of Science, Rehovot, Israel, in a conversation at a Pugwash Conference working group in Turin, Italy, May 1991. Freier has served inter alia, as Chairman of Israel's Presidential Panel for Science Policy.
55. Reilly statement: William Stevens, "Ozone Loss Over U.S. is Found to be Twice as Bad as Predicted," *The New York Times*, April 5, 1991, p. 1. Skin cancer: "Screening Out Good Advice," *Health Letter*, vol. 9, no. 7, August 1990, p. 1. New data "New Data Show Sharp Ozone Drop," *EDF Letter*, April 1988, p. 3. NASA: John Carey with Joseph Weber and David Woodruff, "A Red Alert Over the Ozone," *Business Week*, April 22, 1991, pp. 88–89.
56. Schneider, "Lawmakers . . . ," *op. cit.*, p. A18. Linger: Sharon Begley, "A Bigger Hole in the Ozone," *Newsweek*, April 15, 1991. Vermont: "The States Set the Pace on Global Warming Issues," *Garbage*, July/August 1990, p. 22.
57. The research is led by Drs. Frank and Cedric Garland at the University of California at San Diego. Natalie Angier, "Sunlight and Breast Cancer: Danger in Darkness?" *The New York Times*, December 6, 1990, p. 22.
58. Hans Bos, previously cited (Chapter 1) unpublished paper, May 8, 1990.
59. John Tepper Marlin, *The Book of American City Rankings*, (New York: Facts on File, 1983), pp. 9–10.
60. It could also be measured by the number of people *working* per square mile. In many urban centers the density is very high during the day but not at night. This information is obviously of great importance to transportation engineers, and they maintain records on daytime and nighttime city populations.

Chapter 7: Health Services

1. Craig R. Whitney, "British Health Service, Much Beloved But Inadequate, Is Facing Changes," *The New York Times*, June 9, 1991, p. 16.
2. About $760 billion: Commerce Department estimate, an increase of $80 billion over 1990, cited in Milt Freudenheim, "Surveys Find Americans Satisfied With Quality of Health Services," *The New York Times*, March 7, 1991, p. B9. About 5 per cent above inflation: U.S. Bureau of the Census, *Statistical Abstract of the United States, 1990*, 110th edition (Washington, D.C.: Government Printing Office, 1990), Table 1444, p. 839; Table 691, p. 426; and Table 760, p. 469.
3. 50 percent more: George J. Schieber and John-Pierre Pouillier, "Health Affairs," as cited in Elisabeth Rosenthal, "Canada's National Health Plan Gives Care to All, With Limits," *The New York Times*, April 30, 1991, p. A1, A16. Twice as much: Charles A. Bowsher, Comptroller General of the United States, *U.S. Health Care Spending: Trends, Contributing Factors and Proposals for Reform*, Testimony before the House Committee on Ways and Means, April 17, 1991 (GAO/T-HRD-91-16). 37 million uninsured: Anthony Schmitz, "Health Assurance," *In Health*, January/February 1991, p. 40.
4. Milt Freudenheim, "States Try to Cut Cost of Insurance for Medical Care," *The New York*

Times, December 9, 1990, p. A1, 34. Timothy Egan, "For Oregon's Health Care System, Triage by a Lawmaker With an M.D. [Dr. John Kitzhaber, President of the Oregon Senate]," *The New York Times,* June 9, 1991, p. 18.

5. Examples of Provider categories would be hospitals, physicians and technology. Bowsher, *loc. cit.*

6. Robert Pear, "Democrats Offer Wide Health Plan," *New York Times,* June 6, 1991, p. A22. Philip J. Hilts, "Canadian-Style Health System Gains Support," *The New York Times,* June 4, 1991, p. A18.

7. Robert Pear, "New Cost Control Asked on Medicare," *The New York Times,* June 9, 1991, p. 1. Susan B. Garland, "Terminating the 'Medical Arms Race,' " *Business Week,* April 22, 1991, p. 69.

8. American Medical Association, *Physician Characteristics and Distribution in the United States* (Chicago: AMA, 1987), Table 14, pp. 255–261. The information is collected by the AMA's Department of Data Release Services, Division of Survey and Data Resources. The data on physicians are as of December 31, 1986. No 1988 edition of this source was published. The data cover Doctors of Medicine (M.D.s) only, and exclude, for example, graduates of four-year medical schools who receive a Doctor of Naturopathy degree. Federally employed physicians (e.g., by the military) are also excluded. The calculations relative to population and the rankings were done by the author. A related source on this subject is the American Hospital Association, *Hospital Statistics, 1989–90* (Chicago: AHA, 1990); the AHA counts as "doctors" medical residents, whether or not they are M.D.s; it also adds in dentists and excludes any physicians or dentists who are not practicing at or through a hospital, and covers cities only (not metro areas).

9. The research was conducted by Timothy Lesar and was reported by Erica Franklin, "Diagnosing Bad Doctors," *American Health,* November 1990, p. 11.

10. "6,892 Questionable Doctors," *Health Letter,* August 1990, p. 2.

11. *Ibid.,* pp. 2–5.

12. *Loc. cit.*

13. *Loc. cit.* One source of information the consumer can use is a telephone-book-sized listing of doctors who have been disciplined, published by the Washington-based Public Citizen Health Research Group. The 6,892 medical practitioners are mostly still practicing. One out of eight is a repeat offender. In only one-third of the cases is the precise nature of the malpractice revealed. Some of the doctors on the list are there for reasons that may not be of great concern to patients, such as failing to make a payment on an educational loan. See Franklin, *op. cit.,* p. 11.

14. Relative salaries: From references searched by the Reference Desk of the American Hospital Association. Supplement: John K. Inglehart, "Health Policy Report: Problems Facing the Nursing Profession," *The New England Journal of Medicine,* September 3, 1987, p. 648. By the year 2000, the number of nurses needed in the U.S. is projected to increase by 40 percent.

15. Stressful conditions: Inglehart, *op. cit.,* pp. 646, 648. High turnover: *Ibid.,* p. 646.

16. *Ibid.,* p. 648.

17. Milt Freudenheim, "Rising Number of Hospitals Forced to Close," *The New York Times,* June 23, 1988.

18. Martin Tolchin, "Study Weighs Impact of 69 Hospital Closings," *The New York Times,* May 13, 1989, p. A26.

19. In urban areas, most communities that saw a hospital close had access to emergency services within ten miles.

20. Bruce Lambert, "Flaws in Health Care System Emerge as Epidemic Rages," *The New York Times,* February 8, 1989, p. B6.

21. Jorge C. Rios, "Support Your Local Emergency Squad!," *Cardiac Alert,* September 1990, p. 8.

22. Private hospitals have the option: Judith Nierenberg and Florence Janovic, *The Hospital Experience*, 1978, p. 230. Poor patients wait 6–8 hours: Jorge C. Rios; "Access to Health Care," *Cardiac Alert*, August 1990, p. 7.

23. Massachusetts: Alain Enthoven, "A Consumer Choice Health Plan for the 1990's," *The New England Journal of Medicine*, January 12, 1989, p. 99. Oregon: Timothy Egan, "New Health Test: The Oregon Plan," *The New York Times*, May 6, 1990, p. L31.

24. Martin Tolchin, "U.S. Lists Death Rates for Medicare Hospital Patients," *The New York Times*, December 21, 1989, p. B14. Associated Press, "161 Hospitals Found With High Death Rates," *The New York Times*, May 2, 1991, p. B11. Associated Press, "Uninsured Hospital Patients Found Far More Likely to Die," *The New York Times*, January 16, 1991, p. A20.

25. *Loc. cit.* See also Chapter 3 of John Tepper Marlin, *The Catalogue of Healthy Food* (New York: Bantam, 1990).

26. Hospital ratings as reported in *Health Letter* (Washington, D.C.: Public Citizen Health Research Group), 6:5 (May 1990), pp. 1–4; and Martin Tolchin, "U.S. Lists Death Rates for Medicare Hospital Patients," *The New York Times*, December 21, 1989, p. B14. For detailed information on the 14-volume study of hospitals, contact Sandra Kappert at the Health Care Financing Agency, 301–966–1133; or a regional office of the American Association of Retired Persons; or your local public library.

27. "Choosing the Right Hospital," *The Johns Hopkins Medical Letter: Health After 50*, 2:2 (April 1990), pp. 1–2, and "Death Rates and Type of Hospital Correlated," *The New York Times*, December 21, 1989, p. 14. The Johns Hopkins Medical Letter makes the point that "community hospitals offer the very real advantages of being close enough for family and friends to visit, and because they tend to be smaller, they often provide more personalized and friendly service."

28. Linda Sunshine and John W. Wright, *The Best Hospitals in America* (New York: Avon Books, 1987), p. 7.

29. Neil A. Lewis, "2 Studies Rate U.S. and States On Meeting Children's Needs," *The New York Times*, January 9, 1990, p. A17.

30. *Loc. cit.*

31. "Effectiveness of a Health Education Curriculum for Secondary School Students—United States, 1986–1989," *Morbidity and Mortality Weekly Report*, February 22, 1991, Volume 40, Number 7, pp. 113–115.

32. The *personnel* column used the following weighting system for full-time equivalent employees that is based on relative salaries as provided by the Reference Library of the American Hospital Association: 4 for a physician, 3 for an audiologist or psychologist, 2 for a nurse practitioner, 1.5 for a registered nurse and 1 for a licensed practice nurse, clerks and most other categories. The *programs* column ranks cities based on their total of the following school-health services: (1) *Screens and tests* (we asked how many of 8 were offered): immunizations, mental-health examinations, well-child examinations, hearing tests, vision tests, speech therapy, scoliosis and learning disabilities; (2) *Treatments offered*, if any (medical, dental or psychiatric); (3) Grades in which health education is offered in schools; and (4) *Health-education* topics covered (we asked how many of 7 were offered, and asked for write-ins): nutrition, hygiene, illnesses, sex education, smoking, drugs, AIDS. To calculate the overall ranking, an "NA" in the personnel or programs column was assigned the median value for the column.

33. 1990 U.S. rate: Monthly Vital Statistics from the National Center for Health Statistics as reported in Philip J. Hilts, "U.S. Reports Drop in Infant Deaths," *The New York Times*, April 6, 1991, p. A1; "Death by Red Tape," Editorial, *The New York Times*, May 19, 1991, p. E16. 1989 data on U.S. infant mortality: Lawrence K. Altman, "Infant Mortality Rates in U.S. Fall to a Record Low in 1989," *The New York Times*, August 31, 1990, p. A18. Infant-mortality figures for other countries: from World Health Organization, *1988 World Health Statistics Annual* (Geneva: WHO, 1989), as recorded in U.S. Bureau of the Census, *Statistical Abstract of the U.S. and National Data Book, 1990*, Table 1440,

pp. 835–836, 8th column. Infant-mortality rate for blacks vs. whites: Robert Pear, "Study Says U.S. Needs to Attack Infant Mortality," *The New York Times*, August 6, 1990, p. B9; see also U.S. Bureau of the Census, *Statistical Abstract, op. cit.,* Table 113, p. 78.

34. Hilts, *Loc. cit.*
35. U.S. Bureau of the Census, *Statistical Abstract, 1990, op. cit.,* Table 1440, pp. 835–836.
36. 60 percent: Pear, *loc. cit.* Low-weight infants: Wilkerson, *loc. cit.*
37. Prenatal care: Importance of is attested to by the National Association of Children's Hospitals and Related Institutions. See Jack Moskowitz, *What Lies Ahead: Countdown to the 21st Century* (Alexandria, Va.: United Way of America, 1989), p. 102. Prenatal care programs: Robert Pear, "The Hard Thing About Cutting Infant Mortality is Educating Mothers," *The New York Times,* August 12, 1990, pp. A1, E5.
38. Egan, *loc. cit.*

Chapter 8: Accidents

1. Dropped 21 percent: Trish Hall, "Fatal Accidents Are Down As U.S. Becomes Vigilant," *The New York Times,* October 7, 1990, p. 1. Improved auto safety features: The latest regulation regarding auto safety is a requirement from the Department of Transportation that cars be constructed to better withstand being hit from the side, a ruling that the Department says will prevent more than 500 deaths and 2,600 serious injuries per year; see Barry Meier, "Making Cars Safer in Side Collisions," *The New York Times,* October 25, 1990, p. A23. The 1980s saw more progress: National Safety Council, *Accident Facts,* 1990, p. 1.
2. National Safety Council, *op. cit.,* pp. 2–5.
3. "Deaths in Building-Site Accidents in New York Lead Nation, Study Shows," *The New York Times,* September 21, 1990, p. B4. The Federal Bureau of Labor Statistics now lists construction as the second most risky industry, after mining.
4. In Japan, by way of contrast, workers are considered to be on the job when they leave their front door on their way to work.
5. Linda Mason Hunter, *The Healthy Home,* (New York: Pocket Books, 1989), p. 235.
6. Consumer Product Safety Commission, *1979 Annual Report.* Note that several products are missing from the Commission's list: cigarettes, guns and motor vehicles.
7. Jane E. Brody, "Personal Health," *The New York Times,* May 16, 1991, p. B10.
8. *Loc. cit.*
9. Source: Federal Aviation Administration and National Transportation Safety Board as reported by John H. Cushman, Jr. with Larry Rehter, "Flights That Kill Celebrities Show Risks of Finding Own Way to Fly," *The New York Times,* April 15, 1991, p. 1.
10. The last figure in the table, .01 for scheduled airlines in 1988, appears to be too low, but has been double-checked against the written source. With virtually the same number of deaths in 1987 and 1988, it implies that people increased their airline mileage seven-fold. Similar data are provided annually in the U.S. Department of Transportation, Transportation Systems Center, Cambridge, Mass., *Transportation Safety Information Report.* See also *Statistical Abstract of the U.S.,* 1990, Tables 1065 and 1066, pp. 621–622. For more information, contact the College of Insurance at 212–815–9223 or the Insurance Information Institute, 212–669–9200.
11. Francesca Lyman, "The Future of Transportation in America," *E Magazine,* September/October 1990, p. 37.
12. Insurance Information Institute, Inc., "Auto Safety and Crashworthiness," *Data Base Reports,* July 1990, p. 1.
13. "Alcohol-Related Traffic Fatalities—United States, 1982–1989," *Morbidity and Mortality Weekly Report,* 39:49 (December 14, 1990), pp. 889–891.
14. *Loc. cit.*
15. Jane E. Brody, "Personal Health," *The New York Times,* July 5, 1990, p. B7.

16. Lori Sharn, "South Carolina Leader In Local Traffic Deaths," *USA Today*, September 5, 1990, p. 8A.

17. National Safety Council, *op. cit.*, p. 52.

18. Peter M. Marzuk and J. John Mann, Cornell University Medical College (New York City), *Journal of the American Medical Association* (263:2), reported in "Fatal Attraction," *East/West*, July 1990, p. 11.

19. Debbie Howlet, "Post-Accident Minutes Tick Quickly," *USA Today*, September 4, 1990, p. 6B.

20. Insurance Information Institute, Inc., *op. cit.*, p. 10.

21. Barry Meier, "Device in Air Bags Prompts Recalls," *The New York Times*, October 30, 1990, p. A18.

22. *Ibid.*, p. 1.

23. National Safety Council, *op. cit.*, p. 51.

24. No. 1 cause: *ibid.*, pp. 6–7. 40 percent: Insurance Information Institute, Inc., *op. cit.*, p. 1.

Chapter 10: The Real Truth

1. Survey results reported and summarized by the late Norman Cousins in *Head First: The Biology of Hope* (New York: E. P. Dutton, 1989), pp. 218–221. The best approach to an illness, concluded Cousins, is to tackle it "head first," with a positive mental attitude. The book is a useful attempt to bring together the serious research that supports Cousins's belief that he cured his own cancer through maintaining his ability to laugh.

2. See John Robbins, *Diet for a New America* (Walpole, N.H.: Stillpoint Publishing, 1987), p. 149. Robbins paraphrased Mark Braunstein; I have paraphrased Robbins. For the dietary context, see John Tepper Marlin, *The Catalogue of Healthy Food* (New York: Bantam, 1990), p. 25.